INDIAN
HERBALOGY
OF NORTH
AMERICA

INDIAN HERBALOGY OF NORTH AMERICA

ALMA R. HUTCHENS

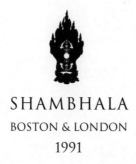

SHAMBHALA

BOSTON & LONDON

1991

Shambhala Publications, Inc.
Horticultural Hall
300 Massachusetts Avenue
Boston, Massachusetts 02115

Shambhala Publications, Inc.
Random Century House
20 Vauxhall Bridge Road
London SW1V 2SA

9 8 7 6 5 4 3 2 1

First Paperback Edition
Printed in the United States of America on acid-free paper
Distributed in the United States by Random House, Inc., in Canada by
Random House of Canada Ltd, and in the United Kingdom by the
Random Century Group

Library of Congress Cataloging-in-Publication Data

Hutchens, Alma R.
Indian herbalogy of North America/Alma R. Hutchens.—1st ed.
p.   cm.
Reprint.
Includes bibliographical references and index.
ISBN 0-87773-639-1 (pbk.:alk. paper)
1. Indians of North America—Ethnobotany. 2. Medicinal plants—
North America. 3. Materia medica, Vegetable—North America.
I. Title.
E98.B7H88   1991
615'.321'097—dc20   91-52511
CIP

Dedicated to

NATALIE K. TRETCHIKOFF and N. G. TRETCHIKOFF

HERBALISTS

for

they hold the key that opened my world of development and service.

Alma R. Hutchens

ACKNOWLEDGEMENTS

Our appreciation of illustrations is acknowledged alphabetically

'Atlas of Medical Plants', Medicina Literatura, Moscow, 1963
Art Academy of U.S.S.R., Moscow, 1960
Bello-Russ. Academy of Science, Minsk, Bello-Russia, 1965 and 1967
Bender, G. A. (Author) and Thom, R. A. (Painter), 'A History of Medicine in Pictures', Parke-Davis, Detroit, Michigan, U.S.A., 1961
Botany, Ministry of Education, Moscow, 1963
Department of Agriculture, Ottawa, Canada
Department of Agriculture, Province of Ontario, Toronto, Ontario, Canada
'Medical Encyclopedia', Moscow, U.S.S.R. 1961, 1966, 1967, 1968, 1969
Medical Plants U.S.S.R. (Lekarstvennye Rastenia), Kolos (Publisher), Moscow, U.S.S.R., 1967
Medicina, Moscow, U.S.S.R., 1965
Moscow University, Moscow, U.S.S.R., 1965
"Misl" Pub. Moscow, U.S.S.R.
Naukova Dumka-Kotukow, G. N., Lekarstvennye Rastenia (Medical Plants); Kiev, U.K., S.S.R., 1966
Thut, Dr. A. J., 'Health from Herbs', Gualph, Ontario, 1941
Teterev, V. A., 'Botanica', Moscow, 1949
Vyashaya Schkola, Moscow, U.S.S.R., 1963
Zdorovie, Kiev, U.K., S.S.R., 1964
U.S. Department of Agriculture, Washington, D.C., U.S.A.

For the review and annotations of the books, refer to the Bibliographv.

CONTENTS

PREFACE

Each book has its own fate and destiny.

While working on material in Windsor, Ontario, Canada, the authoress travelled daily, since June 1964, from Dearborn, Michigan, United States of America, and it is estimated she covered over 100,000 miles before the manuscript was ready for publication. The book was published in 1969 in India.

The first two editions were published far away from North America. This our third edition (Library) and fourth edition (Royal) is published in London, England.

Devotion by, and efforts of the authoress were rewarded in many countries. Letters of appreciation and reviews were received in many languages: Anglo-American, Russian, German, Hungarian, Dutch, Belgian, Lithuanian, Japanese, Talu, Hindi and many others referred to in letters post factum.

There are many favourable factors in relation to the book.

Great progress is evident in Folk Medicine and Medical Botanics in most countries including Japan, China, Russia, India and African countries and Pacific Islands, and all are restoring the Ancient Healing Arts and applying modern methods to further study. Therefore most of mankind is now deeply involved and dependent upon Medical Botanics. In Europe and in the American continent interest in the Medical Botanics is developing greatly, especially in American Indian Medicine.

American Indian problems have been commented on daily in the American press and abroad. This has created interest around the world, not only in the political situations of the American Indian, but in their History, Culture, Arts and Medicine.

The authoress was very objective in her research. She collected, classified, and critically analysed the material and sources, and she found it advantageous to incorporate material which had been specially translated for her book. Material was included which otherwise would not have been available for many years to come.

The book is of great and growing influence. It is used by professionals many of whom have revised their opinions and have become very cautious of using older methods. Gardeners started to grow Indian herbs for their own use. Many people started to grow and collect medical plants commercially: Ginseng (Panax Q), Catnip, Lobelia (Indian Tobacco) Chaga to name only a few. Many projects, excursions, discussions were organized in the high schools, universities and clubs. Eventually Indian Medicine was studied.

The authoress very much appreciated the knowledge that the American Indians recognized her work and gave her advice and encouragement.

We wish to point out some technical points and changes, and we have introduced new material and illustrations. The bibliography was re-arranged. Some publications were omitted but some newly introduced. In re-classifying, the authoress followed the principle that literature and books that are popular and easily available were replaced by the new books, especially in foreign languages, were translated and annotated especially for this book.

Disregarding the bibliography in general, and only considering that which Merco Herbalist has on hand, it is impossible to contain every-thing in one book, so the bibliography was limited to some selective works only. Although the book is now of a slightly smaller format, the economic use of typography has enabled a reduction in size to be made without limiting the contents of this edition.

The misprints and errata of the first edition have been corrected.

The authoress continues to work daily on her study of Medical Botanics. It is our privilege and honour to participate in her efforts; she has put her knowledge, experience and heart into her studies.

The American Indian Medicine was in use for thousands of years before and nothing yet has come to disqualify it. For many generations in the past and many generations in the future we feel that Indian Medicine was and will continue to be used, and Indian Herbalogy of North America will have a *Long Life and Noble Destiny*.

MERCO. Publisher.

GENERAL REMARKS

The subject of our work is Indian Herbalogy of North America, which includes the U.S.A. and Canada, to help us visualize and express the meaning of our Indian Herbalogy—as a study of plants in their economic use.

Herbalogy comes from the Greek—Herba, grass, and Logos, description. Herbalism is the use of medical properties found in non-poisonous plants as used by Herbalists for prevention and correction of diseases and, in general, health tonics.

Our conclusions and judgements are governed and limited to the most popular plants. Sufficient material on the total extremely rich medical botanics of North America is not available.

There are several ways of using medical plants: Home Medicine, Folk Medicine, Clinical and Homoeopathic. Generally speaking, many of the same plants or their family species grow in other countries: Europe, Asia, Africa. We do not feel that this far-reaching, time-approved knowledge about plant life as a food or medicine is a coincident of mankind's accumulated knowledge. Some plants in the past few centuries have gone travelling and in each area, as with our Indians, they are used in a different way other than that of the motherland. This is true concerning the majority, but in each country the poisonous and narcotic properties are well established.

Folk Medicine soon appropriated a symbol of universal natural treatment for those in favour. Then came the Herbalists who classified the uses of their own empirical therapy and gave references systematically. In the middle of the nineteenth century Hahnemann, the founder of homoeopaths, scientifically proved the power of herbal strength. When we speak about this practice of minimum doses, and variety of prescribing, it is not always as simple as thought to be, and we warn the use of caution. The administration of extracts or compounds should be considered either clinical or homoeopathic. Professional diagnosis, as a matter of fact, is only an educated guess, but self diagnosis is even less dependable. Homoeopaths know the power of plants and bio-chemistry, and they use the principle "similar cures similar". You must know precisely the symptoms to give the remedy for sicknesses. From the beginning, homoeopaths used over eighty different ingredients. Today there are a few thousand plants and chemicals comprising the practice. Only the well trained in study, knowledge, and experience can use the field in its entirety.

xv

We will not speak of every function or part of the body, or attempt the thousands of medical terms. N. G. Tretchikoff, Herbalist, has taught through his study and experience to find the malfunction of vital concern affecting the bones, nerves, and glands. Treating conclusively the weakest and supporting the remaining through a combination of herbal preparations.

Herbs and their properties are just one of our essentials. A seed's purpose by itself would have no life or meaning without the changing atmosphere and the right soil conditions. Herbs as internal medicine also need proper environmental conditions. As individuals we are much more than a conceived seed. Every evolving fact contributes careful spiritual, mental, and physical requirement, one for the endurance of the other. People very often think there exists some medicine—herbal or drug—that alone can cure. This is entirely wrong. We shall see that the Indian Nature Healers considered general health, and carefully weighed all possibilities. Only today in our time of scientific proof does Folk Medicine and Herbalogy have a deeper value than we can realize But with everything we have we can only analyse, but not synthesize (create). We could ask: What is the simplest of the simple things— our cell and blood, or life and death? but what this is no scientist of ours can answer.

The sky is populated with many millions of stars, the moon and sun. Their existence has been there since the world was born. These celestials live and exist according to the law precisely established. Our scientists can scrupulously explain how they work and live, nobody in the world can explain how it started and who created this order. Our earth has its own system of processes, of which much is known, but the untold story would occupy many more volumes of microscopic— rather than the telescopic—points of view.

To date, the Indians' knowledge of medical plant food is still being used. Speaking on behalf of Herbalists of the past and present we would like to acknowledge the now admitted scientific art of their trustworthy past.

The main purpose is to attract the attention of general readers and professional groups in this field to the scientific and practical value of Indian heritage, in our case Herbalogy as a field where great possibilities exist. Research abroad has incorporated many old and new facts and figures from Academies of Science, Universities, Laboratories and latest available research material on all Folk Medicine for comparison.

SOURCES AND BIBLIOGRAPHY

Indian medical botanics as compiled authentic information is deniable unwritten, and most of the books and material on the subject in North America is still unreflected. Therefore we had to search many books and field works associated with plant life but without botanics as a conception.

The foundation of this work was from material on Herbalogy compiled by N. G. Tretchikoff, Herbalist, Windsor, Canada. This work of thirty volumes, over 10,000 pages, describing more than 5,000 plants, started with N. G. Tretchikoff while in China (1924–51).

Known in Shanghai, China, as a banker, N. G. Tretchikoff was ill with a tropical skin disease. With all money available and after time and the usual treatment failed, as a last resort he turned to the out-of-date, unorthodox, but simple treatment of a wise Chinese Herbalist. The first three months showed daily improvement and at the end of six months his skin condition had cleared up completely. This personal experience was the starting point of a hobby (1936–51) that led to his collection of material and professional service in Canada (1958).

Out of respect and interest, material has been collected, compiled and systematized for the past ten years of his professional herbal practice. When our research began on Indian Herbalogy (1964) the only other complete set of thirty volumes was presented as an unforgettable gesture, and for organization and ease of work covering Anglo-American, Russian and Oriental Literature on our subject.

Our source was extended by the coast to coast telecast service of the National Library of Ottawa, and the public Library of Windsor. Through this service, books are loaned from other libraries and convenience of research processes is due to the recently established telecast. Herbals and reference books of dictionaries, encyclopaedias, Indian life and history were bought, old, new and revised editions.

A book should not be judged by its title alone. In our search for material we found how difficult the subject is, as there is no special section in the libraries and universities of North America on Herbalogy alone. Therefore bits of information are found a line at a time, book after book. For future readers and students we systematically classified the literature with bibliographical data and annotations.

In the Bibliography we have included books on Herbalogy where material and information on Indian Herbalogy, general literature on Indian life and culture, periodics and reference books were obtained. We also incorporated closely related works on health and medical botanics so our readers and students can appraise the proper significance of Herbalogy in the general field of the healing art. We are not able to

xvii

include all books on the subject as this is impossible, only those we have on hand, or possession of, or in command of, being mentioned.

The Russian medical and herbal books are listed under a separate title. To acknowledge the full co-operation of Natalie K. Trechikoff and N. G. Tretchtikoff, who have an excellent command of the Russian language and authority of Herbalogy, is but a few honoured words in a field of immeasurable thanks. Due to their understanding, experience and success, inspired by love, they took all responsibility to relay the Russian material for translation into English. Our latest scientific data on information on the subject of Herbalogy is from dynamic and prolific Russian literature. Many North American medical plants have more and better scientific uses than in their own country. We bring to your attention only a few of their most publicized or available publications. A complete list of their Folk Medicine and Herbalogy would be a book in itself. As an "on-hand" example, we have more than 500 titles on one subject alone— Ginseng (Panax Q). The information is of monographic character— research, clinical reports, agricultural, botanical and biological data, excluding Russian herbals in which Ginseng always has a prominent place. Up to the present day the medical property of American Ginseng is not officially recognized in North American literature. However, commercially it is highly respected because of Chinese demand.

One purpose of our combined work is to give comparative methods on certain plants and how they were, and still are, used in all other countries. We have separate continents different as to people, culture, history, and geography, but one point in common, their Folk Medicine in the past, and modern medicine of the present, use the same plant for medical purpose brought into use as an individual practice. Also, from this point we have used material on medical botanics from India and we limited ourselves to the material available to us at the moment.

It is a great challenge and rewarding effort to make comparative studies of medical botanics in many countries, but it can be done only on monographic methods, when only one subject is described in all details. Our book is of general character in the initial and pioneering of this field. We only wish to insert the problem and interest students to go farther in this direction. Herbalogy as such is not a one-person project, the horizon is beyond the capability of one person, one institute, or one country.

LANGUAGE BARRIER FOR RESEARCH

To learn more about the Indians we must study each group separately before a general conclusion is made concerning their ways and, in regard to our subject, Herbalogy in particular.

Research has studied and presumed 150 separate tongues. It is estimated by the different authorities as follows: from North America, Canada and U.S.A. 55–56 different stocks of "families", 24–30 in Mexico and Central America and up to 94 in South America. These classifications are already reduced and it is expected that further reclassification will follow after better and extended studies.

Regarding the American Indian language, and many other attributes, a firm opinion was attached—primitive, simple and that their language had no grammar at all. This has since been disproved. The many and unfamiliar sounds were entirely new to the Europeans, but grammatically and morphologically more complex than Indo-European language, and as different from one another as English is from Chinese.

Factual Indian language is a study of limited scientific linguistic, ethnographic, and archaeologist groups, strictly academical and theoretical in character. In practical daily life nobody bothered to study or learn anything about Indians in general, and the language in particular. Once the Indians came in contact with the new profiteers, in one way or the other, be they French, English, Portuguese or Spanish, he slowly adapted to the newcomer's way of life. Everybody taught them how and what to say, or to say it for them. Today Government representatives specialized in Indian affairs speak on their behalf as to how the committees understand their needs. We have mentioned the variety of their language; this alone shows us how rich and different their life was.

To refresh our memory—Canada, Ottawa, Saskatchewan and Ontario are from various Indian linguistic stock. Physiology of language is more than a convenient way of communication, it is logic of thinking, and their logic corresponded to the logic of facts. Since discovery of North America, Indian culture and civilization, we ignore their facts and overlook their logic.

ABORIGINES OF AMERICA

The aborigines of the American continent were thought to be from the islands of the Indies of eastern Asia. This acceptance of landmark and the name, Indians or Red Men, goes back to the days of Columbus (1492). Location and description of the people has been re-evaluated.

Amerigo Vespucci, Italian explorer and controversial venturer from whom the Americas were named, and Cabot "discovered", some years later, that the natives of the land now known as Newfoundland were not red because of blood line, but because they painted their bodies with okra. The popular is often kindled and thus accepted. Before 1492, the so-called pre-Columbus period, an estimate of the total aborigine population in the U.S.A. was 800,000 ("Encyclopaedia

Americana and Canadiana"). The total population of North America and Canada is much more than in 1492, 200,000,000, and it is rapidly growing. At the same time the Indian population in the U.S.A. declined from 800,000 to 240,000 in 1900, but rose slightly to 400,000 in the sixties.

In Canada the total white population rose from zero in 1492 to over 20,000,000 in the late sixties, while native aborigines declined from 220,000 to 135,000, or close to this figure, in the same period. In the overall continent of South and North America around 1960, it was estimated that there was about 30,000,000 Indians of both pure and mixed origin.

Biologically the original Americans were close to the Asiatic groups, as they most resemble the Mongolians of Asia. There is no indication or evidence of sub-human nature, or type of being, as far as archaeological research can reveal today from skeleton finds. We bear the name of Homo Sapiens only, no matter how old the remains, and resemble predominantly Mongolian type or very similar to the Indians of today. We, with our many different approaches to the natives of the American continent, considered these people as savages who needed to be educated. All invaders must teach them their way of life, language, habits, social conception, medicine, art, religion, food, etc.

In the days of long ago a few higher-class Europeans actually abandoned their civilized life after being involved with the Indian way of life and had no desire to return. Adventurous persons such as agents, scouts, missionaries or go-betweens are among the few that ever thought of conforming to their way of life. There always was, and is now, prejudice against the Indians of North America. They are still under protection and they are still outsiders.

Edward S. Curtis, the writer of "Thirty Years of Friendly Understanding", said when asked, "What might we, Americans, have made of the Indians?": "The Indians could have given us physical vigour which must be one of the foundations of any lasting and important strength; they could have helped us in the creation of literature, for they were marvellous in the beauty of their free, poetic thoughts, full of imagery such as white men have never known. Their souls were those of poets. They could have helped us in our music, for their's was a real part of their lives, a genuine expression of emotion. They could have aided us vastly in our decorative art. And in a broad sense, they could have helped us in our morals, for in all their dealings they were fair until we taught them theft and lying."

Our material on Indian life as understood by missionaries, travellers, traders or officials is from appraisal as each man in his own way conveyed it. Fascinating, though incomplete, and only after careful study and analysis, we can see how very wise and practical their moment of significance was.

We feel somehow sad and melancholy when reading and studying habits and enterprises of the oldest travel records of reports. How at first the artist, and then photographers, saw the Aborigines. With few exceptions the material portrays the Indians as physically strong, brave and handsome. When we study their faces after so many centuries we can recognize their proud and strong character, with names like White Eagle, Black Bear, Falconet, men of good sense, etc, we cannot associate them with something less noble and strong.

It would be favourable to compare this time of their lives to the Europeans of the same era. There are so many ways to piece together the rich inheritance of the original aborigines; let it be archaeology or modern science, provided we open our eye of learning instead of a mind full of prejudice.

FROM THE OLD WORLD TO THE NEW

Let us briefly review the beginning of our North American immigrants, which as a historical fact cannot be written before 1492. However, the peoples of North America go much farther back than the Indians the Europeans first encountered.

Some 100 million years ago the seed plants dominated the areas of the earth. Into this carefully balanced creation man was honoured. His dependence on plants for the essentials of his existence has been of paramount importance as the source of nourishment and replenishment. This remains as true in the twentieth century as in the beginning. For men and animals of the universe depend directly or indirectly on seed life for their existence in the Old, or the bountiful North American, world, whose inhabitance seems to be by a gradual population over thousands of years. The four major accountable Ice Ages lasted for thousands of years, with interglacial periods that lasted even longer where the climate probably became much as it is today. These changes from the Ice Age to accustomed conditions drove animals and plants from one part of the world to another, and where there were people they must have been driven also. As the populating of the Americas apparently went on for a very long time. Which will herd along surviving existence, as the requirements for food, water, clothing and shelter is needed.

The where and when of the North American entrance has excited much guesswork, theories, etc., the popular belief being a land bridge from Asia and Siberia to Alaska between the Bering Sea and the Arctic Ocean. The slow movement into the corner of Arctic Siberia followed by a sea passage in small boats, have acted as a sieve. Elements of culture were lost in such a movement—man's knowledge of the Old World was his only means of survival in the unexplored New World and he had to start a few thousand years later.

We must remember that the Bering Straits Route is only one of the numerous assumptions that have been made. The time is estimated from 12000 to 25000 B.C., at which time geologists believe the ice cap started to melt.

The Americans were suspected of being Egyptian, Phoenicians, Greeks, Romans, Chinese, Japanese, Welsh, Irish, or descendants of the lost ten tribes of Israel. Modern science has shown that the American Indians are far more ancient than any of those candidates above mentioned.

Even the last remote Ice Age which drew to a close 10,000 years ago is being pushed back much farther into the past. A recent discovery near Pueblo, Mexico, may push back the horizon to well before 30,000 years ago. These dates can be given with a fair amount of accuracy, long ago as they were, due to the recently developed techniques of Carbon 14. Carbon 14 is present in fixed proportions in most living organisms, and disintegrates at a constant measurable rate after death of its host. It thus acts as a historical "back track" calendar of measurement.

More recently, Dr. John N. Rosholt has developed a dating process by utilizing "daughter" products of uranium. This may prove to be more accurate. An interesting blood type study of our Americans in the above way reveals the purest "A" group in the world, as well as the only known population entirely lacking "A". Also the purest "O" and "B" group in the world. An eminent geographer concludes that the basic peopling of the Americas may have taken place before the primary blood streams of man became mingled.

The New World was a region in which man became separated into small groups and where over a long period of time cultural diversity could and did, develop. In each of these areas the coming of the white man was a cataclysm, its form varying according both to tribal pattern and to the attitude of newcomers. Introduction of iron was everywhere, as a major factor, because there were no tools of material tougher than stone at the time of European contact. Almost equally impressionable and dramatic was the introduction of firearms, steel traps, and of alcohol.

In a different way the coming of Christianity profoundly altered the aboriginal way of life just at the time when these new impacts threw a tremendous strain upon aboriginal culture, and new diseases reduced the native population. Everywhere (with the exception of the arctic) the old skills became valueless in the face of the wheel of metal, tools, clothing, new standards and attitudes.

Within a space of one or two generations the Indian was called upon to adjust to European concepts and to follow a way of life that in

Europe had grown up over a space of thousands of years. Instead of self-sufficiency within the framework of geographical unit, the Indian became dependent upon the whims of an alien market to which he had to conform if he wished to obtain the things that the white man not only offered but pressed upon him with the zeal of the missionary or the trader.

The deficiencies of American Indian culture in comparison with the civilizations of the Old World are not the result of any mental inferiority on the part of American Indians, but are due to the fact that man recommenced his cultural development thousands of years later and had not made up this handicap when Columbus reached the West Indies. Between the sixteenth century and today, the Indian has changed from mastery to a dependency upon strangers in a land that once was his. There have been few cases of a similar reversal within the course of a few generations.

DAILY LIFE AND CULTURE

The outstanding feature of native American culture is its extreme diversity. This is due in part to a varied cultural background from Asia, but far more to New World developments stimulated by the sparseness of population and to isolation under diverse geographical conditions.

In 1960, the Indian population of Canada was 136,000, divided into nearly 600 separate Indian communities known as "bands". Except for a few far northern nomadic groups all others live on more than 2,200 reserves ranging in size from a few acres to more than 500 square miles. They are not amalgamated with the total North American population, and while under protection their rights as citizens are limited. Nearly one-half the total Indian population depend on their traditional trapping, hunting and fishing. Officials encourage natural resource programmes of conservation and rationalization to support their general line of economy and life.

Aborigines are biologically the same group, although conditions and locations vary greatly. Plains and far north groups were predominantly hunters, and the Eskimos, in fact, were entirely dependent on animals for food, clothing, and utilities.

Housing, like elsewhere, is of natural material on hand, in this case being ice and snow igloos.

The north and plains Indians conducted social events and took critical problems to the oldest, and considered the wisest, member in charge.

As we can judge from earlier descriptions, meetings were conducted in traditional solemn manner, young and old participating. New ideas and suggestions were discussed with denial or approval. A definite religion was not established other than each person being his own mediator. They all believed in a higher spirit, "Manittou", associated with Mother Nature, Sun, Moon, Stars and even plants.

Instead of the common acceptance that the Indian has no religion whatever, every single act of his life carries with it some ceremonial function, and his whole being is surrounded by a shining host of devotional spirit. Perhaps the name we give the spirit in man that denotes his inward divinity is different, but the spirit is the same.

As an extreme comparison the farther south we go the more variety and better adaptability we have to natural environment. They used more plants, fish and water products, and in Mexico and South America more than 250 plants were cultivated. Bronze, gold, silver and platinum were artistically in use. Pottery was highly skilful. They had compulsory education; experimental botanical and zoological gardens; astronomy and mathematics had reached a higher plane than that of fifteenth-century Europe. Roads and bridges comparable to those of Rome were built in Peru; whereas in parts of Brazil and northern Ontario scientific and engineering development was of rudimentary nature.

In Mexico the ceremonials were in reign of state priesthood comparable to the great mysteries of Greek and Roman drama, including religion. Their palaces were complicated, stone-cut, architectural achievements. They had simulated all sources of life over thousands of years, and classified social standing of slaves, commoner, aristocrats, princes, and divine kings. It is considered that their old way of life, despite reservation and isolation from the other communities, is gradually vanishing.

This dignity of mankind is inherited, not replaced.

FOODS FROM THE MOTHER EARTH

Our original Americans lived a life of natural dependence in the forests, plains and coastal regions, and existed festively for many generations. Depending on the area, the Indians used wild species as plant food. When weather and season permitted a variety of game and fish were utilized as food, clothing, instruments and decoration. Berries of all kinds were eagerly gathered in the spring and eaten by everyone as a spring medicine or for specific treatment in haemorrhage and pain due to haemorrhage, high fever and convalescents, and as a general blood builder.

Cranberries were a favourite autumn food and were also considered as blood and liver boosters. Blackberry roots were used as an astringent. Nuts were a main source of high nutrition and they used them for making nut bread, crushing them and adding water for nut milks. Acorn and dandelion roots were roasted, pounded and sprinkled over other cooked roots. Pond lily roots are one of the most widely known food roots on the continent, and were eaten from eastern Canada to the Pacific coast. Milk weed roots were gathered while the dew was still on the leaves and a root sugar prepared from them. The white portions of hardwood ashes were used for salt, also certain leaves. Apples and other fruits and vegetables were stored in barrels and buried in winter pits. Some were sliced, strung and dried for later use.

Yucca leaves and Quillaja bark provided soap and shampoo. Although the Indian way of life has vanished, it should be remembered that a considerable number of its elements have been taken over and incorporated by the white man. These included growing of corn, squash, pumpkins and tobacco. The use of canoes and snowshoes and perhaps still more important and half understood idealization of what is assumed to be an Indian way of life.

Man esteems himself happy when that which is his food is also his medicine. The Indians at one time were a people of complete accord, for they practised it daily in many ways.

HEALTH AND SICKNESS

From the earliest days all Europeans were impressed by the robust stamina of the Indians in every location. The original artist and photographer, as previously mentioned also favours the alert, brave, strong and, in many ethnic groups, handsome Indian in every standard of beauty.

Technical study confirms their physical endurance. Archaeology in most cases cannot find any of our modern-day bone deficiency, cavities, arthritis, tuberculosis, etc.

Reviewing the scene from another point of view, our studies on the earliest travellers and missionaries also found the Americans very healthy and comparatively free of disease. From our available sources and varied walks of life we can find only eighty-seven different sicknesses spoken of. It was uncommon for them to have the fatal cancer, TB and heart conditions, all of which have progressed in our time. The figure of eighty-seven sicknesses is really out of date and primitive as compared to our modern list of over 30,000 invented names of disease, which is growing every day.

It is noticed the Eskimos of the north average a sixty-year existence, but in other parts of North America longevity is of 100 years or more. Today's American Indian, especially those living in the city, appear the same as the American or Canadian citizen. They dress, speak and eat the same as we do and they are sick in the same way, only worse. As is explained, the Indians cannot adjust so quickly to the new forms of civilization. For instance, TB is ten times higher with Indians than that of the ordinary American.

Indian women of early history were exceptionally strong. They would often become mother and doctor at the time of delivery and in a few hours resume their daily activity, as their mothers did in the past. On occasions grandmother would assist, leaving the Indian doctor to care for less routine matters. Today, these once self-sufficient women are weaker than the white women and need the most attention, with painful labour lasting for days and the children born weaker.

From 1492 to 1969 we have 477 years, approximately twenty-five generations (averaging one every twenty years). By time: comparitively short; concerning changes: overwhelming in every way when we think of the previous 25,000–30,000 years of life they knew, cherished and respected.

FIRST AMERICANS WERE THEIR OWN PHYSICIANS

Civilization has taught us to build empires for Life Insurance Companies, numerous research, welfare, old age organizations, etc. In comparison, the Indians' protection came from Nature, the "Mother Earth" being the most important. They learned to treat lives with plant life, the medicine from the earth.

After the white man, came they were suddenly introduced to a new way of life which brought them the white man diseases for which they had built no immunity, and thousands died. Self-sufficiency was destroyed as the Indians became dependent on civilized ways.

If we talk to the Indians the years have touched gradually they will remember a few of the family and tribal herbs that we think of as nothing but a troublesome, insignificant weed or shrub. To most of us trees are for beauty alone, but they bring out medical uses from experience we have yet to identify as the same.

The Indians were never at a loss to know which plant was best, or the time it should be gathered to heal them of diseases. They knew how to treat their complaints of physical, surgical and midwifery with a skill that surpasses the medical teachings. For internal and local treatments they used the sources of nature, experienced by a keen sense of knowledge. Local parts were treated by placing parts affected over the roasting pit after being packed in rye grass and earth and subject to almost unbearable heat for as long as possible. They used vapour baths for many ailments. Patients were put into sweat lodges of almost stifling amounts of moist heat to eliminate toxic conditions. Fractured bones were held in splints made of a number of rods tied together at the ends, and covered with leaves and bound with deer skins. Herb roots were pounded fine and used as a poultice for bad cuts and sprains. Sore eyes were treated with a wash consisting of an infusion of a certain root. Our cocaine and novacaine come from ingredients found in the coca plant, the nature healer used to alleviate pain. In this way the original Americans were their own physicians. Sicknesses of civilization like the plague, tuberculosis, typhoid, cancer, ulcers, heart and mental diseases were uncommon among their earlier communities.

Do you know, we spend millions of dollars for weed controls with booklets describing the various plants and how to destroy them? If we were educated as how to use them medically, we could help ourself physically as well as tax wise. We can thoughtlessly ignore our heritage but we should not deny its life-giving truths.

INDIAN HEALER

The Indian art of healing was ceremonial in nature. To us their rituals seem strange and without meaning. They knew physical health often failed without the aid of spiritual means. Dancing, chanting, etc., was conducted, according to conditions, or severity of the patient. Today our get-well cards, entertainment troupes, flowers, prayers are less physical but given in the same manner—to support the spirit. Their health and spiritual source was so closely connected with natural surroundings, they of course were inspired by the significance of nature and to the Sun, Moon, Stars, Rain, Wind, etc., that encouraged it.

Despite all the hardship in their memory and legend, sickness and disaster as was associated with European history and of the status of the Bible did not exist. The Old World was entangled with feelings of inferiority, guilt and sin. The New World legend is not about punishment and sickness, but heroic actions of everyday life. We can read about the ancient interpretations on the art of healing. Praising the temples and cult of Asclepius, Hippocrates and Gallen—establishers of European medicine as a science; Susruta—immortal surgeon of Old India; Phases and Arabia medicine. And others including Egypt, Palestine, Persia, Greece and ancient Asiatic continents, India, Russia, China and Japan. To imagine oneself on the very summit of the mountain and in perspective study of the past and present, a feeling of equal magnetism is in balance.

We admit without our old and new predecessors of genius healers the present and future would be uncertain and fearful. While viewing our panoramic scope we feel as if a heavenly ray or special sign should be seen in reverence. There are no temples and prayers; or songs of legend about the wise Indian medicine man, only a few words of "quack", "Medicine Man" or "Witch Doctor" in neglect.

Training as an Indian healer began very early. Selection was from the family or from signs of devotion, wisdom and honesty. It was more than a career, as is of our time, he was elected by ability. Trusted with all secrets, rituals, habits and legends of their people, while attending all ceremonial celebrations and critical meetings of the people he was at the side of their leader. The trainee must know and remember the many herbal species, their properties and uses. They knew their limitations and that flowers of the garden are not an agent against the fate of death, but there are flowers for sickness and health and flowers to prolong life. All medical plants in the area were used. The flora and fauna differed in each locality, but each knew their immediate supply.

Modern medicine and natural healing still practise their theory. Both used strong steam to create perspiration, isolation of communicable diseases, fasting for health, physiological moments, special diet as to case, and of course herbs. As a healer to all people he was above tribal restriction, he cared for the wounded or needy. The Indian healer was an artist in the best tradition of Hippocrates' principles, so much treasured by us.

INDIAN HERBS FOR THE GLANDS

In the course of the book we will find herbs for the glands and blood. Today we dispense these corrective supplements as routine procedure, as do the European Herbalists, adopted from the generations of Indian usefulness. They depended on the proper function of the system, including all glands and a healthy blood supply, which as a unit is known as the endocrine system of ductless glands, incorporating the pinal and pituitary glands, thyroid glands, parathyroid glands, adrenal glands, thymus gland, islands of langerhans of the pancreas, ovaries and testes. Other structures such as the gastro-intestinal mucus and the placenta also have an endocrine function, which contributes to an internal secreting fluid carried to all parts of the body by the blood and lymphatic system.

The Indians did not care too much about the name of sickness, only physical endurance, "mens sana in corpore sana" (he can not chance a time of failure). Nervous tension, adrenal failure, heart attack, etc., was not a part of their early life; they could overcome a running deer, swim for days at a time, dance ceremonial dances for weeks. They used herbal tonics, and herbs as food for daily nourishment from on-the-spot location.

In our time, news of hunters or persons stranded in remote areas conclusively stress exhaustion from either fear of starving, exposure, or hunger. If for survival alone, identification is worth while for those involved and reassuring for those concerned that stay at home. Due to physical dependence they had to build energy for bravery in hunting, or fighting, which is known in our time as nerve strength, adrenal secretions, and hormone balance.

In our text we will find many herbs used by them for the liver, blood regenerating, nerve tonics, to restore vitality, strengthen the stomach, etc., all of which have a purpose in systemic harmony. By comparison is it fair to say their available source of nourishment surpasses our mechanized, socialized, chemical (synthetic) existence?

SAMUEL THOMSON THE WHITE MAN'S NATURE HEALER

There were many ways and attempts of commercial exploitation, for good and bad, of Indian Herbalism and Folk Medicine use. Study of one Samuel Thomson deserves our attention.

Samuel Thomson (1769–1843) in literature is usually referred to as a doctor. His one month of schooling, lack of formal training and general education did not disparage the man and his ideals.

The encyclopaedia mentions many prominent Thomson legions, but we cannot find a single word about Samuel Thomson and his system. There are many other incidents in world medical history where lack of socially accepted methods go unnoticed. He was first of all a very gifted person with a strong character, a believer in persuasion. He established his own conception, which of late is known and taught in colleges as Physio-Medicalism.

Thomson's practice included only harmless herbs of bodily correction. He was so successful that opposition from the medical profession was strong and uncompromising. They succeeded in prosecuting him, but his name was cleared and he is now universally recognised as an outstanding figure in the medical world.

We reviewed several outstanding "one book authors" formally trained by medical standards but who changed to the Thomson system because of previous unfavourable experience. In England his system was successfully adopted by Herbalist A. I. Coffin (1798–1866), Samuel Westcott Tilke (1794) and many others. Emphasis on his significance was created by knowledge of Indian Herbalogy and Indian Folk Medicine.

It is reasonably estimated that Samuel Thomson effectively treated and helped 2,000,000 people, some say as many as 3,000,000. This of course includes personal analysis and people following his system under guidance. We are not preaching success without education, but to Thomson's critics this was their point, no education, professional training; why he could hardly speak proper English, and his writing was best interpreted by himself.

The acquaintance of Dr. Thomson's review is not for promotion of his theory and practice but to bring to your attention the amount of success possible from even local Indian Herbs and Folk Medicine. Knowledge of plant life was from his immediate area and still the doctor gained more recognition than any single person in the American history of medicine.

An unanswered thought persists: What can we accomplish from total Indian Herbalogy? The arguments and objections because Samuel Thomson could not read and write proper English had little control over Herbal identification, use, and success of dispensing plant life as human correction. It so happens that the Indians had never heard of this language before the white man came. North American natives, with 25,000–30,000 years of pre-Columbian experience in sickness and health, herbs have a positive internal language of their own.

CIVILIZATION VERSUS CULTURE

From across the Atlantic the Europeans arrived and found a condition of "opportunities unlimited". Their civilized ways brought about many changes. From this time hence the New World has progressively depended on a more modern approach. Granted, some things were put here to be improved upon by man for man. Food, as medicine, does not need modernization, for in the natural state it contains all the living chemical elements essential to man. Nobel prizes have been given for medical achievements of serums and formula in the pharmaceutical industry.

Many compounds have been discontinued in the search for improved and effective pathological results only to be replaced by another sincere attempt to redeem the formula, and persons of the administered past. The wonder drugs of ten years ago are seldom used or remembered today, yet the search goes on.

Specialization is so deep and often misleading. We are getting closer to the bacilli than the man himself in our search for an antibiotic to rid the system of unwanted microbes. Very often a different and more complicated type is encountered and the patient slips farther out of reach and we have the modern cliche of "accumulated side affect" or "he or she is allergic".

Our Indians were not trained to our civilized technicalities of the body, and scientific names of malfunctions were uncomplicated. Basically, our original people were constitutionally more fit than we are in our refined, polluted, chemical, tense way of provoking existence. Their nature healers were thought of as inspired individuals with vivid importance to their people. When necessary they administered innocent remedies which never injured their patients. They soon recovered without accommodating the acute or chronic symptoms of modern preparations. These men never claimed to know more than our physicians. They simply relied on the created organic properties of plants and the blood through its circulation, that knows more about individual chemical balance than technical equipment or means. Which in reality, after all is said and done, boils down to how we respond and feel. They never analysed a cell, bacteria, germs or micro-organisms of any kind. Their psychology must have been much as 1 Cor. 12:20–26 refers to: "God hath tempered the body together that there should be no schism in the body but that the members should have the same care one for another, and whether one member suffer, all members suffer with."

Physiological laws of nature and ideas of divine providence concerning our health are abusively unjust. As if health and sickness were previously sanctioned and bestowed according to a Heavenly plan. This ideal is often the beginning of a disillusion, in this case, locking in self pity, sickness because of old age, and misfortunes as if it were meant to be. This may be interpreted as being controversial by those professing to know more about the events of divinity than our individual physical requirements. But for some it is more convenient than to admit that the condition could be due to our own unfavourable indulgence, with or without knowledge of the consequence. Would we agree to: will and duties are ours, events are providence?

Man's conception of nature should be commanded by obeying the vast material fact symbolizing the sovereign creator of the universe. Modern science of civilization will explain the medical culture of the past, as nature and wisdom are one and the same.

EMPIRISM AND DYNAMICS OF HERBALOGY

To the majority, human evolution of 200,000,000 years or more is negligible. Modern medical practice is estimated within the past twenty generations. Folk Medicine and Herbalism are in scrolls of the oldest written histories, after or together with religion.

Our point of view is that after plants became part of our world, animals started to exist with a built-in dependence on the flora of their domain. As plants grow they are able to assimilate and create life from the earth's mineral and chemical substance. From this new, alive creation all living patterns are extended. Therefore, by instinct, or experience, man in all parts of the globe soon distinguished plant life as daily food for man and animal; specifics for medicine; poisonous plants for man and animal, but the same is not always fatal to every specimen.

From time to time we read about new discoveries of what we call forgotten truth. National convention participants often speak about a herb as if it were just discovered for the first time. The written pages of Folk Medicine are yellow and torn with age and use. Social, professional and commercial opinions of the notorious poison oak. marihuana, and jimson weed are an accepted fact. Too few of us credit the residing properties of corrective herbs as being just as effective but in beneficial qualities.

Modern medicine has many good credits, but in medical literature alarming warnings of caution are also given. For the past twenty years actually no new ideas or discoveries are signified in medical science. Yes, there are many spectacular technical demonstrations and improvements, but not valued as a new idea, discovery or approach.

In many fields of our suffering, modern medicine has exhausted all possible chemical approach. We have to admit that many sicknesses by science and law are declared incurable, and the patient is treated to relieve the symptoms, but the condition is still in progress. Every day there is a new-name discovery for sickness; 30,000 was an estimate of disease names a few years ago. It would take a daily world census to keep up with this, and inevitably more sickness lead to a longer list of incurables followed by more and more new medication, which seems to accumulate; and so we have encouraged more and deeper problems.

It doesn't take too long to find that after testing more than 3,000 rats, the medicine is approved and declared safe for women's treatment. But in a short time a terrible and fatal side-effect is announced after treating many with prolonged use of the new miracle medicine. What was safe for 3,000 rats is fatal to women. Which brings us to another twentieth-century discovery. There is finally some difference between women and rats.

Today we can chemically produce sea water which absolutely has the same formula composition according to taste, smell, feel, etc., as sea water, but no sea life can live in this water. When the smallest part of natural sea water is added all life is encouraged immediately.

The rational starting point of the medical world discovery is basically empirism of Folk Medicine.

Today the total plant estimate is over 1,500,000, of which approximately 300,000 are classified as new plants. As about progress in our field, in the early fifties about 8,000 medical botanics were estimated, with new classifications approaching over 15,000 in the late sixties.

HERBALOGY ABROAD

Herbalogy abroad is the most dynamic and progressive. The Orient and Europe, especially Russia, has an army of scientists and practitioners preoccupied with world medical plants research. Whether pathology is from home or foreign soil the field of research holds unlimited opportunity to compare peoples' practical accumulative knowledge concerning history of medical botanics around the world. Every plant has some property that research of our modern science can classify in this endless field of unknown plant purpose and acceptance.

From our Herbalogy book review two names have served more than fifty years: Joseph E. Meyer, "Herbalist" for North America, classified 470 herbals, "Potters Cyclopedia" of drug preparations with 700 plants for the Commonwealth. To date the above books, which have been reprinted, are the only reliable privately published Herbals. There are many other attempts, but they have had only local and temporary fame, despite their excellent value.

We have reviewed Russian literature in the Bibliography. The latest information arrived after our manuscript was in print. Once again as a reminder, Herbalogy abroad is accepted for all known treatment and commands respect in many quarters, including numerous Institutes, Government Bodies, Special Schools, Medical Institutes, Laboratories, Clinics, Universities, Academies of Science, Experimental Stations, Botanic Gardens, School and Youth organizations, for field work in identifying and collecting material for Folk Medicine. The following is from botanical analyses and research for 1968: Alkaloid, over 6,000; Ether Oil, over 4,000; Glucoside (for heart), over 2,000; Saponine, over 3,000; Flavin, about 1,000; Coumarin, 1,000.

Russian Botanics have over 17,000 classified higher flowering plants, of which about 2,500 are used in Folk Medicine. For industrial, commercial (export) and medicine over 600 different plants are worked out by experiments and promoted for over 77 per cent heart and blood circulation conditions; 74 per cent liver and stomach; 80 per cent female corrective; 73 per cent bronchitis; etc., use only plant preparations.

There are over 100,000 accepted medical preparations in the world (Atlas, Moscow, 1963). Of these 30 per cent use pure plants, the other 70 per cent partly plants and partly chemicals. For heart conditions many of the plants cannot be substituted. In Russia, total outlet of plant life is up to 60,000 tons, not including the domestic cultivation by 25,000 Chinese-tea growers and an unknown amount of herbals used as domestic preparations.

In 1967 there were nineteen specialized medical botanic farms with over 250,000 total acres under cultivation belonging to a special state Lekarsprom (Medical Industry), and over 800 collective and state farms (Kolchaz and Sovchoz), working under contract with several state bodies. The over-all amount is still not enough to cover domestic and export requirements. The federal government encourages growth and collection of varied botanics. Educational material on Herbalogy is distributed by and through articles, books, booklets, brochures, encylopaedias, daily publications, magazines and monography.

LITERATURE ABROAD

Dealing with literature on our subject in Russia: publications on botanics are falling short of public request. This is most impressive and encouraging for our concern of the people in all lands.

The following information on their herbal publications is not for statistics but as illustration only. This is but a fraction of total publications Bello-Russ., Academy of Science, 1965, published 50,000 copies of "Medical Plants" priced at 1.73 roubles ($1.50), 380 pages, fully illustrated. Second edition 1966. The third edition, 1967, improved and enlarged issue, 75,000 copies with over 400 pages, 1.63 roubles ($1.80). In 1967 Kolos, Moscow, published "Medical Plants of U.S.S.R., 400 pages, fully illustrated, with 180,000 copies at 1.10 roubles ($1.22). Omitting many others, we have received "Malaya Medicinskay Encyclopaedia" (a small medical encyclopaedia), where herbals take prominent place with latest data. Of the twenty-four volumes we have only seven, all others being in preparation. Each volume is of ordinary encyclopaedia size of folio, with illustrations (some in full colour), and an average of 1,200 pages. The price is 2.20 roubles (about $2.50) a volume. There are 124,000 copies of each volume which means that the first seven volumes give us more than 8,600,000 copies. The set is aimed for general readers, students, teachers, agronomists, scientists, doctors, state organizations, Kolchoz, Sovchos, herb collectors, etc.

The books are difficult to obtain because as soon as they arrive all available stock goes direct to awaiting readers.

The millions of books on health and herbs in use by the army of scientists, researchers and writers is but a small amount compared to the legions of readers and practical businessmen connected with medical botanics. It is not quantity of books published, but the fact that our North American plants and our North American Folk Medicine has had all the attention and credit they deserve.

Publications are available for professions interested in chemical botanical facts, not opinions. Others are less technical for those who can read; can see; and appreciate plant life, sponsored by none other than from the original of origin—creation itself.

Encouraging material from England, Germany and India, as well as from Russia, also followed after printing procedures were set. From all indications the subject under discussion holds world thoughts in steady and undisputed scientific attention.

In most countries primary research is no native flora, not just for abstract scientific knowledge, but for practical purposes of decorating, commercial, and medical powers. Foreign ambition is centred on flora of the American continent for comparison and uses.

Our wish with this modest contribution is to attract attention to our own native treasures which are analysed and admired in distant countries, but so neglected in our own.

CONCLUSION

The beneficial properties of herbs as medicines will often depend upon the greenness or ripeness of the plant. The time for cutting and digging is essential to the peak susceptibility of its known attributes. Whether it be summer, winter, spring or autumn, the timing must be in accord with the plant's protocol. For instance, Cascara, or Sacred Bark, after it has been stripped in the proper season from the tree and made into a powder or tincture is more valuable and effective with age. Nettle is a good food in its earliest stage of growth, but will prove unpleasant with age.

Another great essential of a plant which is to be selected for its medical qualities is its environment. If indigenous to the locality or country wherein it is found, it is the proper one to select. Plants that are introduced from other countries are lessened, or deprived, of their virtues, unless they meet in their new home all the essential conditions possessed in their native place.

It must be apparent to all that herbs are liable to suffer from soil, climate, etc., and from these conditions will vary the medical properties attributed to them. When giving a medical herb be informed as to its proper curative effect upon the system. A herb gathered at the correct time and prepared properly will secure restoration to a patient from disease to health.

There are two terms we use in the action of herbal medicine on the system, they are: Rational Therapeutics, which have a proven scientific course of action within the body, and Empirical Therapeutics, which travel the same circulatory system with unexplained, long established hidden talent. Both have a history of incalculable blessings, and we do not choose one over the other provided both are used intelligently. Many herbal ingredients have great value and strength. But in emergencies they require immediate professional supervision. It is not advisable to take any strong medication on reputation of the past time and individuals.

The parts that make up the world of plants which are used are: Roots, Barks, Twigs, Bulbs, Corms, Rhizomes, Styles, Stigmas, Fruit seed

Juice, Tubers, Herbs, Leaves and Flowers. Supposedly all herbs have a (teleological) identification given by the Creator, and have been called "The Doctrine of Signatures", which indicate the use for which they were intended. Thus a heart-shaped leaf should be used for the heart, the liver leaf, with its three-lobed leaf, for the liver, the walnut as a brain tonic, and so similar shaped plants were named for specific organs of the human body.

We are not suggesting that you make a test project from every leaf, flower or root with this significance, although some of the known plants for bodily correction do correspond this way. There are also plants that do not resemble a part of the body, but have corrective influence over a certain function. Dandelion root has always been used for the liver, but in no way does the signature doctrine apply.

Perhaps in the beginning the resembling plants were planned for our associated awareness, the remaining encouraged by experience. If this is how it was indeed, planned the Indians of all lands displayed noteworthy wisdom before ever a word had been written.

From the first method of analysing herbs to present-day techniques much insight has been obtained as to their content. Much is still unknown, and no doubt many creations will never be fathomed, as the study of goodness and simplicity are indisputably united and often inconceivable. Natural medicine is timeless, it is among the first of creation, and it is as new as today. The past is very rich—the future is promising with all of our scientific "modern discovery of forgotten truths".

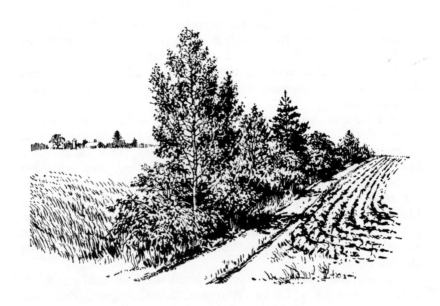

DEFINITIONS

of the medical actions of herbs and herbal medicines

Alterative   Producing a healthful change without perception.
Anodyne   Relieves pain.
Anthelmintic   A medicine that expels worms.
Aperient   Gently laxative without purging.
Aromatic   A stimulant, spicy.
Astringent   Causes contraction and arrests discharges.
Antibilious   Acts on the bile, relieving biliousness.
Antiemetic   Stops vomiting.
Antileptic   Relieves fits.
Antiperiodic   Arrests morbid periodic movements.
Anthilic   Prevents the formation of stones in the urinary organs.
Antirheumatic   Relieves or cures rheumatism.
Antiscorbutic   Cures or prevents scurvy.
Antiseptic   A medicine that aims at stopping putrification.
Antispasmodic   Relieves or prevents spasms.
Antisyphilitic   Having affect or curing venereal diseases.
Carminative   Expels wind from the bowels.
Carthatic   Evacuating from the bowels.
Cephalic   Remedies used in diseases of the head.
Cholagogue   Increases the flow of bile.
Condiment   Improves the flavour of foods.
Demulcent   Soothing, relieves inflammation.
Deobstruent   Removes obstruction.
Depurative   Purifies the blood.
Detergent   Cleansing to boils, ulcers and wounds, etc.
Diaphoretic   Produces perspiration.
Discutient   Dissolves and heals tumours.
Diuretic   Increases the secretion and flow of urine.
Emetic   Produces vomiting.
Emmenagogue   Promotes menstruation.
Emollient   Softens and soothes inflamed parts.
Esculent   Eatable as a food.
Exanthematous   Remedy for skin eruptions and diseases.
Expectorant   Facilitates expectoration.
Febrifuge   Abates and reduces fevers.
Hepatic   A remedy for diseases of the liver.

Herpatic   A remedy for skin diseases of all types.
Laxative   Promotes bowel action.
Lithontryptic   Dissolves calculi in the urinary organs.
Maturating   Ripens or brings boils to a head.
Mucilaginous   Soothing to all inflammation.
Nauseant   Produces vomiting.
Nervine   Acts specifically on the nervous system, stops nervous excitement.
Opthalmicum   A remedy for eye diseases.
Parturient   Induces and promotes labour at childbirth.
Pectoral   A remedy for chest affections.
Refrigerant   Cooling.
Resolvent   Dissolves boils and tumours.
Rubifacient   Increases circulation and produces red skin.
Sedative   A nerve tonic, promotes sleep.
Sialogogue   Increases the secretion of saliva.
Stomachic   Strengthens the stomach. Relieves indigestion.
Styptic   Arrests bleeding.
Sudorific   Produces profuse perspiration.
Tonic   A remedy which is invigorating and strengthening.
Vermifuge   Expels worms from the system.

ADDER'S TONGUE   Erythronium americanum
(N.O.: Liliaceae)

Common Names: DOG TOOTH VIOLET, SERPENT'S TONGUE, YELLOW SNOWDROP.

Features: This beautiful little plant, of the Lily family, is among the earliest of our spring flowers of April and May, growing in moist meadows or thinly wooded areas throughout the United States.

The bulb-like root grows some distance below the surface; the interior is white, with fawn-coloured exterior and feather-like roots extending from the bulb.

The stem supports only two leaves which are lanceolate, pale green with purplish or brownish spots and one almost twice as wide as the other. The leaves are more active than the bulb.

The flower is yellow, with its petals swept away from the face-down centre. The petals partially close at night and on cloudy days and this plant diminishes with the heat of the summer. The fruit is a capsule.

Medicinal Parts: The bulb and leaves.

Solvent: Water.

Bodily Influence: Emetic, Emollient and Antiscorbutic when fresh. Nutritive when dry.

Uses: Made into a tea with the combination of Horsetail grass (Equisetum hyemale) is a good agent for conditions of bleeding or ulcers of the breast, bowels, or for tumours and inflammation therein. Also quick relief for nose bleeding and to aid sore eyes.

The fresh root and leaves simmered in milk is beneficial in dropsy, relieves hiccoughs, vomiting and bleeding from the lower bowels. Juice of the plant infused in apple cider has also been found helpful for the above mentioned.

It is said that the plant boiled in oil is a panacea for wounds and to reduce inflammation. According to Culpeper this herb is under the dominion of the Moon and Cancer and, therefore, if the weakness of the retentive faculty be caused by an evil influence of Saturn in any part of the body governed by the Moon or under the dominion of Cancer, this herb cures it by sympathy.

Dose: 1 teaspoonful of the dried leaves or root to 1 cup of boiling water. Drink a cupful during the day, a mouthful at a time.

Externally: The fresh leaves, bruised and applied as an application three or more times a day, are healing to scrofulous ulcers and tumours. Taken with the tea internally.

1

AGRIMONY   Agrimonia eupatoria, L.
(N.O.: Rosaceae)

Common Names: COCKLEBURR, STICKLEWORT, BURR MARIGOLD.

Features: Agrimony is found in the borders of fields, in ditches and in hedges throughout Asia, Europe, Canada and the U.S.A., flowering in July or August. The seeds ripen soon after.

In Parkinson's "Theatre of Plants" (1640) there are seven varieties of Agrimony; the first and most important is the common Agrimony found in Italy. Second, sweet smelling Agrimony found in Italy. The

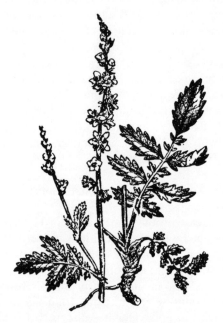

AGRIMONY   Agrimonia eupatoria, L.
(Dr. A. J. Thut, Guelph, Canada)

third is Bastard Agrimony, also found in Italy, which although the resemblance is close is not a variety of this plant. The fourth is Hemp Agrimony, which grows in damp places such as ditches and water courses in England. The fifth, sixth and seventh come from America: the fifth and sixth being varieties of Hemp Agrimony and the seventh known as Water Agrimony. This last named is also known as Burr marigold. It is said to have originated in North America.

The bright yellow star-like flowers are numerous and grow individu-

2

ally from the long, tapering stem. This erect, round, hairy stem reaches a height of 2 ft.

The many pinnate leaves, hairy on both sides, and 5–6 in. long, grow alternately, having three to five pairs of lanceolate, toothed leaflets, with intermediate two sizes of smaller leaves. The taste is astringent and slightly bitter.

The roots are woody and the seeds form little burrs, but it is not the generally known troublesome cockleburr.

Medicinal Parts: Root, leaves, whole herb.

Solvent: Boiling water.

Bodily Influence: Mild Astringent, Tonic, Diuretic, Deobstruent.

Uses: Agrimony is an old remedy of North American and European aborigines for debility, as it gives tone to the whole system. Useful in bowel complaints, simple diarrhoea and relaxed bowels, chronic mucous diseases, asthma, fevers and colds. In chronic affections of the digestive organs, it seems to expel the evil dispositions of the body, including dropsy and yellow jaundice. It opens the obstructions of the liver, loosens the hardness of the spleen, when applied externally as well, with hot damp packs using Turkish towels. The liver is the builder of blood, and blood the nourishment of the body, and Agrimony strengthens and cleanses the liver.

It is healing to all inward wounds, bruises, pains and other distempers. A decoction taken warm before an incontrollable seizure will remove the spell and in time help to prevent another performance. It will kill trouble-making worms and is useful in bed-wetting.

It is cleansing to the blood stream and will assist skin conditions so often complained of these days.

As a gargle for sore throat and mouth, it is very serviceable; also for obstructed menstruation.

The herb has been recommended for dyspepsia, but is probably only useful in the disorder when carefully combined with other more desirable operating agents.

Special note: it should not be used when there is a dryness of secretions.

John Hill, M.D., in "British Herbal" (1751) states that Agrimony was greatly recommended by the ancients but is very much neglected in present-day practice. John Parkinson, in the "Theatre of Plants" (1640), recommended that a decoction of the plant, "made with wine, is good against the sting and biting of Serpents".

Country people give it to their cattle when they are troubled with respiratory difficulties.

Dose: Adult amount (children less according to age) 1 oz. to $1\frac{1}{4}$ pints of water simmered down to 1 pint in $\frac{1}{2}$ teacup or larger doses every four hours. Sweeten with honey or pure maple syrup.

3

Externally: The wine decoction applied to draw out thorns and splinters of wood or any other foreign object in the flesh.

ALDER   Black prinos verticillatus
(N.O.: Aquifoliaceae)

Common Names: WINTER BERRY, FEVER BUSH, BLACK ALDER.

Features: Alder, the common name applied to the genus alnus, of the Betulaceae or Birch family. Ten species occur in the United States, but altogether there are about thirty species of deciduous monoecious trees and shrubs widely distributed throughout the northern hemisphere and ranging as far south as Peru. Most Alders flower in the spring before the leaves appear, with ripe berries in autumn.

Medicinal Part: The bark.

Solvent: Boiling water.

Bodily Influence: Tonic, Alterative, Astringent, Cathartic.

Uses: Very similar in action to Cascara when used for constipation. Alder is an agent used for jaundice, diarrhoea, gangrene, dropsy and all diseases with symptoms of great weakness. It has had success in treatment of dyspepsia, combined with 2 drams of powdered Golden seal (Hydrastis) infused in 1 pint of boiling water and when cold taken in wine glass doses periodically throughout the day and repeated daily.

Make sure you age the outer and inner bark, as the green bark will provoke strong vomiting, pain and gripping in the stomach. Let the decoction stand and settle two or three days, until the yellow colour is changed to black. In this manner it will strengthen the stomach and procure an appetite.

The berries are cathartic and vermifuge when combined with apple cider, a pleasant and effective worm medicine for children. Plan on giving this when the moon is full, as they are most conducive to treatment. Fast the patient before going to bed and give a herbal laxative, fasting again in the morning, and repeat Alder medication. Repeat again after four weeks as the larvae will still be present.

Dose: ½ dram of powdered bark to 1 dram of apple cider; 1 teaspoonful three times a day, for three days in a row, or as above.

Externally: The decoction forms an excellent local application in gangrene, indolent ulcers and in some affections of the skin.

The inner bark boiled in vinegar is an approved remedy to kill head lice and to relieve the itch and take away scabs by drying them up in a short time. For oral hygiene, it is cleansing to the teeth and to take away pain, at the same time firming to the gums.

Homoeopathic Clinical: Tincture of the bark of the young twigs and the bark of Alnus rubra, Tag alder, and Alnus glutinosa, Common Alder

4

of Europe, is clinically used for Ammenorrhoea and Leucorrhoea, Enlarged Glands, Gleet, Haemorrhage, Psora, Rheumatism, Scrofula, Syphilis and many kinds of skin sickness such as Herpes, Impetigo, Prurigo.

Russian Use: Three species of Alnus incanc (Olha), black, grey and white, have a prominent place in Pharmacopoeia and Folk Medicine.

Parts Used: Cones (Fructus Alni), bark of the young twigs (Cortex Alni), leaves (Folia Alni).

These parts of Alder contain 16 per cent of Tannin, which gives predominant characteristics as an astringent.

Uses: As a tea it is used for loose stomach (diarrhoea) and bleeding thereof.

Dose: 3 to 4 cups a day, a mouthful at a time. Can be combined with other herbal teas for astringent and tonic uses.

The extract in alcohol or Russian vodka can be used before meals, 25 to 40 drops three times a day.

ALE HOOF or GROUND IVY   Glecoma hederacea
(N.O.: Labiatae)

Common Names: CAT'S FOOT, GROUND IVY, GILL GO BY GROUND, GILL CREEP BY GROUND, TURN HOOF, HAY MAIDS and ALE HOOF. Various names come from the many localities in which it grows.

Features: The plant is common to North America and Europe. Found in shady places, waste grounds, dry ditches, in almost every part of the land. The green, round leaves endure every season except when the temperature falls below freezing point.

Medicinal Part: The leaves.

Solvent: Water.

Bodily Influence: Stimulant, Tonic, Pectoral

Uses: A singular herb for all inward wounds, ulcerated lungs or other parts indicating the same condition. Either by itself or boiled supplementary with other herbs and drinks.

In a short time it will ease all gripping pains, gas and choleric conditions of the stomach and spleen. Useful in Yellow Jaundice as it opens the stoppage of the gall-bladder and liver; in melancholy, by relieving obstructions of the spleen; expels poisons and also the plague; encourages a release of urine and women's complaints.

A decoction of Ale hoof and the best wine drunk for a length of time will ease a person troubled with sciatica, hip gout or arthritic hands and knees. A decoction with honey and a little Burnt Alum is excellent as a gargle for sore mouth or throat and to wash the sores and ulcers of male and female intimacy. An infusion of the leaves is very beneficial in lead colic. Painters who make use of it are seldom, if ever, troubled with this malady. The fresh juice snuffed up the nose often takes care of most deep-rooted, long-established headaches.

This is one of the most wonderful of all herbs. The mineral content is iron, copper, iodine, phosphorus, potassium. The ancient herbalists praised it greatly, saying it would cure insanity and melancholia by opening the stopping of the spleen. It also regulates the heart beat by making the blood more fluid. An excellent assistant to aid glandular health and prevent premature ageing.

Dose: 1 teaspoonful to 1 cup of boiling water; powder, $\frac{1}{2}$ dram to 1 dram.

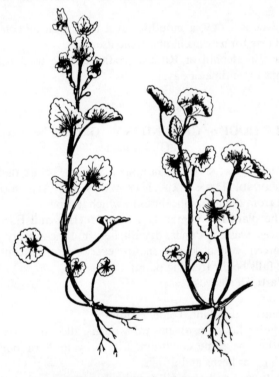

GROUND IVY   Glecoma hederacea
(Department of Agriculture, Ontario, Canada)

Externally: The fresh leaf bruised and bound around a new wound will hasten an early recovery. Ale hoof juice, honey and Marigold (Calendula) boiled together will clean fistulas, ulcers, and control the spreading or eating away of cancers and ulcers, and the less serious effect of the troublesome itching scabs, weals and other skin irritations in any part of the body. The juice dropped into the ear is helpful in noise and singing, and cleansing to decayed hearing.

6

ALFALFA Medicago sativa
(N.O.: Leguminoseae)

Common Names: LUCERN, BUFFALO HERB.

Features: It is native to Asia and did not reach North America until around 1850 or 1860. This deep-growing plant is seen from Maine to Virginia and westward to the Pacific coast in the United States.

North American Indians adapted Alfalfa quickly for human use, as well as for animals. In England and South Africa it is called Buffalo herb.

This is a perennial, herbaceous plant, with two stems. Leaflets: three-toothed above. Flowers: violet. Calyx: five-toothed. Corolla: papilionaceous, six lines long. Stamens: nine united and one free. Pod: spirally coiled and without spines. The small, violet-purple or bluish flowers bloom from June until August. In some regions it is cut every month as cultivated food for both man and animal.

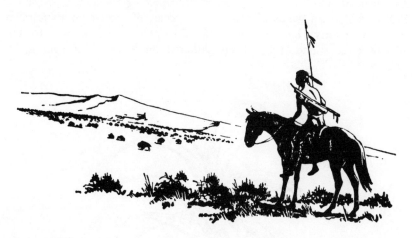

The organic salt is among the richest known, the depth and spread of its roots enabling it to absorb its valuable nutrition as far as 125 ft. below the earth's surface.

Medicinal Part: The leaves.

Solvent: Water.

Bodily Influence: Nutrient, Tonic.

Uses: Alfalfa was discovered by the Arabs and is one of the first known herbs. They called it the "Father of all Foods". This is interesting as they knew only by evidential experience. It is only in recent years that we moderns are rediscovering its valuable nutritive properties, which include organic minerals of Calcium, Magnesium, Phosphorus and Potassium, plus all the known vitamins including Vitamin K and the recently discovered Vitamin B[8] and Vitamin P.

7

It is helpful for every condition of the body whether it be maintaining or regaining health, as the contents are balanced for complete absorption. It may be used by itself or blended with other herbal teas with or between meals.

Claudia V. James (1963) mentions stock farmers of South Africa improving the beauty of ostrich feathers and that cows gave richer milk, chickens laid more often, with the food content of a better quality. State-wise, a turkey farm in Apple Valley, California, has better stock after including Alfalfa as part of the diet.

ALOES   Aloe socotrina
(N.O.: Liliaceae)

Common Names: BOMBAY ALOES, TURKEY ALOES, MOKA ALOES, ZANZIBAR ALOES.

Features: Aloe, a genus of nearly 200 species of mostly South African succulent plants. The properties of this plant were known to the ancient Greeks and it has been gathered on Socotra for over 2,000 years.

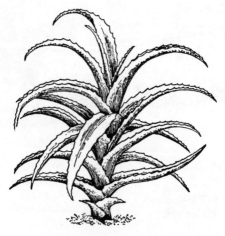

ALOES   Aloe socotrina
(Vishaya Schkolla, Moscow, 1963)

Aloe thrives in warm regions and grows wild in Florida, U.S.A. It is much like succulent cactus in texture. The leaves are usually elongated, of a deep brown or olive colour, frequently pointed, blunt, or spiny-toothed, sometimes blotched or mottled. The stem is commonly short with a basal rosette of leaves; taste: peculiar and bitter; powder:

8

a bright yellow. The red or yellow tubular flowers are found on a stalk in simple or branched clusters.

These properties change somewhat in the different varieties, some species being tree-like with forked branches. Aloe bainesii grows to heights of 65 ft. and 15 ft. wide at the base. Other species of Aloe are often cultivated in gardens of succulents, including the miniature ones grown in homes; they require strong light and careful watering. The "American aloe" is not an Aloe, but Agave americana.

Medicinal Part: The insipid juice of the leaves, which is a greenish translucent salve-like substance.

Solvent: Water.

Bodily Influence: Tonic, Purgative, Emmenagogue, Anthelmintic.

Uses: Aloes are one of the most sovereign agents we have among the herbal medicines, being cleansing to the morbid matter of the stomach, liver, spleen, kidney and bladder. Does not gripe and is very healing and soothing to all the tissue, blood and lymph fluids it obliges.

Aloes should never be used in pregnancy, or by itself when persons are suffering from haemorrhoids, as in haemorrhoids it arouses and irritates the lower bowels. Much used in suppressed menstruation, dyspepsia, skin lesions, disease of the liver, headaches, etc.

Dose: In constipation, in powder form from $\frac{1}{2}$–2 grains, depending on age and condition; for obstructed or suppressed menstruation, 5–10 grains twice daily; to expel thread worms dissolve the Aloe in warm water and use as an injection. The same mixture can be taken internally for several days.

Externally: Powdered Aloes made into a strong decoction and rubbed over the nipples will help wean a nursing child; the association of pleasant experience will soon find other sources due to the disagreeable bitter taste.

Aloes show the same cleansing power for external application. A piece of white linen or cotton saturated in Aloe water and applied to fresh wounds, as well as old ones, are quickly closed.

If ulcers progress to a running stage sprinkle Aloe powder thick enough to cover the open wound and secure with clean gauze, repeating daily. The powder will absorb the morbid, fluid matter, at the same time encouraging healthy, new replacement tissue.

The fresh juice, or solution made from dried leaves, is soothing to tender sunburns, insect bites, over-exposure to X-ray or other emolient uses.

Homoeopathic Clinical: Abdomen (plethora of), Anus (affections of), Bronchitis, Colic, Constipation, Cough, Diarrhoea, Dysentery, Gleet, Gonorrhoea, Haemorrhoids, Hysteria, Lumbago, Onanism (effects of), **Russian Experience:** Aloe vera is cultivated in Russia in many houses Phathisis, Proctitis, Prolapsus uteri, Sacrum (pain in), Tenesmus.

9

as a decorative and medicinal plant. The Soviet Government cultivates Aloe vera for commercial and industrial purposes in the Black Sea coastal area.

Uses: Medical science gives prominent place for this herb and others of the same family. The famous academician, B. R. Fillatow, makes an extract of Aloe for treatment of eye conditions and injections for run-down organisms.

Extract of the leaves, Sabur, is common in hospitals, and in all dispensaries used as a laxative. The influence stimulates the gall-bladder by increasing its secretions.

Warning: Do not give in cases of degeneration of the liver and gall-bladder, as well as menstruation, pregnancy and piles. As a rule it is safe to use Aloe as it is established by Folk Medicine, but in all complicated cases the advice of medical or trained practitioners in this field should be sought.

Externally: In radio and X-ray treatment given on the skin it is important to remember that Aloe leaves prepared with Castor oil or Eucalyptus oil are healing and a moisturizer in prevention against further complications.

ALUM ROOT Heuchera americana
(N.O.: Saxifragaceae)

Common Name: AMERICAN SANICLE.

Features: Alum root is of the Saxifrage family. The long flowering stems have panicles of small rose to purplish white flowers.

The root has a powerful astringent taste and is of yellowish colour. Powdered Alum is the ordinary Alum heated, dried and then pulverized, called also Burnt alum.

Medicinal Part: The root.

Solvent: Water.

Bodily Influence: Astringent, Steptic.

Uses: The spring leaves were used as food by the Indians after being boiled and steamed. The wet, pounded root was taken in small amounts to stop diarrhoea. The boiled root water was given as tea for general debility, and to stop fevers.

Alum is a pure and powerful astringent used effectively in haemorrhage from small bleeding vessels, as of the nose, mouth and surface capillaries, or ulceration of the mouth and throat, also as an injection in bleeding piles, and leucorrhoea. Has been given internally in diabetes, diarrhoea and dysentery.

Dose: $\frac{1}{4}$ teaspoonful of the powdered root to 1 cup of water; drink in $\frac{1}{3}$ amounts three times daily. Do not use extensively.

10

Externally: Our Indians used the fresh pounded root on sores and swellings. Other uses have been for granulated eyelids, or sore eyelids Dip a piece of linen in a weak solution and apply to the closed eye. Dilute Alum water is a proven remedy in mouth conditions where an unhealthy flesh and stagnant blood exists. Suppurated (pus producing) in-grown nails respond to applications of Alum.

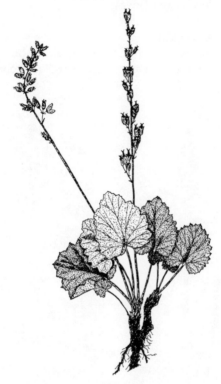

ALUM ROOT   Heuchera americana
(Wild Plants, Canadian Agricultural Department, Ottawa, 1964)

AMAARANTHUS   Amaranthus hypochondriacus
(N.O.: Americanceae)

Common Names: PILE WORT, PRINCE'S FEATHER, RED COCK'S COMB. LOVE-LIES-BLEEDING, VELVET FLOWER.
Features: Amaranthus; the typical genus of herbaceous plants of about sixty species of apetalous plants.
The name is from the Greek, meaning "unfading". In some species the flowers preserve their appearance after they are plucked and dried. Because of this poets have made the plant an emblem of immortality.

11

Chiefly the plant inhabits the tropical countries, and is remarkable for the white or reddish scales of which their flowers are composed. Common garden, ornamental varieties include Love-lies-bleeding, Prince's feather, Cocks comb. The medical properties are of more value in its wild state. They continue in flower from August to the time of Jack Frost.

Medicinal Parts: Flowers and leaves.

Solvent: Water.

Bodily Influence: Astringent.

Uses: Agreeably recognized for menorrhagia (abnormally excessive menstruation), diarrhoea, dysentery, haemorrhage from the bowels.

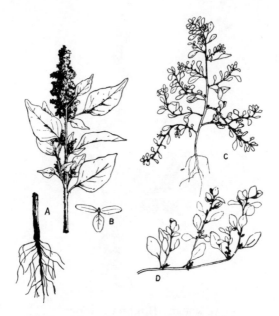

AMARANTHUS   Amaranthus hypochondriacus
A—Redroot pigweed   B—Seedling   C—Tumbleweed   D—Prostrate pigweed
(Ontario Department of Agriculture, Toronto, Canada, 1966)

A decoction is taken in wine-glass doses for the above mentioned. There seems to be some controversy concerning the flower. Culpeper (1616) states: "The flower dried and beated into powder and taken stops the terms in woman, as do almost all other red things." Dalen states, "There can be no compound medicines wherefore they are ill persuaded that think the flower gentle to stunch bleeding because of the colour only, if they had no other reason to induce them thereto." Modern writers àre sceptic of the doctrine of the signature in the plant kingdom; most things have a meaning if we observe them.

12

Dose: 1 teaspoonful to 1 cupful of boiling water. Drink 1 or 2 cupfuls a day, a large mouthful at a time, of the tincture, ½–1 fluid dram.
Externally: For ulcerated conditions of the mouth and throat gargle a warm solution three or four times a day, and apply externally to lesions. 2 tablespoonfuls to 1 quart of water, simmered 10 min. and used as an injection for leucorrhoea, and female conditions.

ANGELICA Angelica atropurpurea
(N.O.: Ammiaceae)

Common Names: MASTERWORT, PURPLE ANGELICA, ALEXANDERS, ARCHANGEL.
Features: Angelica, a genus of herbs of the family ammiaceae. Several species are native to North America. The name Angelica, however, is popularly applied to various other members of the same family.

Angelica atropurpurea is perennial and grows in fields and damp places, developing greenish-white flowers from May to August. Also, it is cultivated in gardens from Canada to Carolina.

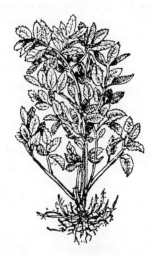

ANGELICA Angelica atropurpurea
(Naukova Dumka, Kiev, Russia)

The plant has a peculiar but not unpleasant odour, a sweet taste, afterwards pungent; but on drying it loses much of these qualities. The cake decoration known as candied angelica is the dried stalks, preserved with sugar.
Medicinal Parts: Root, herb and seed.

13

Solvent: Boiling water.
Bodily Influence: Aromatic, Stimulant, Carminative, Diaphoretic, Expectorant, Diuretic, Emmenagogue.
Uses: The tea taken hot will quickly break up a cold. For general tonic 1–3 cups a day. Angelica should always be remembered in epidemics, as it is said to resist poisons by defending and comforting the heart, blood and spirits.

It is used in flatulent colic and heart-burn. The condition of suppressed liver and spleen causing various digestive malfunctions will yield to this medical herb whose long-standing results have obtained a Heavenly name, "Archangel". Is also serviceable in diseases of the urinary organs.

Dose: 1 oz. of the seed or herb (less if powder is used) to 1 pint of boiling water, taken in $\frac{1}{2}$ cup amounts frequently during the day, or 1 cup after each meal.

Externally: A tea- made of Angelica and dropped on old ulcers will cleanse and heal them. The dry powdered root may also be used for this purpose.

Russian Experience: In Russian literature and pharmacopoeia Angelica occupies prominent attention, prescribed in the form of tablets, extract, powder, all suitably compounded with other herbal ingredients. Latest research and clinical experiments confirms long established, unblemished use of this herb in Folk Medicine.

Uses: Since ancient times Russian people have used Angelica roots, leaves and seeds in tea form for nervous exhaustion, epilepsy, hysteria, as a sedative, for poor digestion, appetiser, stomach and gas bloating, indigestion, heart-burn, atony of the intestines, and as a diaphoretic and expectorant. Extracted Angelica oil used as a pleasant aromatic and tonic.

Other Industries: Veterinary use, as diuretic and diaphoretic. The fresh young leaves, twigs and flowers are artfully used in the food industry for jams, candy, garnish for salad decoration, and baked confections. Especially, Angelica oil (some dry leaves and bark) is used as an aromatic in the wine industry for many varieties of wine, vodka and liquors. The flowering plant is excellent for a good crop of honey, and for this purpose alone cultivation of Angelica archangelica is encouraged.

ARBUTUS, TRAILING Epigaea repens
(N.O.: Ericaceae)

Common Names: GRAVEL PLANT, WILD MAY FLOWER, GRAVEL LAUREL, MOUNTAIN PINK, WINTER PINK, ARBUTUS.
Features: Arbutus, a genus of trees and shrubs in the heath family

(Ericaceae) comprising about twenty species native to southern Asia, the Mediterranean region, and North and South America, as far south as Chili.

Trailing arbutus belongs to the genus Epigaea. This is a small trailing plant, with woody stems, from 6–18 in., which appear early in the spring. An evergreen under-shrub, with a red and brown fibrous root having many tangled rootlets. The stem is 6–18 in. long, woody, rounded and hairy, with a brown bark. The leaves are alternate, and entire, cordate, ovate, petiolate, 2 in. long. The flowers are white, pink or rose coloured, appearing early in the spring in small auxiliary clusters from scaly bracts, and are very fragrant. It is found in woods and sides of hills with northern exposure.

Medicinal Part: The whole plant, especially the leaves.

Solvent: Boiling water.

Bodily Influence: Diuretic Astringent.

Uses: This American plant is said to be superior to Buchu (Barosma crenata) and Uva ursi (Arctostaphylos uva ursi) in all lithic acid diseases of the urinary organs associated with irritation. Useful for gravel, debilitated or relaxed bladder, and in urine containing blood or pus. Successfully used in diarrhoea and bowel complaints of children.

Dose: The infusion of 1 oz. of the whole plant cut small, or the leaves, to 1 pint of boiling water, steep ½ hr. The infusion may be used freely.

Homoeopathic Clinical: Tincture of fresh leaves—Calculi Urinary, Dysuria, Gravel, Dysentery.

ARNICA   Arnica montana
(N.O.: Compositae)

Common Names: LEOPARD'S BANE, ARNICA.

Features: Arnica is of the thistle family, found growing in the northern mountain states of America and Canada.

A perennial herb, with a slender, blackish rhizome 1–2 in. long, from which are given off numerous filiform roots. The stem, 10–12 in. high, is erect pubescent, rough, striated, either simple or with one pair of opposite branches. The leaves, 1½–3 in. long, are few, entire, sessile, opposite, obovate; the radical ones crowded at the base, the upper smaller than the rest. The heads, 2–2½ in. wide, are large and solitary at the summit of the stem and lateral branches. The involucre is cylindrical, dull green, with purplish points and hairy. The disc flowers are yellow and numerous, with tumular corolla with five spreading teeth. The ray flowers are about fifteen in number, yellow in colour. It flowers in July and August.

Arnica is a treasure indeed and has been sought diligently by persons

15

living in accessible localities. The root of Arnica montana, the Mountain tobacco, yields a small quantity of oil and resinous substance.
Medicinal Parts: Rhizome, flowers.
Solvents: Boiling water, alcohol.
Bodily Influence: Stimulant.
Uses: The utmost care should be taken when given internally, as large amounts are poisonous. In emergencies, causing mental or physical shock; pain and swelling after a troublesome dental extraction; sprains of joints; fractured bones; headaches (even concussions), good results follow the internal administration of Arnica. Persons recover much more rapidly than under morphine.

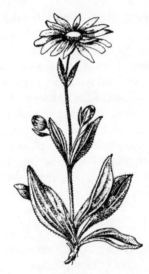

ARNICA   Arnica montana
(Naukova Dumka, Kiev, Russia, 1964)

Administer no more than 5 drops of tincture (children less) every three or four hours, and continue as long as the symptoms seem to require for the above mentioned.

Spirits of Arnica can be made by putting the flowers in brandy or medicinal (internal uses) alcohol. In about three days the tincture may be used: 5 drops every 3–4 hr.

Dose: For infusion, put 2 teaspoonfuls of the flowers to 1 cup of boiling water, simmer for 10 min., cool. To be taken in 5-drop amounts, children less according to age.

Externally: The liquid solution is also used on any unbroken surface to stop pain, such as compresses over rheumatic joints, bruises, painful swollen feet, etc. If bleeding is present a solution of 1–10 dilutions of Calendula (Marigold) is unsurpassed for all lesions or open wounds.

16

Arnica salve is made by heating 1 oz. of the flowers with 1 oz. of cold pressed Arnica oil for a few hours. This is useful for chapped lips and inflamed nostrils, bruises, joint pain, skin rash and acne.

Homoeopathic Clinical: Tincture of whole fresh plants, tincture of root —Abscess, Apoplexy, Back (pain in), Baldness, Bed sores, Black eye, Boils, Brain (affections of), Breath (foetid), Bronchitis, Bruises, Carbuncles, Chest (the affections of), Chorea, Corns, Cramp, Diabetes, Diarrhoea, Dysentery, Ecchymosis, Excoriations, Exhaustion, Eyes (affections of), Feet (sore), Meningitis, Alienation, Miscarriage, Nipples (sore), Nose (affections of), Paralysis, Pleurodynia, Purpura, Rheumatism, Splenalgia, Sprain, Stings, Suppuration, Taste (disorders of), Thirst, Traumatic fever, Tumours, Voice (affections of), Whooping-cough, Wounds.

Russian Experience: At one time Russia had to import Arnica from Central Europe (Germany, Hungary, etc.) for domestic use. Previously thought to be superior to North American Arnica (Arnica chamissonic).

Of late, searching Russian teams scientifically observed both species concerning the medicinal and cultivation contradictory.

Medicinally: The North American variety was the same, if not better in many respects, as the European Arnica.

Uses: Arnica montana has been used since the days of old in Russian Folk Medicine.

The human body responds internationally, and the medicinal properties do not discriminate as to race or nationality. Russian people know of astonishing additions internally. To stop bleeding, boils, inflammation of the genital organs, heart weakness, stimulation of the central nervous system, to promote bile, reduce cholesterol.

Externally: Wounds, black and blue spots (black eye), skin conditions, and many others, the same as above mentioned.

Commercially: The point of view was concentrated on convenient cultivation. From their literature we can learn they have commercial plantations and a very detailed description of their practice.

Arnica is perennial. Once you sow seed, you may harvest for a good many years with little care until flowering season of the next floral medication, which requires some labour to collect. We also found that each acre requires about 5-6 lb. of seed. Total harvest cannot be estimated as it depends on soil conditions, climate, and time for collecting. Due to international demand the price is always increasing. The use of Arnica is limited by the shortage of supply.

North American Herbal Agriculture, and Herbalists, can extend a North American Indian treasure, and Russian experience, from the garden to the patient.

17

ARSESMART   Polygonum hydropiper, L.
(N.O.: Polygonaceae)

Common Names: The hot ARSESMART is called WATER PEPPER (POLY-GONUM HYDROPIPER). The mild ARSESMART is called DEAD ARSSMARE (PERSICARIA MACULATA) or PEACH-WORT because the leaves are just like the leaves of a peach tree, also called PLUMBAGO.

Feature: A well-known plant in America, growing in low lands and about brooks which in most parts are dry in the summer. It flowers in the late summer or early autumn, and the seeds are ripe in August.

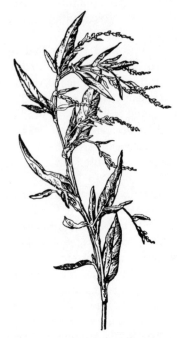

ARSESMART   Polygonum hydropiper, L.
(Vishaya schkolla, Moscow, 1963)

The Arsesmart plants are very much alike, and both have a hot sensation if the broken leaf is touched to the tongue. If seen together the mild water pepper has far broader leaves. Most Herbalists use them together.

The leaves contain essential oil, oxymethyl-anthraquinones; also poly-gonic acid, which has irritant properties, a glycoside which promotes the coagulation of blood and a polygonone-containing ethereal oil which lowers blood pressure. The herb contains formic acid, acetic acid and baldrianic acid, much tannin and a small amount of an essential oil.

18

The fresh plant contains an acrid juice which causes irritation and smarting when brought into contact with the nostrils or eyes. The bruised leaves as well as the seeds will raise blisters if employed as a poultice, as in the case of mustard poultice.

Medicinal Part: The whole herb.

Solvents: Water, alcohol.

Bodily Influence: Stimulant, Diuretic, Diaphoretic.

Uses: Effectual for putrid ulcers in man and beast (internally and externally) having a cooling and drying quality. Swollen injuries, bruises, joint felons, or if the blood has congealed, will dissolve if the juice or the bruised herb is applied. The cold tea will kill worms and cleanse in active putrefied places. Dilute tincture dropped in the ears will kill worms therein. The root or seeds bruised and held on an aching tooth will relieve the pain.

Dose: 1 teaspoonful of the herb cut small or granulated to 1 cup of boiling water; drink cold 1 cup during the day, a mouthful at a time. Of the tincture, 30–60 drops.

Homoeopathic Clinical: Amenorrhoea, Antrum (pain in), Blepharitis, Colic (flatulent), Cough, Diarrhoea, Dysentery, Dysmenia, Dysuria, Eczema, Epilepsy, Gonorrhoea, Gravel, Haemorrhoids, Heart (affections of), Hysteria, Laryngitis, Spleen (affections of), Strangury, Ulcers.

Russian Experience: Arsesmart (Water pepper) is not cultivated commercially but the State encourages its preservation in its natural habitat. In all Russian medical and herbal literature, including general and medical encyclopedias, attention is given to several kinds of Polygonum, and one of them, Polygonum hydropiper (Water pepper-Vodianoy Peretz), is appraised for many things.

Medical research and clinical experiments show that Polygonum contains many minerals and oil, but especially rutin, Vitamins C and K.

Uses: Folk Medicine gives a good account of its use to stop bleeding and sometimes as a diuretic. As a dye that cannot be repeated artificially for rich and beautiful yellow, golden yellow, and golden green colours.

ASH TREE   Fraxinus excelsior, L.
(N.O.: Oleaceae)

Common Names: AMERICAN WHITE ASH, EUROPEAN ASH, WEEPING ASH.

Features: Ash, a genus (fraxinus) of approximately sixty-five species of trees and some shrubs, native mostly of the north temperate zone in North America, Europe and Asia, and extending south into Mexico and Java. It is classified in the Olive family, Oleaceae. There are species thought to be of this family, but are claimed by the popular apple and pear genus.

19

Fraxinus excelsior is easily identified through its composed 7–11 sessile, toothed leaflets, and small flowers coming in panicles from the axils of the preceding year's leaves.

The clustered flowers in many species are imperfect. The flowering ash has two to six (mostly four) narrow white petals, and may grow to over 100 ft. in height. Its use is legendary, from making shoes to musical instruments. Tree yields manna. Bark contains glucoside, fraxin and essential oil.

Of the many species seventeen are in North America, distinguished from each other mostly by detailed characteristic of the fruits.

Medicinal Parts: The bark and leaves.

Solvent: Boiling water.

Bodily Influence: Antiperiodic, Laxative, Purgative, Stimulant.

Uses: The bark is used in intermittent fevers, ague, etc. The young tender leaves are used in gout, arthritis and rheumatic pain, dropsy, and obese conditions.

Culpeper (1616–54) mentions the following: "The decoction of the leaves in white wine helpeth to break the stone and expel it, and cure jaundice." The leaves have a reputation as a preventive measure for snake bites, taken as a tea and the leaves applied to the bite. Foreign species are favoured medicinally over the American White ash. Italy sends to the United States a bark exudation of Fraxinus ornus, more commonly called "Manna", a favourite laxative for children.

Dose: 1 teaspoonful of the leaves or bark to 1 cup of boiling water, steeped for 30 min.; 2–4 cups a day.

Homoeopathic Clinical: American Ash tree is used clinically in cases of affection of the Uterus, Prolapsus and Tumours.

Russian Experience: In Far Eastern Russia, Manchuria and China, Ash leaves and bark are used to stimulate blood circulation, especially in the legs, feet, arms and hands. Usually called old folk's medicine. Used in the form of tea internally and for external poultices, simple and effective.

BALMONY   Chelone glabra, L.

(N.O.: Scrophulariaceae)

Common Names: BITTER HERB, SNAKE HEAD, TURTLE HEAD, SALT RHEUM WEED.

Features: This perennial herbaceous plant is found in the United States in damp soil, and is cultivated in many gardens. It has a simple, smooth, erect stem about 2–3 ft. high. The leaves are shining dark green in colour, opposite, sessile, oblong, acuminate. The ornamental flowers which can be seen in August and September look much like the head of a turtle, and they vary in colour according to the variety of the plant.

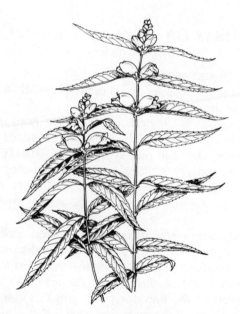

BALMONY   Chelone glabra, L.
(U.S. Agricultural Department, Appalachia, 1971)

The fruit is a capsule.

Medicinal part: The leaves.

Solvent: Boiling water.

Bodily Influence: Anthelmintic, Cathartic and Tonic.

Uses: Balmony is a bitter tonic and among the best medicine there is

21

for improving appetite. When the stomach action is weak, Balmony has a stimulating influence. A tea of the leaves is given to correct the inactivity due to the sluggish flow of liver fluids. Is used for jaundice, chronic malarial complaints, dyspepsia, constipation and during convalescence from febrile and inflammatory diseases.

Balmony is a vermifuge, and is regarded by some physicians as having no superior in expelling worms. When worms are present, we have found they are more prone to treatment each month at full moon. An infusion of 1 oz. of the leaves to 1 pint of boiling water may be taken frequently in wine glass amounts. Purging may be expected.

Dose: 1 teaspoonful of the leaves (according to taste, can be mixed with other herbs), to 1 cupful of boiling water. Of the powdered leaves, 1 dram. Of the tincture, 1 or 2 teaspoonfuls (30–60 drops) with water.

Homoeopathic Clinical: Debility, Dumb-ague, Jaundice, Liver (disease of), Quinine cachexia, Worms.

BALSAM FIR Terebinthine canadensis, L.
(N.O.: Coniferae)

Common Name: CHRISTMAS TREE.

Features: There are nine species of firs in the United States, constituting the genus Abies of the pine family (Pinaceae).

The common name "fir" is probably applied only to the forty or so species of pyramidal or cylindrical evergreen trees found mostly in the mountainous regions of Europe, Asia, north to the Himalayas, and North America, extensively in the eastern states, extending from Virginia and West Virginia in the United States to Labrador and Newfoundland in Canada. It may be 40–60 ft. or more tall, but appears dwarfed near mountain tops.

Members of this genus are characterized by erect cones that mature in one season but drop their scales when ripe (unlike other members of this family). The stems of the cones remain attached to the tree, and fir cones are never found on the ground. The male and female flowers occur on branchlets of the previous year's growth located on different parts of the same tree, the female cones are usually high. The male flowers hang on the lower side of the tree. Both are purplish in colour when young. The variable leaves are sessile are attached singly.

It is a popular Christmas tree due to its persistent leaves. Turpentine and resin are the popular products from Balsam fir.

Medicinal Parts: Bark and twigs.

Solvents: Water, alcohol.

Bodily Influence: Stimulant, Expectorant.

Uses: Very much like Balm of Gilead in its action. The bark and twigs are filled with a season's storehouse of Materia Medica, produced only by the elements of nature.

As in all herbal practice we use the plant in its original state. The unanimous and ancient recognition for rheumatism, kidney conditions, gleet, inflammation of the bladder, urinary difficulties, typhoid fever, capillary bronchitis, etc., may find a year-round meaning in your home other than the seasonal, Christmas adornment.

Dose: From J. H. Greer, M.D.: "Balsam Fir, 1 oz., Glycerin, 4 oz., Honey, 4 oz. Mix thoroughly, 1 teaspoonful four times a day." The bark and twigs may be added to other herbal teas for the above.

Externally: The resin is healing to external wounds. Used as a liniment for rheumatic pain. The twigs, bark and leaves are a refreshing and beneficial addition to steam cabinets for sore muscles, and sluggish skin action.

Homoeopathic Clinical: Oil of turpentine—Albuminuria, Amblyopia, Asthma, Back ache, Bladder (irritable), Bronchial neuralgia, Bronchitis, Chordee, Chorea, Ciliary neuralgia, Cystitis, Dropsy, Dysentery, Dysmenorrhoea, Enteric fever, Epilepsy, Erysipelas bullosa, Erythema, Fibroma, Gallstone colic, Glands (inguinal swelling of), Gleet, Gonorrhoea, Haematuria, Haemorrhoids, Hernia (strangulated), Herpes labialis pudendi, Hydrophobia, Hypochondriasis, Insanity, Intestines (ulceration of), Iritis, Jaundice, Kidneys (congestion of), Lumbago, Neuralgia (supraorbital), Ovaries (pain in), Dropsy of. Pityriasis, Strangury, Stricture, Tetanus, Tympanites, Uremia, Urine (suppression of), Worms (retention of).

BARBERRY   Berberis vulgaris, L.
(N.O.: Berberidaceae)

Common Names: BARBERRY, PIPPERIDGE BUSH, BERRY.

Features: One hundred and seventy-five species of shrubs make up this large family of Berberidaceae, many of which are used in ornamental planting and for hedges. The plant is native to the temperate climates and grows wild in the New England States, on the mountains of Pennsylvania and Virginia.

The flowers grow in small yellow clusters in April and May, are succeeded by red, dark-blue, or black fruit which in some species is used for making jellies of beautiful colour and distinct taste; also used like raisins when dry.

Barberry is an erect deciduous shrub, from 3–8 ft. high. The leaves are obovate, oval form, terminated by soft bristle, about 2 in. long and one-third as wide. The yellow root was an important dye for baskets, buckskins and fabric among the Indians. The Spanish-Americans used the yellow root to make neck-crosses (crucifixes). The active principle is Berberine.

Medicinal Parts: Root, bark, berries.

Solvent: Water.

Bodily Influence: Antiseptic, Laxative, Stimulant, Tonic.

Uses: The Indians knew by experience the use of Barberry for ulcers, sores, consumption, heart-burn and rheumatism. Root tea was prepared as a blood tonic, cough medicine and for kidney ailments.

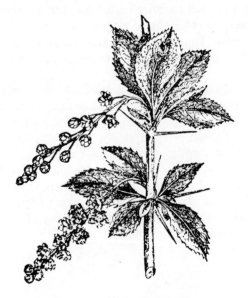

BARBERRY   Berberis vulgaris, L.
(Dr. A. J. Thut, Guelph, Canada)

Barberry is indicated in the chronic ills of the stomach and the early stages of tuberculosis, general debility, liver and spleen derangements. The agent is excellent to cleanse the body of choleric humours, and free it from such diseases as cholera and its associated malicious oddities such as scabs, itch, tetters, ringworm, yellow jaundice, bile, etc. It is also frequently prescribed in catarrhal conditions of the bronchial tubes, Barberry has a history of being an "old woman's medicine" because of its general use in infusion as a stomach and liver agent. As a tonic it will help convalescent patients recouperate.

Barberry bark is the most active anisian intensely bitter stimulant. The berries can be eaten and the juice is an agreeable acridulous refrigerant, useful in· fevers, and will generally stop the bloody flux and diarrhoea that often accompany typhus fevers.

Barberry can be effectively combined with Golden seal (Hydrastis canadensis), Burdock (Lappa minor), Yellow dock (Rumex crispus), Fringe tree (Chionanthus virginica) and Wild cherry (Prunus serotina). **Dose:** ½ oz. to 1 pint of boiling water, steeped 10 min., 1–4 cups a day before meals, made fresh daily. Of the tincture, ½–1 fl. dram.

Externally: Liquid from chewed root was placed on injuries and on wounds, while cuts and bruises were washed with a root decoction. A preparation of the bark or berries will be of service as a gargle for sore mouth and chronic ophthalmia.

Homoeopathic Clinical: Tincture of the bark of the root—Biliary colic, Bilious attack, Bladder affections, Calculus, Duodenum (catarrh of), Dysmenorrhoea, Fevers, Fistula, Gall-stones, Gravel, Herpes, Irritation, Jaundice, Joint affections, Knee (pain in), Leucorrhoea, Liver disorder, Lumbago, Opthalmia, Oxaluria, Polypus, Renal colic, Rheumatism, Sacrum (pain in), Side pain, Spermatic cords (neuralgia of), Spleen (affections of), Tumours, Urine (disorders of), Vaginismus.

Russian Experience: Since 1950 the official Pharmacopeia recognized two species of Barberry—Berberidis amerenis (Amur barberry) and Berberidis vulgaris (Barberry common).

In extract form for female genital organs, inflammation of gall-bladder pain and to increase bile. Also helpful to reduce high blood pressure.

Folk Medicine: Since olden days Russian people have used the same two, now recognized officially, for inflammation, excess of menstruation, and to stop bleeding in general and gall-bladder conditions.

BARLEY   Hordeum distichun and Hordeum vulgare, L.
(N.O.: Gramineae)

Features: Barley, a cereal of the genus Hordeum.

There are several species of barley. The two cultivated are H. vulgare, or six-rowed barley. H. distichun, the so-called two-rowed barley. Others are herbs, slightly similar to barley in general appearance.

Barley seeds have been found in tombs in Asia Minor dating from about 3500 B.C. Believed to have had its origin in western Asia and used as food for man and beast and was the chief grain for making bread in Europe until replaced by wheat and rye. In the United States, North Dakota, Minnesota, South Dakota and California are the major producing states. In Canada, Saskatchewan, Alberta, Ontario and Manitoba.

The vegetative parts of the barley plant are similar to those of wheat and oats, being distinguished by the auricle at the base of the leaf which clasps about the stem, extending farther than in other cereals with

25

pointed projections which overlap at the side opposite the leaf. Each barley seed is enclosed in a strong hull which remains intact even during threshing. The naked barley seed within this hull is similar in shape to a kernel of wheat.

Solvent: Water.
Medicinal Part: Decorticated seed.
Bodily Influence: Demulcent, Nutritive.

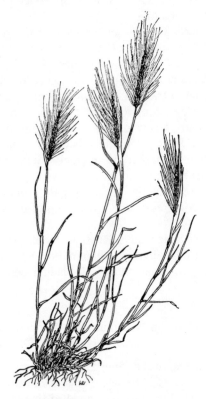

WILD BARLEY   Hordeum jubatum, L.
(Weeds, Canadian Agricultural Department, Ottawa, 1955)

Uses: The earliest settlers brought barley to North America continent. Indian keen judgement taught them that this, as with other whole food that has not been deprived through soil degeneration and refinement and thus robbed of their natural elements, had the original composition created for maintaining the ultimate health of mankind.

Barley is more cooling than wheat and due to the sodium content it is valuable for persons suffering from rheumatic and arthritic symptoms by keeping the calcium in solution. Barley water gives relief in fevers,

26

children's re-occurrence diarrhoea, catarrhal inflamed bowel and stomach irritation. Barley water is a good addition to any diet of harmonious intestinal flora.

Dose: Boil 2 oz. of pearl barley for a few minutes in a little water, strain and to the barley add 4 pints of boiling water, which is reduced by boiling to 2 pints; lemon juice or raisins may be added to suit patient's taste, 10 min. before complete cooking time.

Externally: The water distilled from the green barley fresh from the fields is prepared for film over the eyes or when in pain. Saturate white bread in the distilled barley water, squeeze gently and apply to the eyes, while relaxing.

BAYBERRY   Myrica cerifera, L.
(N.O.: Myricaceae)

Common Names: AMERICAN BAYBERRIES, CANDLE BERRY, WAX BERRY, WAX MYRTLE, TALLOW SHRUB, AMERICAN VEGETABLE WAX.

Features: From the Myricaceae family we have Bayberry, popular as an ornamental shrub because of the attractive fruit masses that persist all winter. The stiff shrub or small slender tree grows to 40 ft. tall, but is usually low and spreading, forming dense thickets. Native in sandy

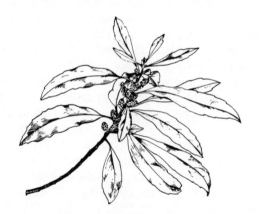

BAYBERRY   Myrica cerifera, L.
(U.S. Agricultural Department, Appalachia, 1971)

swamps, marshes and wet woodlands from southern New Jersey to Florida and the West Indies, west to Arkansas and Texas.

The bark is brownish-grey and smooth; leaves narrow at the base, oblong or lanceolate, 1–4 in. long, much reduced towards the tip of the branches, often sparingly toothed, dark green and shiny above, paler and sometimes hairy beneath. The flowers appear in early spring, March and April, before or with the new leaves. The fruits, borne against the stems. The green berries are covered, when mature, with a pale blue, lavender or greyish-white aromatic wax in microscopic rounded particles used in making candles which burn with a pleasing fragrance.

The root bark should be gathered in the fall. Cleanse it thoroughly and while fresh separate the bark with a hammer. Dry the bark completely and keep in a dry place; when dry enough to pulverize do so and store in a dark glass or pottery sealed container.

The berries or berry wax, which possess mild astringent properties, can be obtained by boiling the berries. The wax will come to the surface and can be removed when cool and hard. The fragrant wax makes a delightful scented candle, so popular at the Henry Ford Greenfield Village, Dearborn, Michigan, U.S.A.

Medicinal Part: The root bark.

Solvent: Boiling water.

Bodily Influence: Astringent, Stimulant, Tonic.

Uses: Bayberry is considered one of the most useful in the Medical Herbal practice. Its popularity has had respect for generations.

Myrica has the most effective influence in diseased mucous accumulation of the alimentary canal, which in this morbid soil is an incubator for bronchopulmonic diseases; sore throat or scarlet fever; dysentery and symptoms such as chronic catarrhal diarrhoea, cholera, goitre, scrofula, toxic seepage from the stomach and intestinal tract, gastritis, leucorrhoea, typhoid, etc. Myrica is both a general and special stimulant to the mucous membranes, without increasing a rise in temperature; at the same time an aid for digestion, nutrition and is blood building.

For female weakness and where better contraction is indicated in the uterus, it is indispensable. This applies in cases of uterine haemorrhage whether due to miscarriage or other causes. The uterus can be packed with cotton saturated with a tea solution and will assist excessive menstruation and haemorrhage from associated functions during this time. In all haemorrhages, from the stomach, lungs, uterus, or bowels, Bayberry should be remembered. In case of coldness of the extremities, chills and influenza a compound of the following will encourage circulation and promote perspiration.

> Bayberry bark (Myrica cerifera), 1 oz.
> Wild Ginger (Asarum canadense), $\frac{1}{4}$ oz.
> Cayenne (Capsicum), $\frac{1}{2}$ oz.

A teaspoonful of the powdered compound to 1 pint of boiling water (sweetened with honey), taken in mouthful amounts throughout the day. Be sure to stay indoors and away from draughts as you may perspire and a draught or cold conditions at this time will only delay treatment.

Galen mentions the berries wonderfully helping all colds and rheumatic distillations from the brain to the eyes, lungs and other parts. Dr. O. P. Brown tells us, "the wax possesses mild astringent with narcotic properties".

Dose: 1 teaspoonful to 1 cup of boiling water. Of the tincture, ½–1 fl. dram.

Externally: For nasal stoppage or inflammation, sniff, holding one side of the nose and then the other. Gargle the solution for sore throat and spongy bleeding gums. Skin ulcers and all kinds of sores, boils, carbuncles will all benefit greatly if bathed often with the freshly prepared solution.

Homoeopathic Clinical: Tincture of fresh bark of root—Catarrh, Conjunctivitis, Heart (affections of), Jaundice, Leucorrhoea, Liver (affections of), Pharynx (affections), Tendo-achillis (pain in), Throat (sore), Urticaria.

BEARBERRY Arctostaphylos uva ursi, Spreng.
(N.O.: Ericaceae)

Common Names: UPLAND CRANBERRY, ARBERRY, MOUNTAIN CRANBERRY, MOUNTAIN BOX.

Features: Found in dry, sterile, sandy soil and gravely ridges of North American south to Mexico in 3000–9000 ft. altitudes.

The perennial evergreen shrub is recognized by large mats of low-growing ground cover. The urn-shaped flowers are white and sometimes tinged with red, flowering from June to September, followed by red lustrous berries of the winter season. The green leaves should be picked and dried in the autumn.

The name is also applied to other plants, such as Ilet decidua, a shrub of southern United States.

Medicinal Part: The leaves.

Solvents: Alcohol, water.

Bodily Influence: Astringent, Diuretic, Tonic.

Uses: The leaves were mixed with smoking tobacco leaves by the Indians and they called it Kinnikinnick. More important was their use as medicine to treat inflammations of the urinary tract, especially cystitis.

Bearberry is among the herbs useful in diabetes for excessive sugar. Particularly useful in chronic diarrhoea, dysentery, profuse menstruation, piles, spleen, liver and the pancreas. The outstanding results of curative influence for diseases of the urinary organs, more especially in chronic affections of the kidneys, mucous discharges from the bladder and all derangements of the water passages, it is undisputed. Old cases of leucorrhoea and chronic urethritis will be relieved by its use, a valuable assistant in the cure of gonorrhoea of long standing, whites, ulceration of the cervix uteri (neck of the womb), pain in the vesicle region, etc. Can be used internally and also as a douche.

Cover and steep 1 heaped teaspoonful in 1 pint of boiling water for 30 min., cool, strain and use warm as a douche for the above mentioned. If too strong, dilute as required.

Dose: Can be taken internally as follows. Soak the leaves in sufficient alcohol or brandy to cover, for one week or more. Place 1 teaspoonful of the soaked leaves in 1 cup of boiling, or cold, water, drink 2–3 cups a day. Quantity of the tincture to be given in the same manner, 10–25 drops in water three or more times a day, according to symptoms. The tea can be made without the brandy or alcohol, if desired, preparing as you would ordinary tea. Effective if mixed with tincture of Quaking aspen (Populus tremuloides) 2–15 drops, tincture of Bearberry (Arcto-staphylos) 10–20 drops.

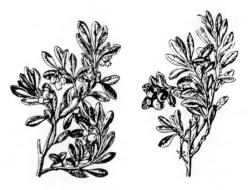

BEARBERRY   Arctostaphylos uva ursi, Spreng.
(Kotukov, Lekarstevennye Rastenia, Kiev)

When used in the treatment of diabetes Vaccinum myrtillus (Blue-berry) should be combined with it. Tincture of Blueberry leaves (Vaccinum myrtillus) 20–40 drops. Tincture of Bearberry (Arctostaphy-los) 10–20 drops in water three or more times a day.

Homoeopathic Clinical: Cystitis, Dysuria, Haematuria, Urinary affections.

Russian Experience: The pharmacopoeia uses Uva ursi (Bearberry) extracts or combined with other Herbals as antiseptics, or in diuretic conditions.

Folk Medicine: The tea of Uva ursi is used especially for female complaints, kidney and bladder disorders.

Veterinary: Successfully useful as indicated above.

BEAR'S FOOT   Polymnia uvedalia, L.

Common Names: LEAFCUP, BALSAM RESIN, YELLOW LEAFCUP, UVEDALIA.

Features: Bear's foot, a member of the astor family, is a large perenial 3–6 ft. high. Native of North America from New York to Michigan; south to Florida, Texas and Canada in ravines, and edges of the woods.

The leaves are the size of a man's hand, but shaped like a bear's foot. The root is like that of a small sweet potato, with a much darker skin.

Medicinal Part: The root.

Solvent: Water.

Bodily Influence: Stimulant, Anodyne, Laxative, Alterative.

Uses: Bear's foot is called the mammitis (inflammation of the breast) remedy. The affect on non-malignant indurated swellings such as mammitis and enlarged (engorged) cervical nodules will respond by breaking up accumulations when other medication fails.

Given internally for enlarged spleen and has considerable value in certain malarial conditions. It is used as an alterative in scrofula and a good remedy in old chronic cases of rheumatism.

Dose: 1 teaspoonful of the granulated root to 1 cup of boiling water. Drink 1 cup during the day, a large mouthful at a time. Of the tincture of Uvedalia alone, 10–25 drops three or more times a day. Dosage and frequency depends on condition for which it is prescribed.

Externally: The root is boiled in coconut oil, or an agent of salve consistency, and applied to swollen areas, two or three times a day, followed by a flannel cloth and water bottle held in position for better absorption of medication. The ointment is also used for scalp massage, as a hair tonic.

BEECHDROP   Epiphegus americanus, Orobanche virginiana, L.
(N.O.: Orabanchaceae)

Common Name: CANCER ROOT.

Features: A parasite of the family Orabanchaceae (broom-rape family). The name Cancer root is applied to several of the root parasites but more specifically to the Beechdrop or cancer drops of the beech tree roots.

The low wiry plant has pale brown, dull red, or light brown stems usually marked with fine brown purple lines. The stem has leaf scales but no leaves. The root is scaly and tuberous. Altogether the taste is disagreeably astringent. The August and September flowers are white in the upper corolla, about 1 cm. long, striped with brown-purple and are sterile; the less conspicuous lower flowers bear seeds.

31

Medicinal Parts: Tops, stems, root.

Solvents: Water, alcohol.

Bodily Influence: An eminent astringent.

Uses: This plant has been used by the teaching of the Folk Medicine and homoeopaths for cancer, hence the name is commonly known as Cancer root. It has other attributes, especially for asthma and is valuable in the treatment of obstinate ulcers of the mouth or stomach and diarrhoea.

Dose: Mainly a Folk Medicine, the amount to be taken is not mentioned in herbal practice in English or Russian literature. Unless given by persons of experience, it is best prescribed by the medical profession.

Further research is needed both in North America and abroad. The long established homoeopathic practice makes use of its properties in the form of extracts and tinctures.

Externally: Of use for all dermatitis inflammations, broken or unbroken skin conditions.

Homoeopathic knowledge has added: Tincture of whole fresh plant in full flowers—Diarrhoea, Gonorrhoea, Headaches, Palpitations—to our list of effective but little published medicine from the earth. They also mention cancer in this homoeopathic clinical.

BEECH TREE   Fagus sylvatica, L.
(N.O.: Fagaceae)

Common Names: AMERICAN BEECH, BEECHNUT TREE.

Features: The American beech (F. grandiflora) and the European or common beech (F. sylvatica) are closely similar.

They are handsome forest trees of the family Fagaceae. Both species thrive in light, limey loams; they do not grow in damp locations. (Blue or water beech, better known as American hornbean, Carpinus americanus, is not a member of this genus.) F. sylvatica has grey bark and shining leaves which persist during most of the winter.

The tree scarcely bears fruit before the fiftieth year. When about 250 years old and when matured to the fruit-bearing age both species yield pleasant edible, three-angled nuts in September, usually in pairs in prickly involucres, nourishing and enjoyable to both man and animal. The beech tree is used in ornamental planting due to their symmetrical forms.

Medicinal Parts: Bark and leaves.

Solvent: Water.

Bodily Influence: Tonic, Astringent, Antiseptic.

Uses: Beech, a medical tree of internal and external value. The bark and leaves contain effective substance for the action of the stomach, ulcers, liver, kidney, bladder and the weakening inflammation of dysentery. Beech is among the herbal tree medication for improving conditions of diabetes. The leaves are soothing to the nerves and stomach and are astringent. As a tonic for all, used to clean and tone up the entire system and improve appetite.

Dose: 1 teaspoonful of the crushed leaves or ¼ teaspoonful of the granulated bark to 1 cup of boiling water, 3–4 cups daily.

Externally: Culpeper (1616): "The water found in the hollow places of decaying beeches will cure both man and beast of any scurf, scap, or running tetter if they wash there with."

The leaf tea is antiseptic, cleansing, cooling and healing to old sores, feverish swellings or skin diseases. Bath often with the fresh tea, or applications of the boiled leaves. Can be applied, or made into an ointment by boiling in coconut, or other suitable oil.

Homoeopathic Clinical: Trituration of the nuts: Epilepsy, Headache, Hydrophobia, Vertigo.

Russian Experience: Beech tree in Russia is called "Buk" (pronounced, book). Medically they use creosote, distilled from Beech tar, as antiseptic, cleansing, disinfectant. The odour is very aggressive and when given internally for catarrh of the lungs, throat, etc., it is combined with more acceptable tasting herbs. Also used widely for industrial and commercial purposes.

BETH ROOT   Trillium pendulum, wild, Trillium edectum, L.
(N.O.: Liliaceae)

Common Names: BIRTH ROOT, WAKE ROBIN, INDIAN BALM, AMERICAN GROUND LILY.

Features: Trillium, a genus of the family Liliaceae, common to temperate North America and eastern Asia. This flowering herb has twenty-five to thirty perennial species that thrive in the acid mould of rich, moist woods.

The root has the faint fragrance of turpentine and a peculiar aromatic and sweetish astringent taste when first chewed, but becomes bitter and acid, causing salivation. Its shape is remindful of the popular Ginseng root. The simple stems range from 3–30 in. high, rising from the apex of a blunt tuber-like rhizome from ½–1½ in. thick. The leaves are from 2–15 in. long, and are net veined and somewhat mottled. Varying in colour according to species, the three sepals and petalled flowers are identified in May and June from white to pink and sometimes rose-maroon, red-brown, purple, green, yellow-green, or bright yellow. The fruit is a pink or red three- or six-angled berry.

Medicinal Part: The root.

33

Solvents: Diluted alcohol, water.

Bodily Influence: Astringent, Tonic, Antiseptic, Alterative, Pectoral.

Uses: The American Indians use Beth root as an aid to lessen pain and difficulty at the time of delivery, hence the synonym, Birth root. Taken internally, Beth root has a soothing tonic impression. The properties of Trillium are due to its active principle and it is used for all forms of haemorrhages, such as bleeding from the nose, mouth, stomach, bowels and bladder.

In female disorders it is especially valuable as a general astringent to the uterine organs and should be used in fluor albus, menorrhagia (profuse menstruation). It is considered almost a specific for female weakness, leucorrhoea, or whites.

Dose: Useful in pulmonary conditions, Beth root with the accompanying herbs Slippery elm (Ulmus fulva) and a small portion of Lobelia seed (Lobelia inflata), in powder form 10–20 grains.

One teaspoonful of the powdered root boiled in 1 pint of milk is an expedient help in diarrhoea and dysentery. For the above mentioned 1 teaspoonful of the powdered root to 1 cup of boiling water; two to three cups a day, or more often in wine-glass amounts, as case requires.

Externally: The root made into a poultice is very useful in tumours, indolent and offensive ulcers, stings of insects and to restrain gangrene. The leaves boiled in lard makes a good external application in ulcers and tumours.

Homoeopathic Clinical: Tincture of the fresh root—Bladder (catarrh of), Climacteric, Diabetes, Dysentery, Fainting (with flooding), Fibroma (haemorrages from), Haemorrhages (post-partum, ante-partum), Menorrhagia, Metrorrhagia, Writer's cramp.

BILBERRY   Vaccinium myrtillus, L.
(N.O.: Ericaceae)

Common Names: HUCKLEBERRY, WHORTLEBERRY, HURTLEBERRY.

Features: Bilberry, any of the several species of shrubs belonging to the heath family Ericaceae; genus Vaccinium. Some members are found in the cooler areas of both Eurasia and North America. One of the principle species is V. myrtillus, known simply as Bilberry, which is found in acid soil, in forests, heaths, rocky barrens, bog and tundra.

The Blueberry-like Bilberry is an edible fruit, growing in twos or threes at the bases of the leaves instead of in clusters terminating the branches as in true Blueberries. The seeds resemble currants in appearance, with a dark blue or black colour. The leaves are obovate, about 1 in. long, upper surface dark green and shiny. Depending on location, May through July is the flowering season for the reddish pink, white, or purplish blossoms.

Medicinal Parts: Leaves and berries.

Solvents: Dilute alcohol and boiling water.

Bodily Influence: Diuretic, Refrigerant, Astringent.

Uses: The fresh berries are enjoyed by most as a cooling, healthful dessert. For medication out of season, the dried berries have proven beneficial to cool feverish liver, and stomach conditions; they are arresting in vomiting and a useful agent for dropsy and gravel.

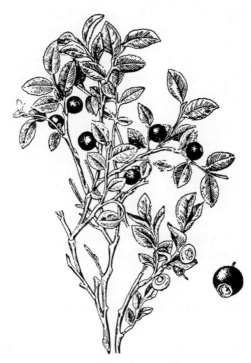

BILBERRY   Vaccinium myrtillus, L.
(Medicina, Moscow, 1965)

To make your own private stock, place two or three handfuls of Bilberry in a bottle and pour a good, real brandy over them. Secure with a good fitting cap or cork. The longer the tincture stays the more powerful a medicine will this berry spirit be.

Violent, continuous diarrhoea accompanied by great pain, sometimes with loss of blood, is stopped by taking 1 tablespoonful of Bilberry brandy in ¼ pint of water; may be repeated in 8 or 10 hr. For diarrhoea, dysentery and derangements of the bowels, a decoction of the leaf tea will bring relief. Also as a gargle for sore throat, and feminine hygiene of leucorrhoea.

At one time Bilberries were used in the treatment of scurvy in Norway and other northern countries.

Dose: Of the leaves, 1 teaspoonful to 1 cup of boiling water. In the Herbalist by J. E. Meyers: "A mixture of equal parts of Bilberry leaves, Thyme, and Strawberry leaves makes an excellent tea." Of the tincture, 10–30 drops, varying according to seventy of the case and age.

Externally: The tea decoction is used for sores, wounds and ulcers: apply the freshly made tea freely.

Russian Experience: Chernica (Bilberry) in Russian Folk Medicine is used mainly as an astringent for gastric colitis and other stomach conditions.

It may be of interest to know that in Russia, Bilberry has a well-established reputation as being similar to insulin for sugar diabetes. Used as fresh or dried berries and leaves as tea, decoction, syrup and for poultice.

Clinical: Research and clinical experiments confirm value as first recognized by Folk Medicine for practical home use. Extracts and tinctures are given clinically alone or combined with other suitable herbs when a tonic and astringent is required. Dose 1–2 teaspoonfuls to 1 cup of boiling water, taken warm in ½ cup amounts four times a day on an empty stomach.

Industrial: A home and industrial leather dye of brown and yellow colours. Combined with other chemicals to produce violet, red, green and blue for wool, cotton and linen material.

BIRCH Betula alba, L.
(N.O.: Cupuliferae)

Common Names: BLACK BIRCH, CHERRY BIRCH, SWEET BIRCH, MOUNTAIN MAHOGANY, SPICE BIRCH.

Features: Nearly forty species in the family Betulaceae of trees and shrubs are given the common name of Birch.

This is an ancient tree; in fossil form it goes back to the upper Cretaceous, and remains abundant and widespread in the northern hemisphere, in both the Old World and the New. In North America they range from the Arctic circle to Florida and Texas; usually found in woods; domestically in landscape decor throughout the United States.

Birch, an eye-catching tree, reaches heights of 45–50 ft. It may be white, yellow, brown, or almost black; frequently the trunk is smooth in young trees, later becoming marked with horizontal lines. The alternate leaves are characteristically simple, bright green and toothed. The

36

flowers develop in worm-like catkins of two types. The staminate appear near the ends of the branches in late summer or autumn and elongate the following spring into pendulous structures, exposing the brownish bracts. In the axils of these the minute flowers are located. Seen in the temperate zones in April and May. The ovaries mature into minute winged nutlets which are scattered in autumn or can be seen flecked on the winter snow.

Medicinal Parts: Bark and leaves.

Solvents: Alcohol, boiling water.

Bodily Influence: Aromatic, Stimulant, Diaphoretic.

Uses: As a food and medicine; the Indians tapped the Birch for its sap as a beverage and syrup. Oil of wintergreen is distilled from the inner bark and twigs.

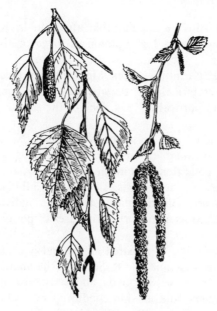

BIRCH Betula alba, L.
(Bello-Russ. Academy of Science, 1965)

The common Birch has a purpose in our family of medical trees. When we see them used for landscaping we may like to remember, with pleasure, the fore-ordained thought of their creation.

Traditionally the Birch is appropriate in treatment of diarrhoea, dysentery, cholera and all maladies of the alimentary tract. The natural properties are cleansing to the blood and it is used specifically for rheumatism, dropsy, gout, stones in the kidneys and bladder, and to expel worms.

37

Dose: A teaspoonful of the leaves and/or bark infused in 1 cup of boiling water for 15 min., 3–5 cups daily; mixes well with other herbal teas.

Externally: Drink the tea freely when troubled with boils or skin eruptions. The oil of Birch is applied to the skin for eczema and cutaneous diseases; the tea is an effective when gargled for canker and mouth sores.

Russian Experience: Belaya Bereza, Birch, is inseparable from the Russian people as it is their most poetic tree. In some way or time of life the Birch will be known to them through their history, literature, poetry, songs, art and fairy tales. They consider it the most attractive and beautiful of all the trees in the world. Besides emotional and spiritual popularity, the use as medicine from time immemorial goes back to the oldest tale of Russian history and their witness of Folk Medicine and Birch.

The American Birch has admirable attention in Russian botanical literature and they have a high opinion as to decorative and industrial use.

Folk Medicine: For centuries Folk Medicine has used Birch in many preparations for empirical and therapeutic results, long before clinical achievements and approval in 1834. One of the serious conditions being Cardial Dropsy.

Birch Buds: Gathered and preserved with vodka (Nastoika) for out-of-season use is an invaluable home medication. This is used for Colds, Pain, Rheumatic conditions, Stomach ulcers and pain, Vitality, Blood purifying, Appetiser, Avitaminosis, Liver and Gall-bladder, to dissolve stones of Kidney and Bladder and many other individual complaints.

Birch Charcoal: Used as an absorbent in cases of poisoning, gas bloating and indigestion.

Birch Sap: In the spring is prepared as tea and is considered a vitamin treat as a tonic for Anaemia, Gout, Scurvy, Rheumatism, etc.

Externally: Extract of leaves, buds and bark are applied to ulcers, wounds, boils, eczema and all skin conditions of broken and unbroken surfaces; rheumatic pain, swelling, albuminuria.

Russian history and life is unthinkable without a steam bath, Bania. Once a week this is the accepted routine. The stout-hearted race prepare a room with leaves placed over the hot rocks which expel the cleansing vapours of moist heat as hot and as long as the person's health will stand, and Russians excel in physical endurance. When perspiration is established, if the leaves were not placed over the rocks a Beresovy Venic, Birch Broom, is used to vigorously thrash the body. They know any trouble will be taken care of, whatever it is, if the person can stand the heat and the thrashing. In our condition we can do something similar, but not as severe. Boil 2–5 lb. of leaves with enough water to cover for 1–2 hr. in a pillow case or cotton cloth, pour this along with enough hot water in the bath tub to reach the waist when seated. Drench the shoulders, neck, back, face and arms with the container for as long as you feel comfortable. In this case your heart will be your doctor; if you feel weak, or relaxed to the point of falling asleep, make yourself get out. This type of herbal bath done once or twice a week for thirty times consecutively will prove most beneficial for internal and external complaints, as the proper function for both will be improved.

BIRD'S NEST   Monotropa uniflora, L.

Common Names: ICE PLANT, FIT PLANT, OVA-OVA, INDIAN PIPE.
Features: Found in North America from Maine to Carolina, and westward to Missouri, growing in shady, solitary places in rich moist soil composed of decayed wood and leaves.

Dr. O. P. Brown (1875) says: "It is evidently a parasite of the roots at the base of trees." The whole plant including the stem and flowers is of a clear white colour and the jelly-like substance melts away when rubbed a little. It flowers from June to September.
Part Used: The whole plant.
Solvent: Water.
Bodily Influence: Antispasmodic, Tonic, Sedative.
Uses: The root of this plant is regarded as almost an infallible remedy for fits in children and has been used with great success in St. Vitus dance.

Instead of employing opium for restlessness, pain, nervous irritability, etc., Bird's nest is effective without any dulling properties. A triumphant gain over remittent and intermittent fevers and an excellent replacement for the tissue retentions of Quinine. The juice of the plant is an excellent remedy in gonorrhoea and ulceration of the bladder, used as an injection.
Dose: The powdered root, $\frac{1}{2}$ teaspoonful, two or three times a day.
Externally: For tired, swollen or sore eyes, saturate a piece of cotton in a tea made from equal parts of Bird's nest and Fennel seed, squeeze gently and apply to eyes; serviceable added to vaginal douche water.

BITTER ROOT   Apocynum androsaemifolium, L.
(N.O.: Apocynaceae)

Common Names: DOG'S BANE, MILK WEED, WESTERNWALL.
Features: Indigenous to North America, growing in many of the States, and Canada, depending on the species, of which there are many. In North America there are sixty of them.

The large milky root is quite bitter (the bitter outside slips off when boiling, as for food) though edible, starchy, but nutritious and was an important food among the Indians. Bitter root is perennial, almost stemless with a rosette of oblong fleshy leaves. The flower appears in the centre, is rose or white coloured, and generally remains open only in the sunshine from May to August.

Montana State of U.S.A. claims Bitter root (Lewisia rediviva) as its State flower.

Medicinal Part: The root.
Solvents: Alcohol, though more especially water.

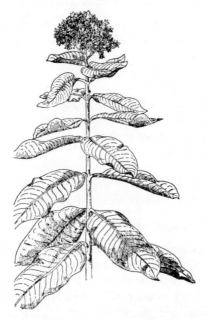

BITTER ROOT   Apocynum androsaemifolium, L.
(Weeds, Canadian Agricultural Department, Ottawa, 1955)

Bodily Influence: Emetic, Diaphoretic, Tonic, Laxative, Expectorant.

Uses: Bitter root is a celebrated remedy among the Indians for the treatment of venereal diseases and is regarded as almost infallible. Has been recommended in the treatment of Bright's disease. It is also highly praised for rheumatic gout of the joints and has been known to relieve cardial dropsy when everything else has failed. Parkinson quotes it is a "sovereign remedy against all poisons and against the bites of mad dogs"; hence it derives it's name Dog's bane.

Bitter root will help to rid the system of other impurities, including expelling worms, and is influential in treating Diabetes.

40

Bitter root is a very bitter stimulating tonic, acting chiefly upon the liver, emptying the gall ducts, securing a free discharge of bile and thereby causing activity of the bowels. For jaundice, gall stones and chronic sluggish conditions of the liver Bitter root is unequalled. It should not be employed in irritable conditions of the stomach.

When used as an alterative to act on the liver, or for dyspepsia, a dose would be 10 grains twice a day (5–6 grains of the extract). This remedy has been employed by some practitioners for nervous headache, for which it is said to be one of the most prompt and effective remedies in use. Large doses cause vomiting but tendency to gripe can be eliminated by adding Peppermint (Mentha-piperita), Calamus (Sweet flag), Fennel (Foeniculum officinale) or other carminatives. Take 2–5 grains thrice daily as a general tonic.

Externally: In the spring the milk of Bitter root will remove unsightly warts (if the circulation is active within the system) if applied fresh two or three times daily. Be sure to apply only on the raised area. You will notice a burning and, perhaps, swelling, this is to be expected. If the area forms a scab, let it drop off of its own accord, underneath will be a smooth unelevated surface. (Do not regard moles as warts.)

Homoeopathic Clinical: Tincture from the root—Diarrhoea, Dropsy, Nausea, Neuralgia of the face, Vomiting, Wandering rheumatism, Worms.

Russian Experience: American Bitter root does not grow wild in Russia. After extensive research on medical purpose and cultivation, they commercially cultivate Kendir Konoplevy (Bitter root) in the European part of Russia and West Siberia. In all herbal and agronomical publications they encourage and promote the use of the rhizome and root for medical aid.

Dr. A. Nelubin in his Pharmacography (Medical Botanics) first described American Bitter root in 1850. This credit aroused interest and was clinically proved in many cases of heart diseases and dropsy. Up to 1930–33 it was imported from the United States of America, but since this time plantations have been cultivated which yield an estimated 500–700 lb. of dried material for each acre.

Clinically: No side effects can be found from the proper administration of Bitter root. Clinically used in many cases of heart deficiences, high blood pressure, Cardiac-sclerosis and blood circulation disturbance of second and third degree. It is prescribed in ampules only.

BITTER SWEET   Solanum dulcamara, L.
(N.O.: Solanaceae)

Common Names: BITTER SWEET, NIGHTSHADE, VIOLET BLOOM, FELON-
WORT, MORTAL, FEVER TWIG.
Features: Naturalized in the United States of America from native
Europe and Asia. The zigzag, sprawling, slender vine climbs along trees,
hedges, thickets and fences, especially in moist places, seldom exceeding
7 or 8 ft. in length.

In June and July the purplish or blue flowers can be seen arranged
in cymes which are succeeded in the autumn by attractive bright red
juicy berries that hang on the vine for several months. The attraction
is for decoration only, they should not be eaten. The leaves are acute

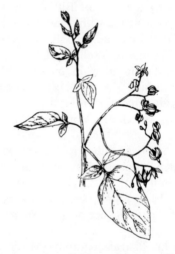

BITTER SWEET   Solanum dulcamara, L.
(Ontario Department of Agriculture, Toronto, Canada)

and generally smooth, of a dull green colour. When fresh, the leaf stems
have an unpleasant odour, which is lost by drying. The root is long
and almost orange-coloured. Twigs and root bark should be collected
after the foliage has fallen. Taste is first bitter, then sweet.
Medicinal Parts: Bark of the root and twigs.
Solvents: Diluted alcohol, boiling water.
Bodily Influence: Alterative, Diaphoretic, Discutient, Diuretic, Deobstruent, Narcotic, Resolvent.
Uses: Known to the original people of North America, Folk Medicine
and Herbalists for skin conditions of which the symptom is obvious, but
the source of the real culprit is usually large in the glandular system and
blood stream.

It is serviceable in cutaneous diseases and syphilitic conditions, as it excites the venereal functions, and is in fact capable of wide application and use in Leprosy, Tetter and all skin diseases, Eczema, Scrofula, etc. Also for rheumatic and cachetic affections, ill-conditioned ulcers, glandular swellings, and in obstructed menstruation it serves a good purpose.

Dr. O. P. Brown (1875): "The Complete Herbalist regard this plant as important as any in the Herbal Kingdom, and too little justice is done to it by those under whose care the sick are intrusted." Recent information from "Rodale Health Bulletin", September 1966: Dr. Kupchan said, "We're using Folk Medicine and Herbalism as source of leads. One of the plants we're studying, Solanum dulcamara, also called 'Bitter sweet' or Woody nightshade, was recommended by Galen in A.D. 150 as a treatment for Tumours, Cancer and Warts." He added, "A substance from red milkweed or 'Cancerillo' used for centuries by Central American Indians to treat Cancer inhibits the growth of lab-cultured human cancer tissue." When asked whether the cure for cancer would come from the greenhouse rather than the laboratory, Dr. Kupchan answered, "There probably won't be a single cancer cure, but cancer cures for the different types of cancer." He told reporters that the possibility of cancer treatment from plants should not be overlooked, particularly since "the synthetic medicinal chemists have almost exhausted the possibilities for anti-cancer drugs". Most Herbalists combine Bitter sweet with other Herbal agents as individual case requires.

Dose: Boil 1 teaspoonful of cut or powdered Solanum in 1 pint of water for a few minutes, cover and steep for $\frac{1}{2}$ hr., 1 teaspoonful in 1 cup of boiling water as required. Of the tincture alone, 10–20 drops in water three or four times a day. Caution: Large doses produce vomiting, faintness, vertigo, convulsive muscular movements, dryness and constrictions of the throat, thirst, diarrhoea, weakened heart action, paralysis.

Externally: One pound of the cut bark of Bitter sweet slowly heated in 1 lb. of lard for 8 hr. makes an excellent ointment to scatter painful tumours, and is one of the best preparations available for application to ulcers, irritated skin conditions, piles, burns, scalds, etc., involving pain and social awareness.

Homoeopathic Clinical: Not to be confounded with "Deadly nightshade", Belladonna, or with "Climbing Bitter-sweet", Celastrus. Tincture prepared from fresh green stems and leaves, gathered just before flowering.

Uses: Adenitis, Angina faucium, Aphonia, Bladder (affections of), Blepharophthalmia, Catarrh, Cholera, Crusta lactea, Diarrhoea, Dropsy, Dysentery, Emaciation, Exostosis, Haemorrhage, Haemorrhoids, Hayfever, Meningitis, Myalgia, Myelitis, Nettle-rash, Neuralgia, Ophthalmia, Paralysis, Pemphigus, Rheumatism, Scarlatina, Scrofula, Stammering, Stiff neck, Tibiae (pains in), Tongue (affections of), Tonsilitis, Tumours,

Typhoid, Urine (difficulty in passing) (incontinence of), Warts, Whooping-cough.

Russian Experience: Several kinds of the Bitter sweet family known as Paslen Kisoladky (Solanum dulcamara, Solanum lacitum) are used for medical and industrial purposes.

Anglo-American medical research has attracted much attention to Solanum dulcamara. Russian experience and laboratory research informs us as to the same and other importance. This endeavour should not be neglected.

Agro-technic and laboratory experiments have worked out many details. In western Siberia 1½–2 lb. of seed is used for 1 acre. Depending on weather conditions they cut three or four times a season; four or five weeks apart. Packages of 50 kg. are delivered to factories where extract is prepared for synthesis of progesterone, cortisone and other hormone preparations.

Uses: Home medicine for many families favours Palsenovaya Nastoika (herbs with vodka) for heart disease, a few drops at a time. One to two cups of the tea taken a mouthful at a time has proven successful for skin and hair diseases and very effective for worms.

Clinically: In use for disturbances of the liver, spleen, gall-bladder, catarrh, asthma and chronic skin disease.

India and Pakistan Experience: Solanum nigrum (Garden nightshade and their native Solanum xanthocarpum, which is Indian Kantakari, Kateli, Katai, and English name, Indian Solanum, grows throughout India and Pakistan. They find the whole plant useful as Expectorant, Bitter Stomachic, Aperient, Diuretic, Astringent, Anthelmintic, Alterative, Anodyne, Febrifuge. The root used for Fever, Cough, Asthma, Flatulence, Costiveness, Dropsy, Heart disease, Chest pain, Gonorrhoea, Dysuria, Stones in the bladder, Liver and spleen enlargement. Given in decoctions of ½ to 2 oz., or its juice in doses ½–2 drams; also as a confection.

BLACKBERRY   Rubus villosus, A.t.

Common Names: DEWBERRY, BRAMBLE BERRY, GOUT BERRY.

Features: There are numerous species of Rubus (Blackberry), two types are recognized. The trailing blackberries or dewberries and the erect blackberries. However, both in the wild and under cultivation there are many intermediate forms. This particular variety is native to the northern United States of America and Canada, other centres being central and western Europe.

The Blackberry has a root that lives for many years and a top that grows one year, fruits the next with juicy, black, delicious berries, which in contrast adheres to the core when ripe rather than separating from the receptacle as does the ripe raspberry. This trailing vine dies back to the ground when out of season. Spring finds new, prickly tips forming rootlets in sandy or dry soil. The flowers are white.

Medicinal Parts: The root, leaves and berries.

Solvents: Water, alcohol.

Bodily Influence: Astringent, Tonic.

Uses: As a remedial agent Blackberries are classed as astringents and are far more serviceable medicinally than most of our generation is aware of. The berries were used as food and medicine by our Indians, and today we know by their experience, and by scientific proof, that the plant is exceedingly valuable in chronic Diarrhoea, Dysentery, Cholera and summer complaints of children and is often the only thing which gets results.

A decoction of the root or leaves, or both (the root being more astringent than the leaves) may be used freely, four to five times a day.

Being pleasing to the taste, this agent is useful in excessive menstruation, and very effective in fevers and hot distempers of the body, head, eyes and other parts.

The berries have cordial properties and can be made into jello, brandy, jam, jelly and also vinegar.

Dose: 1 teaspoonful of the root or leaves to 1 cup of boiling water, steeped 15 min.; three or four cups a day depending on age and condition. Of the tincture $\frac{1}{2}$–1 dram, three or four times a day.

Externally: The leaves, bruised and applied outwardly, will act as an astringent to haemorrhoids. For sore mouth and inflamed throat, gargle the tea of the roots and leaves often; they can be used green or dried.

BLACK COHOSH   Cimicifuga racemosa, L.
(N.O.: Ranunculaceae)

Common Names: RATTLEROOT, SQUAWROOT, SNAKEROOT, BLACK SNAKE-ROOT.

Features: The plant is a genus of the Crowfoot Family, comprising about twenty species, native to North America, Asia and Europe.

The best-known American species, because of their medical properties, are the bugbane (Cimicifuga racemosa), Cimicifuga, from the Latin "to drive away", so named because certain species are used to drive away bugs and other insects. Can also be used as an antidote for the venom of serpents. Black cohosh can be seen in upland woods and hillsides. A perennial herb with a large knotty root, having a few short roots. The stem is simple, smooth and furrowed, from 3–9 ft. high, with irregular leaves. The small white flowers are numerous in wand-like racemes, flowering from May to August. The root contains a resin known as cimicifugin (macrotin), starch, gum, tannic acid, etc.

Medicinal Part: The root.

Solvent: Boiling water enhances the properties of the root but dissolves only partially; alcohol dissolves wholly.

Bodily Influence: Alterative, Diuretic, Diaphoretic, Expectorant, Antispasmodic, Sedative (arterial and nervous), Cardiac stimulant (safer than Digitalis), Emmenagogue.

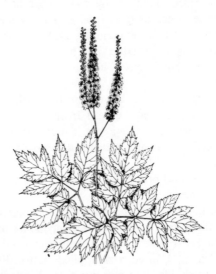

BLACK COHOSH   Cimicifuga racemosa, L.
(U.S. Agricultural Department, Appalachia, 1971)

Uses: The American Indian women knew of Black cohosh for relieving pain during menstrual period and used its properties extensively during childbirth.

Dr. Young introduced Cimicifuga racemosa to the medical world in 1831. It was adapted as a cardiac tonic in fatty heart, chorea, acute and chronic bronchitis, rheumatism, neuralgia, hysteria, phthisis, dyspepsia, amenorrhoea, dysmenorrhoea and seminal emission. It is also admirable treatment for scarlet fever, measles and smallpox. Regarded by some physicians as one of the best agents in use for whooping cough.

2 tablespoonfuls of tincture of Black cohosh (Cimicifuga racemosa)
2 tablespoonfuls of tincture of Blood root (Sanguinaria canadensis)
2 tablespoonfuls of tincture of Lobelia (Lobelia Inflata)
2 tablespoonsful of syrup of Squill (Sea onion)
Dose: 15–30 drops every three or four hours.

The above tinctures have been successfully employed in St. Vitus

46

dance and in asthma, delirium tremens, consumption, acute rheumatism, scrofula and leucorrhoea. Large doses cause vertigo, tremors, reduced pulse, vomiting, prostration.

Dose: The tincture should be made from the fresh root, or that which has recently been dried; 2 oz. to $\frac{1}{2}$ pint of alcohol (96 per cent proof) taken 5–15 drops four times a day. As a tea 1 teaspoonful of the cut root to 1 cup of boiling water three times a day, or 15–30 drops of the tincture added to 1 cup of water, sweetened with honey.

Externally: The bruised root was used by the Indians as an antidote for snake bites, which was applied to the wound, and the juice, in very small amounts, was taken internally.

Russian Experience: Cimicifuga Dahurica, not poetic in name, but known by all aborigines of the Far East and Mongolia as Klopogon Daursky or Bug Chaser Daurian. Lately Russians recognize the medical value of native American Black cohosh.

Clinically: The extract, tincture, straight or in combination, has of late been discovered and clinically approved for cardial asthma, high blood ·pressure, anaemia of the intestines, tonic for central nervous system. They vividly advise that even in large doses it does not create intoxication.

Folk Medicine: Used as a tea decoction and poultice for high blood pressure, headache, tonic, sedative, hysteria, neuralgia, asthma and migraine, in female disorders, painful menstruation and to ease labour pain.

BLACK HAW   Viburnum prunifolium, L.
(N.O.: Caprifoliaceae)

Common Names: AMERICAN SLOE, STAGBUSH.

Features: Black haw is found in most of the North American states, more abundantly from New York to Florida.

This is an erect, bushy shrub or tree from 10–25 ft. tall, with a 10 in. trunk diameter. The bark is irregular, transversely curved and greyish brown, or where the outer bark has scaled off brownish-red; inner surface reddish brown. The root bark is cinnamon colour and tastes bitter and astringent. The deep-green leaves are broadly elliptical or obovate, finely and sharply toothed, the under-surface smooth, 1–3 in. long. The flowers bloom from May to June in small white clusters 2–4 in. across and 3–5 lobes in each flower. The fruit known as Black haw is edible, but to some unbearably sweet. They are shiny black; cadet blue on red stems.

Parts Used: Root bark (preferred), bark of stems and branches.

Solvents: Water, alcohol.

Bodily Influence: Diuretic, Tonic, Antispasmodic, Nervine, Astringent.

Uses: To expectant mothers in cases of threatened abortion Black haw is an almost infallible remedy and therefore of special value to women who are subject to miscarriage, acting as a specific tissue bracing Materia Medica for the womb.

The preparation for this purpose should be anticipated two or three weeks before the expected reoccurrence of the misfortune and continued for about two weeks after any disturbance. If there are no symptoms of the above mentioned during the last weeks, discontinue until after delivery. To allay the severity of after pains and to arrest bleeding, Black haw is also administered.

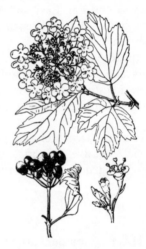

BLACK HAW   Viburnum opulus, L. (Kalina)
(Bello-Russ. Academy of Science, Minsk, 1965)

A decoction of this plant will generally alleviate chills and fever and usually gives speedy relief in palpitation of the heart and is a valuable agent in diarrhoea and dysentery. Notice that the herbs that have healing qualities on the stomach and intestinal tract are also influential for the complaints of the mouth and throat.

Dose: 1 oz. to 1 pint of boiling water taken in tablespoonful amounts three or four times a day; 1 teaspoonful of the tincture, three or four times a day.

Homoeopathic Clinical: Tincture of fresh bark—Abortion (threatened), Dysmenorrhoea, Menorrhagia, Tetanus, Tongue (cancer of).

Russian Experience: Kalina (Viburnum opulus) is the words and melody used by the Russian Folk singers and responds medically as well. Many years ago Black haw was used in the home before it was recognized clinically and given the credit it deserves.

48

As we are all inclined to believe, imports are not always desirable. Russia at first imported American Black haw and long afterwards revalued their own Folk Medicine and found the contents to be the same as the American herb. Today it is used in clinics and hospitals as extracts and compounds, concentrating mostly on heart treatment.

Uses: As a tea and decoction it is used for female complaints: painful menstruation, excess of bleeding, cramps and hysteria.

Sometimes associated with and used for heart tonic, blood circulation, kidney and bladder, and many other ailments, as there is seldom an isolated condition. Bark decoction for cramps. Berries for ulcers. Leaves as tea and decoction, also Nastoika (a kind of brandy), or better still, extract with Russian vodka. Nastoika with Kalina Yagoda (Black haw berries) is the best home medicine for ulcers.

BLACK INDIAN HEMP   Apocynum cannabinum, L.
(N.O.: Apocynaceae)

Features: Native to North America, of the Dogbane family, growing wild in pastures and fields.

It is one of several species called Indian hemp. The root grows deep in the soil, supporting a plant 1–5 ft. tall with erect, smooth and pointed leaves and resembling Bitter root (Apocynum androsaemifolium). They are distinguishable by their leaves and flowers. The leaves of this species are oblong and sharper pointed at both ends, while those of the Bitter root are pointed only at the outer end and quite round at the stalk end.

The flowers of this species are greenish-yellow, a light pink or purple inside, while those of the Bitter root are white, tinged with red. Poisonous to stock, but usually avoided due to the bitter, rubbery juice. The seeds, oil and fibre of hemp have uses for paint, bird preparations and clothing.

Indians made nets and rope from the fibres of pounded stems and roots.

Medicinal Part: The root.

Solvent: Water.

Bodily Influence: Anodyne, Hypnotic, Antispasmodic, Diuretic, Diaphoretic, Expectorant, Cathartic, Tonic.

Uses: The dried rhizomes and roots were used as a heart stimulant and for kidney complaints by the Indians. The root should be used with caution as too large an amount will cause vomiting, etc. This plant has the same attributes as Bitter root for the relief of dropsy.

A quote from the book by Dr. G. Wood and Dr. E. H. Ruddock, M.D. on Vitalogy: "It is an infallible remedy for the cure of thread or pinworms. For this purpose take twenty drops of the tincture three times a day for three successive days, then use an injection of cold water and the worms will be dislodged." If after this there are still symptoms, take a laxative tea a day before the full moon, and repeat the above each month until the pests have disappeared. We have found they are more active at this time and respond more completely to treatment.

Black Indian hemp root produces sleep without derangement of the digestive organs, principally allaying spasmodic pains of nervous origin where there is marked nervous depression.

Dose: 1 teaspoonful of the root to 1 pint of boiling water; take a tablespoonful of the tea three to eight times a day. Of the tincture, 2–5 min. four times a day.

Homoeopathic Clinical: The whole fresh plant, root included, should be used for making the tincture or infusion—Ascites, Catarrh, Coryza, Diabetes (insipidus), Diarrhoea, Dropsy, Enuresis, Heart (affections of), Hydrocephalus, Menorrhagia, Metrorrhagia, Nausea, Neuralgia, Snuffles, Tobacco-heart, Urinary difficulties, Vomiting.

Russian Experience: Indian hemp is known as Kendir konoplevy in Russia. The plant does not grow wild, but by their laboratory research and clinical experiments cultivation of North American Hemp is encouraged.

Agro-Technic solved detailed requirements. One acre yields up to 1,500 lb. of dry root and rhizome, which should yield $1,500 an acre by the latest price list of dealers and factories.

Uses: Used clinically for many heart conditions and blood circulation. Disturbance or congestion of second and third degree resulting from rheumatically affected heart, cardiac sclerosis, blood pressure and many other conditions depending on the normal flow of blood.

India and Pakistan Influence: India and Pakistan contribute greatly in the use of Hemp, as their knowledge has a history that exceeds ours. They use preparations of the whole plant.

Charas: The resinous exudation that collects on the leaves is a valuable narcotic. They found it has great value when Opium cannot be used. To encourage sleep and effectively administered in Malaria, Periodical Headache, Migraine, Acute mania, Insanity, Delirium, Whooping cough, Cough of T.B., Asthma, Brain Anaemia, Tetanus, Convulsion, Nervous exhaustion and Dysuria. Acts as anodyne in severe pain of Eczema and Neuralgia. Anaesthetic in Dysmenorrhoea also as an aphrodisiac.

Hashish: A special preparation of the dry leaves and flowers for Dyspepsia, Gonorrhoea, Appetizer, Nervine, Stimulant and Bowel disorders. They do not consider the seeds as a narcotic, infusions are given when treating Gonorrhoea.

Dose: Powder of Indian hemp is usually given in $\frac{1}{6}$–$\frac{1}{4}$ grain. The agent is far reaching and complicated and should be administered under supervision of authorized persons only as it requires great caution and consideration.

Externally: To resolve Tumours: paste of fresh leaves. To remove dandruff and head lice: juice of the fresh leaves. Dressing for wounds, ulcers and sores: powder of the leaves. Opthalmia and other eye diseases: poultice of the leaves applied to the closed lids. Haemorrhoids and Orchitis: poultice of the leaves applied to affected parts.

BLACK ROOT   Leptandra virginica, L.
(N.O.: Scrophulariaseae)

Common Names: CULVER'S PHYSIC, TALL SPEEDWELL, LEPTANDRA, CULVER'S ROOT.

Features: Black root is indigenous to North America and is from the Figwort family.

The soil in which the plant is grown is important as to its virtues. It can be seen in new soil, moist woods, swamps, etc. Limestone soil improves the medical value assuring the user of its attributed influence. Taste very bitter acrid. Autumn of the second year is the proper time for gathering. The dried root is the most accepted procedure (fresh root being too irritable) but it has to be used with extreme care.

The plant obtains heights of 2–5 ft. with simple, straight, smooth, herbaceous stems. Leaves are short and finely-serrated, whorled in fours to sevens. The flowers are white, nearly sessile, and very numerous; calyx, four-parted corolla, small and nearly white; stamens, two. The fruit is a many-seeded capsule.

Part Used: The dried root.

Solvents: Water, alcohol.

Bodily Influence: Emetocathartic, Cholagogue, Alterative, Tonic, Antiseptic.

Uses: Black root, long established Indian remedy, as white man's medicine was introduced as a medicinal agent by Dr. Culver and is admirably called Culver's physic.

The leading significance of Black root acts chiefly on the intestines in chronic constipation when insufficiency of biliary flow, and very much used in chronic Hepatic diseases. It operates with mildness and certainly without producing the depression of the powers of the system so common to other purgative medicines.

In fevers, it removes the morbid matter from the bowels without weakening their tone, or leaving behind that poisonous sting so often remaining after the use of Calomel. It is used very effectively in the care of pleurisy and also in some forms of dyspepsia. As a cathartic in dysentery, it is one of the best medicines known when given in moderate

51

doses. In such cases combine with a little Rhubarb root (Rheum palmatum) and give the decoction in doses of 3–4 tablespoons, repeating every three hours until passively relaxed.

Formula for Liver Disorders
1 oz. of Black root (Leptandra virginica)
2 oz. of Golden seal (Hydrastis canadensis)
2 oz. of Senna (Cassia marilandica)
2 pints of distilled or boiled water.

Boil until reduced to 1 pint. Take two tablespoonfuls three or four times a day increasing the quantity if it fails to operate gently, or decreasing if it operates too much. Bowel action should not be more than perceptible.

In this you have a herbal medicine superior to most of the popular preparations and one that has been used for generations.

Dose: Lepthandrin is the extract made from the root; it should be used in lesser amounts, from $\frac{1}{4}$–1 grain, adjusting according to age and case. Dose of the powder, as a cathartic, 20–40 grains.

Homoeopathic Clinical: Tincture of resinoid Lepthandrin, tincture of second-year fresh root, trituration of dried root—Ascites, Bilious attack, Bilious fever, Constipation, Diarrhoea, Dysentery, Dyspepsia, Headache, Jaundice, Liver (affections of), Remittent fever, (infantile), Yellow fever.

BLACK WALNUT   Juglans nigra, L.
(N.O.: Juglandaceae)

Features: Six species of the walnut, genus Juglan, are native to the United States. Black walnut is among them, widely distributed in the eastern states and extending to adjacent Canada. Their deciduous hardwoods have rough furrowed bark, alternate pinnately compounded leaves with a distinctive odour when bruised, and greenish flowers, the male in drooping catkins.

Black walnut is one of the best-known, largest and most valuable native hardwoods. Though not plentiful, the tree grows rapidly in mixed forests on rich, moist well-drained soil such as is found in valleys. They sometimes exceed 100 ft. in height with trunks 3 ft. in diameter. Planted for roadside shade, ornamental and shelter belts.

The wood is figured beautifully and used as panelling, for cabinet making and in salad bowls.

The nut is a popular food for candy, ice cream and cake flavouring. The husk does not split open like that of the Hickory nut; it is covered with a green pulp coating while on the tree, which turns black when on the ground and in storage. This outside pulp is used for dyeing and tanning, if you have ever gathered or hulled Black walnuts you will recall the lingering walnut stains.

Parts Used: Bark, leaves, rind, green nut.

Solvents: Alcohol, water.

Bodily Influence: Vermifuge, Tonic.

Uses: Materially, Scrofula has had harmonious results with 1 cup of the leaves boiled in 1 quart of water, made fresh daily and used often, with honey. This should be continued for several months. The dry leaves may be used when the green cannot be had. A strong tincture of the leaves and nuts is highly extolled as a remedy in the treatment of bilious and cramp colic.

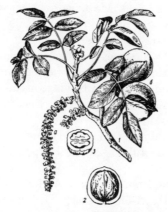

BLACK WALNUT   Juglans nigra, L.
(Vishaya Schkolla, Moscow, 1963)

Dose: 1–2 teaspoonfuls every twenty or thirty minutes until relieved. Also a decoction as a vermifuge is effective. The rind of the green fruit removes ringworms, tetter, and is given in diphtheria. The distilled fresh walnuts in spirit alcohol will calm hysteria, cerebral and pregnant vomiting.

The Black walnut is one of the foods rich in manganese, important for nerves, brain and cartilage. Nutritionally, the Missouri Black walnut is of high manganese content. All nut fruits should be fresh, as rancid oil is detrimental.

One teaspoonful of the inner bark or leaves and rind cut small or granulated to 1 cup of boiling water. Drink 1–4 cups a day often, a large mouthful at a time.

Homoeopathic Clinical: Tincture of leaves and of rind of green fruits— Acne, Anus (burning in), Auxiliary glands (suppuration of), Chancre, Ecthyma, Eyes (pain over), Favus, Flatulence, Headache, Herpes, Herpes preputialis, Levitation (sensation of), Menorrhagia, Purpura, Ringworm, Scurvy, Spleen (pain in), Syphilis.

53

Russian Experience: Black walnut is known in Russia by the common name of Greek nut (Juglan regia) which grows in Kaukaz and Middle Asia of Russia.

Uses: Long before vitamins were discovered Folk Medicine knew by experience and results that botanical treatment was reliable.

In Russia they prepared a walnut jam in a way that 90 per cent of the vitamins were still intact. This pleasing food as body repairing material is now known to contain a rich supply of Vitamin C, carotin and many important minerals. As a tea (external and internal) in home medical use for scrofula, ulcers, wounds, gargle and rickets.

Externally: Since the seventeenth century Russian military hospitals have used this well-established Folk Medicine for cleasing and quick healing medication of wounds and ulcers. Now clinically it is used for many kinds of skin diseases, especially tuberculosis.

Indian and Pakistan Experience: By the local Indian name Akhort or Akshot, the Black walnut would be a stranger to North Americans. Some of the uses are familiar, with advantageous additions.

Bark: Astringent, Anthelmintic, Detergent, Lactifuge. Successfully used as a bark decoction in skin diseases.

Leaves: Astringent, Alterative, Tonic, Detergent. A decoction of the leaves is specific in Scrofulous, Sores, Herpes, Eczema, Syphilis and Intestinal worms.

Green Hull: (separated from the hull) Anthelmintic, Antisyphilitic.

Kernel: Is given in Heart-burn, Colic, Dysentery and considered as Aphrodisiac. Immature nut rich in Vitamin C.

Walnut Oil: Mild laxative Cholagogue, Anthelmintic. Especially effective for tape worm and as a dressing for Leprose type skin disease.

BLOOD ROOT   Sanguinaria canadensis, L.
(N.O.: Papaveraceae)

Common Names: RED PUCCOON, INDIAN PLANT, TETTERWORT, SANGUINARIA.

Features: Indigenous to eastern North America, Bloodroot, a monotypic genus of the Papaveraceae family.

The small herb is often difficult to find in its woodland home, where the sheltered places and leaf mould is ideal for its survival. The thick, palmately lobed leaf is lapped around the bud, which swiftly outgrows its protector, loses its two fugacious sepals and opens into a star-shaped flower, one to each stem, with several fleshy white petals and a mass of golden stamens in the centre.

The flower closes at night or on shady days and is among the early spring flowers. Often cultivated in gardens. The leaves continue to grow during the summer, becoming nearly 7 in. long. The seeds are contained in spindle-shaped capsules.

The whole plant is very brittle and succulent and when broken, especially at its thick, fleshy root, an acrid red juice bleeds from the divided sections: The root is about the size of a man's little finger. The taste is bitter and harsh. The whole plant is medicinal, the root being the part chiefly used. Age and moisture impair the properties.

Medicinal Part: The root.

Solvent: Alcohol, water.

Bodily Influence: Systemic emetic, Stimulating expectorant, Sialagogue, Alterative, Tonic, Diuretic, Febrifuge.

Uses: Used by the aborigines for all blood conditions and as a stain for their skin and dye for decoration. The action of Blood root varies according to administration. In small doses it stimulates the digestive organs, acting as a stimulant and tonic, in large doses it is an arterial sedative. The properties are useful in chronic bronchitis, laryngitis, croup, asthma, whooping cough and any complaints of the respiratory organs. The tincture has been used with success in dyspepsia and dropsy of the chest, in cases of gastro intestinal catarrh, or enlarged, morbid or jaundice liver conditions. Blood root excites the action of this large glandular organ of which its correct function is so necessary to the complete physical and mental make-up of our everyday life.

Dose: 1 level teaspoonful of grated root steeped in 1 pint of boiling water for $\frac{1}{2}$ hr. Cool, strain, take a teaspoonful three to six times a day. Powder as an emetic, 10–20 grains, powder as a stimulant and expectorant, 3–5 grains, powder used as an alterative, $\frac{1}{2}$–2 grains. Of the tincture, 20–60 drops.

Externally: For leucorrhoea and haemorrhoids, injections of strong tea is excellent. As an external remedy the powdered root or tincture acts energetically in cases of fungoid tumours, ringworms, tetter, warts, etc., at the same time to be taken internally as mentioned. Nasal polypus is often treated by using a snuff of powdered Blood root.

Homoeopathic Clinical: The resin, leaves, seeds, capsules, powdered root and expressed juice and tincture of fresh root—Alcoholism, Aphonia, Asthma, Breast (tumour of), Bronchitis, Cancer, Catarrh, Chest (pain in), Cold, Croup, Deafness, Diphtheria, Dysmenorrhoea, Dyspepsia, Ear (polypus of), Flushes, Climacteric, Gleet, Granular lids, Haemoptysis, Headache, Influenza, Keratitis, Liver-cough, Menstruation (breasts painful during), Nails (ulceration of), Neuralgia, Oedema of glottis, Opthalmia, Pharyngitis, Phthisis Florida, Physometra, Pneumonia (acute), Polypus, Pregnancy (affections during), Pyrosis, Quinsy, Rheumatism, Rhus poisoning, Shoulder (rheumatism of), Smell (illusions of; loss of), Stomach (neurosis of), Syphilis, Tinnitus, Tumours, Vomiting, Whitlow, Whooping cough.

BLUE COHOSH   Caulophyllum thalictroides, Mich.
(N.O.: Berberidaceae)

Common Names: PAPPOOSE ROOT, SQUAWROOT, BLUE GINSENG, YELLOW GINSENG.

Features: This handsome perennial grows in all parts of the United States near running streams and in low moist rich grounds. The plant is 1–3 ft. high, purple when young, with 1–3 in. long leaves.

May or June finds the yellowish-green flowers in bloom which ripen to seeds in August, these being used for a decoction which closely resembles coffee. Its active principle is Caulophyllin.

Medicinal Parts: The root, rhizome.

Solvent: Water.

Bodily Influence: Antispasmodic, Diuretic, Emmenagogue, Demulcent, Sedative, Oxytocic, Spasmodic, Dysmenorrhea, Diaphoretic, Parturient.

Uses: The old-established Indian uses were for cramps during difficult menstruation periods promoting the flow and administering relief. It is especially valuable and has been found in many cases to almost entirely relieve the patient of pain in childbirth and promote prompt delivery. For assurance, a tea of Blue cohosh should be used for the last three or four weeks of pregnancy. A decoction is also useful for colic (thus the common name of Pappoose root), cramps, hysterics and rheumatism.

In their book "Vitalogy" (1925) Dr. Geo. P. Wood and Dr. E. H. Ruddock, M.D. found Blue cohosh "especially valuable in epileptic fits and ulcerations of the mouth and throat". Among other therapeutic properties, Blue cohosh contains the following vital minerals: Potassium, Magnesium, Calcium, Iron, Silicon and Phosphorus which helps to alkaĺize the blood and urine.

Dose: Steep 1 oz. of the root in 1 pint of boiling water; dose, 2 tablespoonfuls every three hours. For nervous and sluggish cough it will act as an expectorant, for spasms it may be given more freely.

Homoeopathic Clinical: Tincture or trituration of root—Abortion (threatened), After-pains, Amenorrhoea, Barrenness, Bearing-down pains, Chloasma, Cholera morbus, Dysmenorrhoea, False conception, Feet (affections of), Gonorrhoea, Hands (affections of), Intramammary pain, Labour (abnormal; false pains of), Leucorrhoea, Menstruation (disorders of), Ovarian neuralgia: Pityriasis, Pregnancy (disorders of), Rheumatic gout, Rheumatism, Uterine spasm, Uterine atony.

Russian Experience: On the Russian Far East Amur river and Sakhalin the same family called Caulophyllum robustum, or in Russian, Steblelist moshny, is found growing wild.

Blue cohosh has many good medical properties, including antibacterial properties for T.B. Taspin (Acetan) is used in proportions 1–1,000,000. This is a strong irritant and limited strictly to clinical use for female disorder and as a tonic for blood circulation. Further experimental research required.

BLUE FLAG   Iris versicolor, L.
(N.O.: Iridaceae)

Common Names: IRIS, FLAG LILY, LIVER LILY, WATER FLAG, SNAKE LILY, FLOWER DE-LUCE.

Features: This Lily-like flower is recognized by most of us for beauty alone. About 800 species belonging to more than fifty genera have been described from temperate and tropical climates, mostly from South Africa and tropical America.

The common wild iris or Flag (I. pseudacorus) is also found in the eastern United States and common in Europe. Several wild species are found in the United States. They are characterized by two rows of leaves, the outer of which fit over and protect the inner. The flowers are various shades of blue and purplish-blue, with yellowish markings at the base of the sepals, flowering from May through July. In some areas the Iris is cultivated for ornamental purposes and perfume, and some species have been used as food in countries where they are native.

Beauty alone is not the only quality possessed by the Iris. The underlying tissue of the root and rhizome hold unbelievable corrective influence on the human tissue. The root and rhizome should be sliced transversely, dried and placed in a dark vessel well covered and in a dark place. It will then preserve the oleo resin which is called Iridin, its active principle.

Parts Used: The root and rhizome.

Solvents: Water, alcohol.

Bodily Influence: Alterative, Cathartic, Sialagogue, Vermifuge, Diuretic, Resolvent.

Uses: From the booklet "Early Uses of California Plants", by Edward K. Balls: "It is said that long ago the Yokia squaws of Mendocino Country wrapped their babies in the soft green leaves of I. douglasiana while on the hot dry hillsides collecting Manzanita berries. This wrapping retarded perspiration and saved the babies from extreme thirst."

Blue flag has a special influence on the lymphatic glands and the necessity of active, pure lymphatic circulation is spontaneous to longevity. Recognized for endrocrine physiological active fluid in the thyroid imbalance, scrofula, and is regarded by some practitioners as one of the most miraculous Herbal Medicines in secondary Syphylis.

Traditionally a valuable substance in all diseases of the blood, chronic hepatic, kidney and spleen affections. Has been known to relieve all symptoms of chronic hip disease. It should be combined with Mandrake

57

(Podophyllum peltatum), Poke (Phytolacca decandra), Black cohosh (Cimicifuga racemosa), Ginseng (Panax quinquefolium), Sarsparilla, Yellow dock (Rumex crispus), etc. If it causes salivation do not be apprehensive as it is distinguished from mercurial salivation by absence of stench, sponginess of the gums and loosening of the teeth.

In "Nature's Healing Agents", Dr. Clymer says it's one of the very few remedies that has any influence in correcting milk-coloured, clay-coloured stools in adults.

Dose: Tincture alone, 10–25 drops in water three times a day. 1 teaspoonful of the powdered root to 1 pint of boiling water, drink cold, 2 or 3 tablespoonfuls six times a day. Iridin, 1 grain.

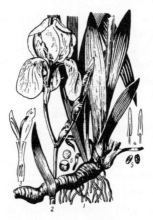

BLUE FLAG   Iris versicolor, L.
(Naukova Dumka, Kiev, 1964)

Homoeopathic Clinical: Tincture of fresh root, collected in early spring or autumn, trituration of resinoid, Iridin or Irisin—Anus (fissure of), Bilious attack, Constipation, Crusta lactea, Diabetes, Diarrhoea, Dysentery, Dysmenorrhoea, Dyspepsia, Eczema, Fistula, Gastrodynia, Intermittent Headache, Impetigo, Liver (affections of), Migraine, Neuralgia, Nocturnal emissions, Pancreas (affections of), Parotid glands (affections of), Pregnancy (morning sickness of), Psoriasis, Rectum (burning in), Rheumatism, Salivation, Sciatica, Vomiting, Whitlow, Zoster.

Russian Experience: Kasatik is the Russian name given to the Iris with all their fondness and tender love, of which the true meaning is difficult to convey by translation. The encouragement and promotion of cultivation has had strong propaganda. Agro-technic skilfully planned agricultural methods for medicinal, commercial and industrial business. It is used for internal and external medicine, cosmetics, perfume, aromatic and taste in confectionery; widely used in wine industry; praised highly by gardeners and florists for floral decor.

Clinically: Recognized for bronchitis and teething babies.

Folk Medicine: Used medically in Russia for many serious cases of dropsy when the heart is involved, inflammation of the lungs, angina, calming to reduce involuntary emission. Root and rhizome used by Folk Medicine as tea, decoctions and poultice.

Externally: Successfully used in infected wounds, ulcers, fistula and to take away freckles.

BLUE VERVAIN   Verbena hastata, L.
(N.O.: Verbenaceae)

Common Names: WILD HYSSOP, SIMPLER'S JOY, INDIAN HYSSOP.

Features: Native to temperate and tropical America; Mediterranean region and the Near East; introduced elsewhere in the Old World.

This complex perennial has 352 known specific and sub-specific natural and artificial hybrids. Numerous species have been employed medicinally in various localities. The herb reaches heights of 3 or 4 ft., usually with a four-square stalk; branching limbs, whitish flowers, followed by long slim tassels of seeds.

Growing usually in dry, hard soils along roadsides and fields. For medicinal purpose Vervain should be collected when in flower from June to September.

Medicinal Parts: Root, leaves, stems.

Solvent: Water.

Bodily Influence: Diaphoretic, Expectorant, Emetic, Antiperiodic, Nervine, Tonic, Sudorific, Antipasmodic.

Uses: Vervain expels worms and is a capable, capital agent for invoking all diseases of the spleen and liver. If given in intermittent fever in a warm infusion or powder, the results are considerable. In all cases of cold and obstinate menstruation it is a most complete and advantageous sudorific.

When the circulation of the blood is weak and languid, it will increase and restore it to its proper operation. The infusion, taken cold, forms a good tonic in cases of constitutional debility and during convalescence from acute diseases. Its value has been found to be apparent in scrofula visceral obstructions, stones, gravel, etc., but its virtues are more wonderful still in the effect they produce upon epilepsy, or falling sickness and fits.

Dr. O. P. Brown in "The Complete Herbalist" (1875): "I found after close investigation and elaborate experiment that prepared in a certain way and compounded with Boneset (Eupatorium perfoliatum), Water pepper (Polygonum punctatum), Chamomile blossoms (Anthemis nobilis) in best whiskey has no equal for the cure of fits, or falling sickness, or anything like fits; also for indigestion, dyspepsia and Liver complaints of every degree. A more valuable plant is not found within the whole range of the Herbal Pharmacopoeia."

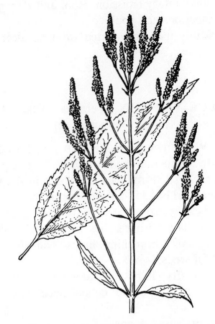

BLUE VERVAIN   Verbena hastata, L.
(U.S. Agricultural Department, Appalachia, 1971)

It is also an antidote to Poke (Phytolacca decandra).
Dose: 2 teaspoonfuls of the herb to 1 pint of boiling water. Drink cold 2 or 3 teaspoonfuls six times a day. Of the tincture, 10–20 min.
Homoeopathic Clinical: Tincture of entire fresh plant—Ague (chronic), Epilepsy, Rhus poisoning.

BONESET   Eupatorium perfoliatum, L.
(N.O.: Compositae)

Common Names: BONESET, THOROUGHWORT, INDIAN SAGE, AGUE WEED.
Features: Boneset grows plentifully in all parts of the United States, in low, moist and damp lands, reaching heights of from 2–5 ft. The stem has the appearance of penetrating the leaves through the centre and standing them out crosswise. Flowering in August and September, the

60

large bushy white flowers top the lavish green plant. It has a feeble odour, with a bitter taste.

Medicinal Parts: Tops and leaves.

Solvents: Alcohol, water.

Bodily Influence: Stimulant, Tonic, Diaphoretic, Emetic, Aperient, Antispasmodic.

Uses: As is true of other plants, Boneset is dual in action, depending on how it is administered, when cold a tonic, when warm emetic diaphoretic. As a tonic it is very useful in remittent fever, intermittent and typhoid fevers, dyspepsia and general debility. Give the infusion as hot as can be comfortably swallowed, this including profuse perspiration and sooner or later evacuation of the bowels.

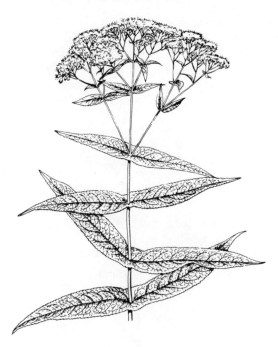

BONESET   Eupatorium perfoliatum, L.
(U.S. Agricultural Department, Appalachia, 1971)

Likewise in febrile diseases, catarrh, colds and wherever such effects are indicated. Dropsy, intemperance, acute and chronic rheumatism, bilious fevers, influenza and especially where there is aching of the bones. Its powers are manifested upon the stomach, liver, bowels and uterus. It is extremely bitter to the taste and is disliked by children, but in these cases a thick syrup of Boneset, ginger and anise is used by some for coughs of children, with good results.

Dose: Of the powder from 10–12 grains; of the extract from 2–4 grains. Infusion, 2–4 wineglassfuls.

Homoeopathic Clinical: Anus (herpes of), Back (pain in), Bilious fever. Tincture of whole plant—Bones (pains in), Cough, Dengue, Diarrhoea, Fractures, Gout, Hiccough, Hoarseness, Indigestion, Influenza, Intermittent fever, Jaundice, Liver (soreness of), Measles, Mouth (cracks of), Ophthalmia, Relapsing fever, Remittent fever, Rheumatism, Ringworm, Spotted fever, Syphilitic pains, Thirst, Wounds.

BURDOCK   Arctium lappa, L.
(N.O.: Compositae)

Common Names: LAPPA, LAPPA MINOR, THORNY BURR, BEGGAR'S BUTTONS, CLOTHBURR.

Features: Naturalized in North America, from Asia and Europe, this plant grows from 2–5 ft.; can be found along roadsides and in all vacant lots. Hunters will remember Burdock burrs adhering to their clothes and being troublesome to their game dogs. The stems are stout with wide

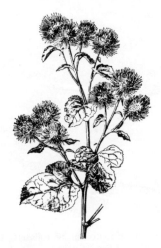

BURDOCK   Arctium lappa, L.
(Vishaya Schkolla, Moscow, 1963)

spreading branches carrying alternately elongated heart-shaped leaves. The purple flowers bloom in July and August, after which they dry out and the base becomes the troublesome burr. The root, which should be dug in the autumn or early spring, is thick, brownish-grey externally, with white pith-like tissue inside. The root and seeds have a sweetish, slimy taste, the leaves and stems being bitter. Common Burdock is sometimes

62

planted in Japan, where it has been improved by cultivation, for its enlarged parsnip-like roots, which are eaten as a boiled vegetable.

Parts Used: Root, seed, leaves, stems, the whole herb.

Solvents: Diluted alcohol, boiling water (partially).

Bodily Influence: Diaphoretic, Diuretic, Alterative.

Uses: Herbalists all over the world use Burdock. Such an effective and ultimate blood purifying plant has well earned the unpretending authentic value for which we know it is capable. The root and seed of Arctium lappa is a soothing demulcent, tonic, alternative; it slowly but steadily cleanses skin, soothes the kidneys and relieves the lymphatics; eliminates boils, carbuncles, canker sores, styes, felons, etc. Soothing to the mucous membrane throughout the entire system, and is also used for gout, rheumatism, scrofula, syphilis, sciatica, gonorrhoea and kidney diseases. It is best combined with more stimulating agents.

> Tincture of Burdock root, 10–20 drops
> Tincture of Golden seal, 8–12 drops
> Tincture of Buchu, 10–15 drops.

The above can be made into a herbal tea preparation reducing the formula by a quarter and using ounces instead of drops. The leaves shredded fine in aged wine will help if bitten by a mad dog.

Externally: The leaves will be found very useful in fever, by bruising and applying to the forehead, or to the soles. For burns, shred the bruised leaves fine and fold into a stiffly beaten egg white; it will relieve the pain and hasten healing.

Homoeopathic Clinical: Tincture of fresh root—Acne, Bunion, Dupuytren's contraction, Eczema serpeginosa, Eruptions, Glands (affections of), Gonorrhoea, Gout, Impotence, Leucorrhoea, Phosphaturia, Rheumatism, Ringworm, Scrofula, Sterility, Ulcers, Uterus (prolapsus of).

Russian Experience: As in North America, herbs have several common names. Burdock is very popular scientifically and as a home medicine; it is known as Repeinik or Lopuh, very close to the official Latin name of Lappa.

Burdock roots contain from 27–45 per cent inulin, and up to 12 per cent protein, as well as oils and other trace minerals. Therefore it is easy to understand why they consider food as medicine, and medicine as food. It is best to collect the roots of one or two-year-old plants in the autumn.

Folk Medicine: The use of Burdock in Russia can be traced back many generations both as a table herb and a medicine cabinet herb. Especially valued as a diaphoretic for dropsy, gout and rheumatism.

Clinically: Used in the form of extracts, ointments, tinctures and oils for the same purpose as Folk Medicine administered for generations.

Food: If you happen to see persons digging a hole in Russia it could very well be they are preparing a pit for fish or game to be wrapped in Burdock leaves (they do not use any added seasoning). A fire is made in the pit and when the ground is hot enough they take away the ash and charcoal, place the carefully wrapped morsel in the bottom and cover with the surrounding sides, which have reached a very high temperature. In a short time they have a delicacy that barbecuing cannot equal.

As a kitchen preparation the roots are roasted and used for coffee; the fresh root in soup instead of potatoes; fried as cuttlets, and pancakes. Cut very fine and boiled with apple cider vinegar and Yellow dock with appitionic sour cream, they make a tasty and nutritious jam.

Externally: From the olden days of Russian experience, Burdock oil, called Repeinoe Maslo, has a reputable lifeline as a hair tonic to strengthen and encourage the growth of new hair. This can be done if the hair follicles are just dormant and not completely destroyed. It usually takes from six to eight months for a noticeable change. Many conditions of eczema-type skin diseases are forgotten after several applications of Burdock, externally, and Burdock taken internally. Persistent black (comedo) and white heads (milia) are treated with a facial steam bath. Also as a poultice for boils.

BUTTER NUT   Juglans cinerea, L.
(N.O.: Juglandaceae)

Common Names: OIL NUT BARK, WALNUT, LEMON WALNUT, WHITE WALNUT.

Features: Butter nut, of the family Juglandaceae, native to America where it ranges from New Brunswick to Georgia westwards to the Dakotas and Arkansas.

A handsome, spreading tree with smooth, light-grey bark, varying from 50–80 ft. in height. Male and female small flowers are on the same tree followed by oblong, pointed, ribbed green nuts. The ripe nuts have very hard shells and are highly prized for deserts in regions where the trees grow; the green nuts are used for making pickles. An inferior sugar can be made from the sap.

Solvents: Alcohol, water.

Medical Parts: The dried inner bark and leaves.

Bodily Influence: Cathartic, Tonic, Vermifuge.

Uses: The active principle of Butter nut is juglandin, one of the most certain and efficient cathartics that can be used for dysentery, diarrhoea and worms, leaving the bowels in better condition than almost any other medicine.

This old-fashioned, natural Materia Medica improves assimilation, promoting a steady improvement on the structure of any protracted febrile disease. It is usually prepared by adding water to a quantity of the bark and boiling it down until it is reduced to a thick extract. Sweeten with honey or pure maple syrup to taste. Use the concentrates as a hot tea or take by teaspoonfuls three times a day, or as required. As a cathartic it is somewhat harsh and drastic, though effective, and should not be used by delicate invalids, or large amounts persisted in, as it could produce inflammation. It is a mild and certain remedy in consumption, when combined with Apocynum (Bitter root). This combination has proven an effective compound for expelling thread and pin worms.

Dose: 1 teaspoonful of the inner bark of the root, cut small or granulated to 1 cup of boiling water. Of the tincture, 5–20 min.

Externally: For chronic skin diseases the dilute tincture is charitably applied, at the same time taken internally.

Homoeopathic Clinical: Tincture of root bark, triturations of resinoid juglandin—Acne, Angina pectoris, Axilla (pain in), Chest (pain in), Coryza, Ecthyma, Eczema, Erysipelas, Erythema nodosum, Headache, Herpes, Hydrothorax, Impetigo figurata, Lichen, Migraine, Pemphigus, Ringworm, Rodent ulcer, Scapula (pain in), Scarlatina, Tetters, Vision (lost).

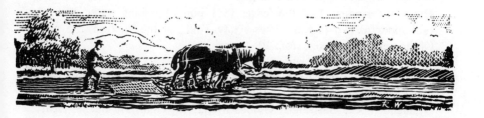

CALICO BUSH   Kalmia latifolia, L.
(N.O.: Ericaceae)

Common Names: SHEEP LAUREL, SPOONWOOD, LAMBKILL, MOUNTAIN LAUREL.

Features: The Calico bush can be found in rocky hills and elevated ground in most parts of the United States, standing 4–8 ft. high with crooked stems and rough bark. The leaves are evergreen and are 2–3 in. long. The flowers are white and numerous, appearing in June and July.

The leaves have the reputation of being a poison to the animals that eat them, sheep, birds, etc., and can be a poison to those who eat the animals that have been feeding on the plant.

The Indians brought attention to this plant by their use of the decoction they made from it, namely, to say hello to another world.

Medicinal Part: The leaves.

Solvent: Water.

Bodily Influence: Sedative, Astringent.

Uses: By medical practioners only. The preparation should be employed with great care and prudence as extra amounts are poisonous. The plant, in medicinal doses, is antisyphilitic, sedative to the heart, and somewhat astringent. It is a most efficient agent in syphilis, fevers, jaundice, neuralgia and inflammation. A quote from Dr. Brown (1875), "The Complete Herbalist": "In case of poisoning with this plant, either man or beast, whiskey is the best antidote."

Dose: 1 teaspoonful of the leaves to 1 pint of boiling water. Take 1 tablespoonful two to four times a day, cold. Of the tincture, 2–5 min. Of the powdered leaves, from 10–20 grains.

Externally: Stew with lard as an ointment for various skin irritations.

Homoeopathic Clinical: Tincture of fresh leaves when the plant is in flower—Angina pectoris, Blindness, Bright's disease, Dropsy, Dysmenorrhoea, Gastralgia, Globus hystericus, Gout, Headache, Heart (diseases of), Herpes zoster (neuralgia after), Keratitis, Leucorrhoea, Locomotor ataxia, Lumbago, Neuralgia, Paraplegia, Ptosis, Pregnancy albuminuria, Retinitis bulism, Sun-headaches, Syphilitic sore throat, Tinnitus, Tobacco (effects of), Vertigo, Vomiting.

CAPSICUM   Capsicum minimum (Roxb), Capsicum frutescens, L.
(N.O.: Solanaceae)

Common Names: CAYENNE, RED PEPPER, BIRD PEPPER, AFRICAN PEPPER.
Features: This plant is indigenous to Asia, Africa and the parts of the United States beyond the southern line of Tennessee. The African Bird pepper is the purest and the best known medically. It is a small, oblong, scarlet, membraneous pod, divided internally into two or three cells containing numerous flat, white, reniform seeds. It has no odour, its taste is hot and acrid.
Solvents: 98 per cent alcohol, considerable extent vinegar or boiling water.

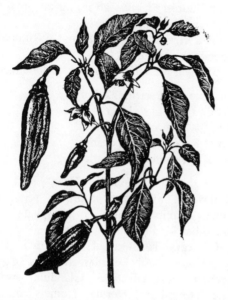

CAPSICUM   Capsicum minimum Roxb., Capsicum frutescens, L.
(L. Y. Sklyarsky, Lekarstevennye Rastenia, Moscow, 1968)

Medicinal Part: The fruit.
Bodily Influence: Stimulant, Tonic, Carminative, Diaphoretic, Rubefacient, Condiment.
Uses: The all-supporting, stimulating effect of Capsicum is the infallible action of internal success. Capsicum taken with Burdock, Golden seal, Ginger, Slippery elm, etc., will soon diffuse itself throughout the whole system, equalizing the circulation in all diseases that depend upon an increase of blood, and unlike most of the stimulants of allopathy, it is not narcotic.

67

It acts mainly upon the circulation, giving immediate action to the heart and then extending to the capillaries, giving tone to the circulation without increased pulsation, but giving equalized power to it.

Remember that it is an agent that is seldom used alone, as by itself the power is soon extinguished.

Cayenne has many unwanted accomplishments to its credit. Indigestion, dyspepsia, atonic gout, alcoholism, delirium tremens, intermittents, flatulence, colic, low fever, diphtheria, haemorrhoids; it is useful in cramps, pains in the stomach and bowels, causing peristaltic action of the parts previously contracted. Bleeding of the lungs is easily checked by the use of Cayenne and the vapour bath. By this means circulation is promoted in every part of the body and consequently the pressure upon the lungs is diminished, thus affording an opportunity for a coagulum to form around the ruptured vessel.

Capsicum is not a cure-all and we do not recommend its continual use beyond the obtainable results.

Externally: As a liniment for sprains, bruises, rheumatism and neuralgia:

> Tincture of Capsicum, 2 fl. oz.
> Fluid extract of Lobelia, 2 fl. oz.
> Oil of Wormwood, 1 fl. dram
> Oil of Rosemary, 1 fl. dram
> Oil of Spearmint, 1 fl. dram

According to the analysis in "Back to Eden", by J. Kloss, Capsicum contains the following: albumen, pectin, a peculiar gum, starch, carbonate of lime, sesquioxide of iron, phosphate of potash, alum, magnesia, and a reddish kind of oil.

Homoeopathic Clinical: Tincture of the dried pods—Amaurosis, Asthma, Brain (irritation of), Delirium tremens, Cough, Diarrhoea, Diphtheria, Dysentery, Ear affections, Glandular swellings, Haemorrhoids, Headache, Heart-burn, Hernia, Home-sickness, Intermittents, Lungs (affections of), Measles, Mouth (ulcers in), Neuralgia, Nose (affections of), Obesity, Oesophagus (stricture of), Paralysis, Pleuropneumonia, Pregnancy (disorders of), Rectum (diseases of), Rheumatic gout, Rheumatism, Sciatica, Scrofula, Sea-sickness, Stomatitis, Throat (sore), Tongue (paralysis of), Trachea (tickling in), Urine (disorders of), Whooping cough, Yellow fever.

Russian Experience: Krasny Peretz, Kayansky Peretz (Red Pepper) is common home medicine in many families. Besides its use as a hot seasoning it is always handy as Nastoika in vodka (one or two pods in a bottle of vodka). They drink this decoction in wineglassful amounts by those tolerant of the kick of vodka spiked with the hot peretz.

Uses: Diaphoretic for colds, Appetiser, Rheumatism, and stomach disorders.

Externally: Nastoika is used as a poultice and liniment with other compounds.

Clinically: There is a warning that dose should not exceed 1–2 grains at a time, as it can produce a burning sensation in the stomach and disorders, with undesirable effect on the heart. The oil is clinically used; powder most always in composition with other herbals.

CASCARA SAGRADA   Rhamnus purshiana, D.C.
(N.O.: Rhamnaceae)

Common Names: SACRED BARK, CHITTEM BARK, PERSIAN BARK.

Features: The flowering Cascara can be found in North Idaho, and west to the Pacific, Northern California. This is a species of the California Buckthorn, also known as Sacred bark.

The small tree, Cascara sagrada, has dull green leaves, with black fruit, three lobed seeds and purplish-brown bark, changing to dark brown with age.

The bark should be obtained from the young trunk and large branches in the springtime, as taken from other parts and out of season it will have a different taste and characteristics. Age at least one year before using.

Medicinal Part: The aged, dried bark.

Solvents: Diluted alcohol and boiling water.

Bodily Influence: Laxative, Bitter tonic.

Uses: This plant has had early recognition from the Indians and has gained a mutual consummate as a tasteful Cascara cordial prepared by the Parke Davis Co.

A thoroughly established agent for habitual constipation, dyspepsia, indigestion and haemorrhoids. 1 oz. of the fluid extract in 8 oz. of syrup of Yellow dock (Rumex crispus) makes an excellent preparation for engorged liver and blood disorders with constipation. As a laxative 1 teaspoonful of the fluid extract at bedtime. Of the tincture, 40–60 drops with water, morning and evening, according to the individual.

Homoeopathic Clinical: Extract of bark used in constipation and rheumatism.

Russian Experience: Cascara sagrada in Russia is known as Krushina or Joster. It grows in Siberia, Kozahstan and central Russia.

Uses: Folk Medicine first used the leaf or berry extract in herbal combinations as a laxative. Clinical use soon followed.

CASTOR BEAN   Oleum ricini, L.
(N.O.: Euphorbiaceae)

Common Names: CASTOR OIL, PALMA CHRISTE (from supposed shape of leaves resembling Christ's hand).

Features: The variety is variable as to continent and conditions. In the United States the hollow stems are high with purplish bloom above, bearing bluish-green leaves which are one or two feet broad; flowers in July; capsule expelling the various tinted, shining bean. The plant is decorative and is regarded as a mosquito repellent if planted in presumable direction of entry. Native to India, but cultivated extensively in the U.S.A.

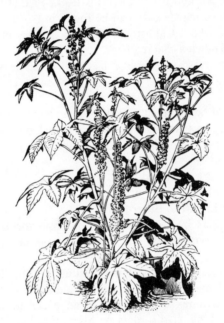

CASTOR BEAN   Oleum ricini, L.
(G. N. Kotukov, Lekarstvennye, Kiev, 1964)

Medicinal Parts: The bean; the fixed oil, expressed from the seeds. The first settlers make a traditional laxative from it; Europe—American Indians found it useful as well.

Bodily Influence: Cathartic, Purgative.

Uses: Expect purging from 4–6 hr. after 1 tablespoonful for adults, and 1 teaspoonful for children, has been taken, followed by the feeling of sedative effect on the intestines. The mildness of action is acceptable for young children, child-bearing women, and in cases of constipation, colic, diarrhoea due to slow digestion, tape and lumbricoid worms.

Not recommended for dyspeptics, where contraindicated, as it is oppressive to the digestive powers. If the taste is disagreeable, flavour with equal parts of oil, and either heavy sarsparilla, peppermint or cinnamon syrup, and mix thoroughly. To relieve the lower bowels an injection of 4 tablespoonfuls is thoroughly mixed with a mucilage of Slippery elm bark.

Externally: For aid in ringworm, itch and cutaneous complaints if applied assiduously. The leaves are said to be galactagogic when applied to the breast. The Canary Island women know of its effect as they have increased the secretion of milk with the leaves for centuries.

Homoeopathic Clinical: Albuminuria, Aphthae, Cholera, Cholera infantum, Diarrhoea, Duodenum (catarrh of), Dysentery, Eruptions, Gangrene, Gastroenteritis, Jaundice, Lactation, Peritonitis.

Russian Experience: Castor oil has many uses in Russia and is known as Kastorka. Industrial for lubricating oil in commercial equipment and aeroplanes, as it does not freeze in the severe Russian climate. They use the stems in the textile industry, and oil for paints and cosmetics. Agro-technic deserve attention for commercial cultivation. Depending on climate and soil they harvest from 500–2,500 lbs. of beans from each acre.

Folk Medicine: As a laxative, plus gynaecology, ulcers, eye treatment, and hair restoring preparations.

India and Pakistan Experience: From our daily experience we associate Castor oil as a laxative. Many varieties are in use of this valuable home medicine. Locally named and easy to remember as "Erand".

Uses: In general practice for Constipation, Enteritis, Peritonitis, Dysentery, Spasmodic diseases of the bowels, Inflammatory disorders of the urogenital organs, Gonorrhoea, Stricture of Urethra, Milk fever, Amenorrhoea, Asthma, Dropsy.

The juice of the leaves is a strong emetic, and is very serviceable in cases of narcotic poisoning. Decoction of the leaves, purgative, lactogogue, emmenagogue. The root bark, strong purgative. The seed contains the alkaloid ricinine; also ricin, a potent vegetable toxin. This stays in the oil cake after the oil is extracted.

The Castor oil plant is given with combinations of carbonate of potash; if not available the kernels without the embryo is boiled in milk and water and given for Lumbago, Rheumatism and Sciatica.

Caution: When the patient cannot strain the stool as in colitis, prolapsus, weakened structural tissue, the oil is given in very small doses. Can be used as an enema with soap suds and water.

Externally: Poultice of the leaves for boils and swellings, also applied over the breasts of nursing mothers as a lactogogue, and over inflamed breasts during lactation to soften the mammary glands. To relieve flatulence or to promote menstruation, cover the abdomen with the

71

boiled leaf poultice. and stay warm. The oil is locally applied in conjunctivitis.

CATNIP Nepeta cataria, L.
(N.O.: Labiatae)

Common Names: CATNIP, NEP, CATMINT, CAT'S WORT.
Features: This perennial herb is naturalized in the United States and
found in all parts. The square erect branching stems are covered with
fine whitish hairs; leaves 1–2½ in. long with heart-shaped or oblong
pointed apex, the top side green with greyish-green and whitish hairs

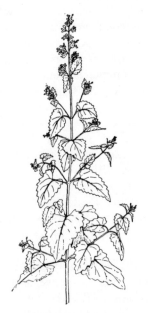

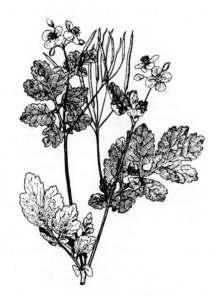

CATNIP Nepeta cataria, L.
(Ontario Department of
Agriculture, Toronto,
Canada, 1966)

CELANDINE Chelidonium majus, L.
(Bello-Russ. Academy of
Science, Minsk, 1969)

underneath. Flowering in June to September with whitish corolla, purple
dotted sectioned lips, and lobes make up the conformation of the bloom.
Faintly mint aromatic, with bitter taste.
Solvents: Diluted alcohol, boiling water.
Medicinal Part: The whole herb.
Bodily Influence: Carminative, Stimulant, Tonic, Diaphoretic,
Emmenagogue, Antispasmodic, Aphrodisiac (cats).

72

Uses: When most of us think of Catnip, unfortunately it is only associated with the cat family. Its uses are many, and mild in the proper amounts, for both infants and adults. When troubled with flatulence and digestive pains, the American physio-medical practice recommends "blood warm bowel injection of the infusion for babies with intestinal flatulence". All Herbalists find Catnip useful for feverish colds. It will produce perspiration without increasing the heat of the system, and induce sleep. It has proved efficacious in nervous headache, for allaying hysteria and insanity and other forms of nervous diseases of an acute character, without any effect of withdrawal from its use.

Equal parts of Catnip and Saffron are excellent in scarlet fever, small-pox, colds, etc. The fresh expressed juice of the green herb taken in tablespoonful amounts three times a day will encourage suppressed menstruation.

Due to its transient action, Catnip is more serviceable in tea form. Always steep the herb in a closed container, never boil.

Dose: 1 oz. Catnip to 1 pint of boiling water.

Adults: 2–3 tablespoonfuls, children 2–3 teaspoonfuls, frequently, for the above mentioned. When taken in very large doses when warm, it frequently causes emesis.

Externally: Culpeper states the green herb bruised and applied to the part for 2–3 hr. eases the pain arising from piles. The juice made into an ointment is effective for the same purpose. There is an old saying that if the root be chewed it will make the most quiet person fierce and quarrelsome.

CELANDINE Chelidonium majus, L.
(N.O.: Papaveraceae)

Common Names: GARDEN CELANDINE, GREATER CELANDINE, TETTER-WORT, CHELIDONIUM.

Features: Celandine is a pale green, evergreen perennial, with stems from 1–2 ft. in height, leaves round and smooth from $1\frac{1}{2}$–$2\frac{1}{2}$ in. long; the flowers are bright yellow, umbellate on long, often hairy, stocks.

Indigenous to Europe and naturalized in the United States. It grows wild along fences, roadsides and in waste places, etc., flowering from May to October. When the plant is cut or wounded a noticeable, unpleasant yellow sap flows out, and is of offensive odour, nauseous, bitter tasting with a biting sensation when put to the mouth.

The fresh reddish-brown root is the part most used; drying diminishes its activity.

Celandine is often considered the same as Lesser celandine, which is Pile wort; they are different medicinally and botanically.

Solvents: Alcohol, water.

Parts Used: Herb and root.

Bodily Influence: Cathartic, Diuretic, Diaphoretic, Expectorant, Purgative, Vulnerary, Alterative.

Uses: It is used internally in decoctions or tinctures for hepatic affections or liver complaints, and has a special influence on the spleen. It is often used in dropsy and skin complaints.

Culpeper knew of its virtues long ago and we quote: "The herb or root boiled in white wine and drunk, a few aniseeds being boiled therewith, openeth obstructions of the liver and gall, helpeth the yellow jaundice."

Celandine has had much recognition. The herbalist of ancient times cleansed the eyes of film and cloudiness that darkened the sight with the juice of this plant diluted with breast milk. Of the powdered root, $\frac{1}{2}$–1 dram; of the fresh juice, 20–40 drops (in some bland liquid); of the tincture, 1–2 fl. drams; of the aqueous extract, 5–10 grains.

Externally: Application for progressive spreading ulcers, malignant running sores, and other spreading skin conditions such as tetters, ringworm, or cancers will show a speedy recovery if used daily. The fresh juice rubbed on warts will take them away. If persons of sensitive skin notice itching, equalize the area with diluted vinegar and water.

Homoeopathic Clinical: Antrum of Highmore (inflammation of), Cancer, Chest (affections of), Chorea, Constipation, Cough, Diarrhoea, Dyspepsia, Gall-stones, Gonorrhoea, Haemoptysis, Haemorrhoids, Headache, Influenza, Jaundice, Lachrymal fistula, Laryngismus, Liver (affections of), Nephritis, Neuralgia, Nose-bleed, Pleurodynia, Pneumonia, Rheumatism, Scald-head, Stiff neck, Taste (altered), Tumours, Warts, Whooping cough, Yawning.

Russian Experience: Chistotel Bolshoy (Clean Body—Large) Chelidonium majus. Clinically the fresh extract and compound complex is used in many cases of spasmatic conditions involving the liver, and closely associated with gall-bladder, kidney and bladder. For domestic use the above administration should be in the hands of the medical practitioners, or carefully trained persons. Chelidonium is poisonous and cannot be eaten up by animals.

Russian Folk Medicine: The effects of Chelidonium seem to be universal in the treatment of liver, gall-bladder, kidney and bladder. The time-honoured properties of this herb brings us unalterable use for malignant swellings and stomach conditions, used in the form of tea.

Externally: The fresh leaves and stems have a milky juice that quickly turns orange-red when exposed to the air. This fluid can burn the skin, as if coloured by iodine, causing blisters that are very painful. Experimentally, treatments have shown excellent results for stopping malignant swellings and it is effective in TB, especially skin tuberculosis. For small cuts, ulcers and warts a special liniment or fresh juice can be used if very careful.

CELERY   Apium graveolens, L.
(N.O.: Umbelliferae)

Common Names: SMALLAGE, GARDEN CELERY.

Features: Southern Europe, Asia and Africa have the honour of origin. In the older civilized parts it was cultivated prior to the Christian era. It is now cultivated in the British Isles, India and North America (U.S.A. and Canada). The wild biennial, or annual, herb grows in marshy places and has qualities resembling domestic celery, although it is smaller in every way and has a less agreeable taste. The seeds are dark brown; with five slender ribs; odour characteristic, agreeable; taste, aromatic, warm and pungent. Seeds and plant contain volatile and fixed oil.

Solvent: Alcohol.

Medicinal Parts: Root and seed.

Bodily Influence: Carminative, Stimulant, Nerve Sedative, Diuretic, Aromatic, Tonic.

Uses: Have you ever given thought to the seed world that is accepted as food? When we stop to think, a seed has the power to reproduce (when given the proper elements). Without debatable research, we realize that within the unit is balanced chemistry, alive with a meaningful existence.

The importance of regular uric release is not often thought of, and over a period of time can slowly diminish in amount. Celery seed is one of the herbs used in incontinence of urine, dropsical and liver trouble, rheumatism, neuralgia and nervousness, combined with suitable alteratives such as Red clover, Burdock, Iris versicolor, Mandrake, etc.

Dose: 5–30 drops of the fluid extract; can be combined in herbal tea with lesser effect.

Homoeopathic Clinical: Tincture of seeds, tincture of sticks—Nervous headache, Heart-burn, Otorrhoea, Post-nasal catarrh, Vomiting, Toothache, Urine (retention of), Urticaria.

India and Pakistan: Ajmoda is India's Celery, and they use the plant for many ailments—Asthma, Bronchitis, Liver, Spleen, Amenorrhea, Urinary discharges, Rheumatism, Hiccough, Rectal trouble, Ascites, Flatulence, Nasal catarrh, Fever with cough.

Root: Considered an Alterative and Diuretic.

Seed: Carminative, Diuretic, Stomachic, Aphrodisiac, Tonic, Astringent to the bowels, Cordial, Laxative, Appetizer, Stimulant, Emmenagogue, Anthelmintic, Abortifacient, Antispasmodic.

75

CENTAURY   Sabbatia angularis, Pers.
(N.O.: Gentianaceae)

Common Names: ROSE PINK, BITTER BLOOM, BITTER CLOVER.

Features: This plant is common to most parts of the United States. There are many species and colours: the English distinguish between them by using the red Centaury in diseases of the blood, the yellow in choleric diseases, and the white in those of phlegm and water. Variety and habitat is not only limited to colour; the Centaury family will grow in many soil conditions—moist meadows, among high grass, on the prairies and in damp ditch soil. It flowers from June to September and is best gathered at this time. The flowers close at night and the American variety is considered preferable to the European.

Solvents: Water, alcohol.

Part Used: The whole herb.

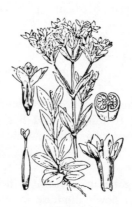

CENTAURY
Centaurium erytraea, Pers.
(Naukova Dumka, Kiev,
1965)

Bodily Influence: Tonic, Febrifuge, Diaphoretic.

Uses: Excellent, old American remedy, bitter tonic, preventive in all periodic febrile diseases, dyspepsia, and convalescence from fevers; it strengthens the stomach and promotes digestion. An aid to rheumatic and all joint pains. The following in a warm infusion is a domestic remedy for expelling worms and to restore the menstrual secretions: Of the powder, $\frac{1}{2}$–1 dram; of the extract, 2–6 grains.

The loose dried herb, 1 teaspoonful to 1 cup of boiling water. Although bitter, this effective herb is a good accompaniment to all herbal teas and preparations. For taste, combine with other herbs such as Anise, Cardamom, Peppermint, Ginger, Fennel, etc.

Homoeopathic Clinical: Used as tincture of root in cases as follows: Coryza, Diarrhoea, Inflammation of the eyes, Fever, Home-sickness, Influenza intermittents, Vanishing of sight.

Russian Experience: Russian Centaury, Centaurium erytraea, (Zo-lo-to-ti-sia-chnik) "A thousand golden leaves", and many other beautiful names given to it by Folk Medicine with all respect. Official medicine very often prescribes Centaury alone, but also with other herbal preparations.

Folk Medicine: Centaury tea and a home extract, usually prepared with vodka, is given in cases of high blood pressure, liver and gall-bladder malfunctions. The bitter tonic is antiseptic in stomach sickness, working with nature without destroying the necessary secretions which stimulate desirable digestion and appetite. The parasitic tape worm cannot hold its circlet of hooks and suckers which enable it to maintain livelihood in the mucous membrane of the intestines of its host when Centaury is taken persistently.

CHAGA   Inonotus obliquus, (Pers.) P.L.
(N.O.: Polyporaceae)

Common Names: CHAGA, BIRCH MUSHROOM.

Features: In North America and Canada the Birch is well known for its beauty alone. The unthinkable medical purpose can be found in the older trees in what is known as a mushroom, or fungus-type growth (also grows on beech and other trees). This growth is rough, dry, porous, crusty, with deeply cut and crooked separations having the appearance of dull charred wood on the outside. The surface is almost black in colour. When this projection is sawn off the tree, it is as if the tree was having cosmetic surgery or the removal of an out-of-control wart. The matured and most desired Chaga is 30–40 cm. in width, 10–15 cm. thick and up to 4–5 ft. long, and from 4–5 lb. in weight. There are three layers: (1) outside, rough with some old bark and possibly twigs, must be cleaned; (2) inside, soft, very close to the tree trunk, must be cut off; and (3) middle part, granulated and not spoiled, which is the part to use. It can be collected at any time of the year.

Always keep Chaga in a dry and dark place (dark covered jar) as dampness and strong light dissipate its power.

Part Used: Inside granulated parts of the three layers.

Solvents: Boiled (not boiling) water, alcohol, vodka.

Bodily Influence: Tonic, Blood purifying action, Anodyne, Restorative.

Uses: It is well known that our early Indians knew all plants and how they were best used—for food, medicine, or if they be poisonous. In Anglo-American literature we know that treatments of many sicknesses were kept as tribal knowledge. We know they used the properties of many fungi, but from our research work we cannot find a definite record of Chaga being identified; we are poorly informed.

The existence of Chaga and its uses are mentioned in Russian literature, in sources such as monographies, medical books, encyclopaedias and popular herbal books.

Folk Medicine of European Russia and Siberia gives unlimited credit to Chaga. From year to year scientific medical literature carefully gives more credit to this mysterious Chaga, which for generations has been thought of as magic. Chaga has a long list of uses by persons of

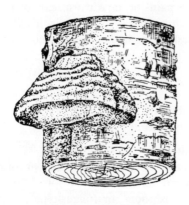

Ganoderma applamatum
(Flat Trutovik Russian)
(Not to be confused as Chaga
because of different properties)

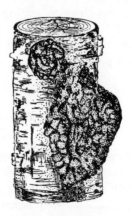

Chaga   Birch mushroom
Inonotus obliquus (Pers.) P.L.
(Bello-Russ. Academy of
Science, Minsk, 1965)

experience and faith in Herbal Folk Medicine. Chaga was used for all stomach complaints, from gastritis, pain in the stomach, ulcers; cancer, TB of the bones, and glandular organs where operations were not possible due to the network of blood vessels.

Folk Medicine, as a general impression, may be unlimited in its credit and belief, but science is reserved and careful. The aspect of this plant life has confirmed commitments subject to further research, laboratory and clinical tests. Refer to Bello-Russ. (White Russia) Academy of Science.

In 1864 Prof. G. Dragendork gave laboratory research a chance to explain why Chaga was so wonderfully praised. Scientifically they could not find anything of importance. Meanwhile Folk Medicine was still using Chaga successfully despite the fact that medicine and science could not unlock its virtues. Dr. Froben was also successful in clinical treatment. His cases of cancer still remained positive, despite this de-fact of science. Clinically used in solid extract, powder and tablets dissolved in water, used as directed.

Since 1955 the Medical Academy of Science, Moscow, has promoted Chaga for clinical and domestic medicine, encouraged it commercially, and collected it for medical use.

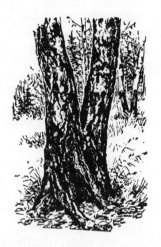

Old Birch, where Chaga can usually be found. The tree must be alive.
(Botany, Ministry of Education, Moscow, 1963)

In the "Atlas of Medical Plants", Medical Academy of Science, Moscow (1962) (see bibliography), Chaga is carefully recommended but definitely approved, administered as a tea, extract, nastoika (Chaga in vodka), for malignant indications. It is directed to cases when the patient cannot stand operations or radio therapy. Chaga is confirmed as a very old Folk Medicine with highest credit for stomach gastristis, ulcers and especially cancer, TB, or conditions of malignancy unfavourable to operations due to the intricacy of nerve and blood vessels.

It should be understood that not all advanced forms of cancer can be controlled, but Chaga will reduce pain, give comfort and stop or slow down growths. The beginning of cancer and some cases of less advancement are arrested and can prevent the spreading processes. In swelling of the lower bowel, Chaga decoctions are prepared for colonics in addition to oral medication.

The diet is very definitely restricted to milk products and vegetables—no meat, conserves, sausages or strong spices (Saratov University, 1932).

79

Chaga is blood purifying and regenerates deteriorated organs and glands, "Medical Encyclopaedia" (Moscow 1965). Time must be given for Chaga. Recommended treatment is from three to five months, with seven to ten days intervals.

Domestic Use: The bark and middle portion which have been carefully separated and cleaned must be crushed or shredded then soaked in warm water (not over 50 degrees). When preparing Chaga think of it as yeast, water too hot will kill the living fungus. For 1 part of crushed Chaga pour over 5 parts of boiled (not boiling) water, let stand covered 48 hr., strain pour more boiled (not boiling) water, say twice as much, then drink three cups a day 30 min. before each meal.

The above statements are for the attention of the healthy, sick and scientists of human concern.

CHAMOMILE   Matricaria chamomilla, L.
(N.O.: Compositae)

Common Names: ROMAN CAMOMILE, GARDEN CAMOMILE, GROUND APPLE, PINHEADS.

Features: The favoured Chamomile comes from southern Europe and is officially known as Anthemis nobilis, possessing medicinal qualities superior to ours.

This yellow or whitish small daisy-like perennial, with its strong fibrous root, pale green thread-shaped leaflets, has a very bitter taste, with the strong aromatic smell of the apple. It is interesting to note that the name "Chamomile" is derived from the Greek, meaning "ground apple".

Parts Used: Flowers and herb.

Solvents: Water, alcohol.

Bodily Influence: Stomachic, Antispasmodic, Tonic stimulant (volatile oil), Carminative, Diaphoretic, Nervine, Emmenagogue, Sedative.

Uses: Chamomile is one of the widely known herbs. Perhaps its livelihood is established through its early use in childhood ailments such as colds, infantile convulsions, stomach pains, colic, earache, restlessness, measles, etc. If children were treated like this today, we would have fewer of the accumulative diseases that trouble us in later years.

When given warm, Chamomile will favour perspiration and soften the skin. The cold infusion acts as a tonic, and is more suitable for stomach difficulties, and as a drink during convalescence from febrile disease, dyspepsia, all causes of weak or irritable stomach, intermittent and typhoid fever. Take 2–3 tablespoonfuls, or cupfuls, adjusted according to age, two or three times a day.

Syrup made of the juice of Chamomile, using the white flowers (fresh or dried) with the best white wine, is a tonic for jaundice and dropsy. Old fashioned but worth remembering for hysterical and nervous affections in women, and will promote the menstrual flow, relieve dysmenorrhic spasms, and promote the menses when due to exposure to colds, uterine spasms or nervous tension, bilious headache, and aids digestion. A specific for uterus pains of mother at nursing time.

Externally: The flower of Chamomile, beaten and made into oil, will comfort side pain of liver and spleen; at the same time drink the tea of the fresh or dried herb. Culpeper states: "A stone that hath been taken out of the body of man, being wrapped in Chamomile, will in time dissolve, and in a little too."

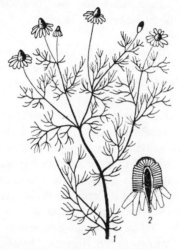

CHAMOMILE   Matricaria chamomilla, L.
(G. N. Kotukov, Lekarstevennye, Kiev, 1964)

The flowers combined with crushed poppy head make a good poultice for allaying pains when other means have failed. As a lotion, it is also excellent for external application in toothache, earache, neuralgia, etc.

A poultice of Chamomile will often prevent gangrene and remove it when present. For sprains and bruises, the herb bruised and moistened with vinegar is excellent in the pulverized form. It may be made up with Soapwort (Saponaria) into shampoo, especially for keeping fair hair light and alive.

Homoeopathic Clinical: Acidity, Anger, Asthma (from Anger), Blepharospasm, Catarrh, Coffee (effects of), Colic, Convulsions, Cough, Cramp, Croup, Dentition, Diarrhoea, Dysmenorrhoea, Dyspepsia, Earache, Eyes (blepharitis, ophthalmia), Eructations Erysipelas, Excitement, Excoriation, Fainting fits, Fevers, Flatulence, Flatulent colic, Gout, Gum rash,

81

Headache, Hernia, Hysterical joint, Influenza, Jaundice, Lienteria, Labour (disorders of, after-pains), Mastitis, Menstruation (disordered), Miliary eruption, Milk fever, Miscarriage, Mumps, Neuralgia, Parotitis, Perichondritis, Peritonitis, Pregnancy (disorders of), Red-gum, Rheumatism, Salivation (nocturnal), Sciatica, Screaming, Sensitiveness, Spasms, Speech (affections of), Toothache, Ulcers, Uterus (disease of), Waking (screaming on), Whooping cough.

Russian Experience: In Russia Chamomile has the tender-sounding name of Romashka. The demand is so great that supplements are imported from Europe. Details on how to plant, cultivate and prepare for shipment have been worked out. They estimate that one acre can yield 500–1,000 lb. of dried Romashka. The North American market depends on imports from Europe, and for the last decade the demand has exceeded the supply. Chamomile Damasky, or Persian Chamomile, is highly praised.

Uses: No family can stay without this simple aromatic home medicine. It is used as a tea from the cradle to the grave for Colds, Stomach trouble, Anaemia, Gargle, Sedative, Nervine, Calming, Colitis, Eczema and Antiseptic for all inflammations.

Clinically: Widely used as oil extract in compositions.

India and Pakistan Experience: The rhythmic Babunah or Babuni-kephul is India's local name. Indian Chamomile grows wild and they consider the herb second best to the European imported flower.

Uses: India's knowledge gives added variety and credit to the popular miniature, daisy-like flower. As a Carminative, Stimulant, Emmenagogue, Diaphoretic, Attenuation, Discutient. Special interest is given to Babunah (Chamomile) for uterine reflex disturbance of women. Also for dyspepsia, flatulent-colic, fever, menstruation disorder, hysteria, and conditional debility. Popular as a children's remedy for nervine and sedative, tonic, stomach disorders, earache, neuralgia pain, convulsion and dentition. A weak infusion is a tonic and febrifuge. Strong warm infusion as an emetic and for periodic headaches. Dose of the flower oil, 1–3 drops for flatulence and colic.

Externally: The oil is especially helpful applied to rheumatic joint pain.

CHAPARRAL   Larrea divaricata, (D.C.) Cov.
(N.O.: Zygophyllaceae)

Common Names: CHAPARRAL, CHAPARRO (Mexican name), CREOSOTE BUSH, GREASEWOOD, GOBONADORA, DWARF EVERGREEN OAK.

Features: Chaparral belongs to a group of desert Artimesia. It is an Indian term referring to over one hundred different botanical plant types growing in alkali soil, from narrow strips to over 100 sq. miles in the south-western part of the United States. Beginning at La Joya, California, extending eastward through California, across Nevada, Arizona and New Mexico.

The dark-green stems and leaves (if drought season, pale or yellowish-green) provide a 4–8 ft. miniature desert-forest. Distinguished from the usual grey green colour of the other desert species. The strong-scented leaves are opposite and are divided into two leaflets. The bright yellow, five petal flowers, $\frac{1}{2}$ in. or more across, appear in spring and winter. The fruit is rounded, up to about $\frac{1}{4}$ in. long, and is covered with white hairs.

Australia has a similar plant, also northern Argentina in South America.

The leaves and stems of Chaparral contain a generous supply of gums and resins, protein, partially characterized esters, acids, alcohol, a small amount of a mixture of sterols, sucrose, and a very small amount of volatile oils. No alkaloids were detected and it is non-toxic.

Medicinal Parts: The leaves and stems.

Solvent: Hot water (partially).

Bodily Influence: Antiseptic, Diuretic, Expectorant, Tonic.

Uses: In 1848 the U.S.–Mexican boundary commission is reported to have brought Chaparral to the attention of the medical profession as treatment for internal conditions of rheumatism; mixed with Sarsaparilla for venereal nodes and chancre. Generations previous to the above recognition, Indians of the south-western areas used the plant as varied symptoms prevailed. More recently, in October 1967, after three previous surgically removed growths, an eighty-five-year-old man refused medical treatment on the same; fourth-recurrent growth, documented as malignant melanoma, in favour of "Chaparral tea", an old Indian remedy. Of this tea he drank 2–3 cups a day. In September 1968 he was re-examined by the Medical Centre, Utah, U.S.A. They found the growth had decreased from the size of a large lemon to that of a dime. No other medication was used, only the Chaparral tea. In eleven months he gained a needed 25 lb., with improvements in general health, as previous to Chaparral treatment, he was pale, weak and lethargic.

The above case seems to be the re-awakening of the desert plant through publications of health magazines using natural sources.

Personal and professional cases appearing in the magazines have added to its modern list of usefulness as follows: Acne and skin conditions of warts and blotches, Arthritis, Cancer, Chronic backache, Increases hair growth, Improvement of eye sight, Increases bowel elimination (though not laxative), Kidney infection, Leukaemia, Prostate gland trouble, Skin cancer, Sinus, Stomach cancer, Throat, Bronchial and pulmonary conditions, Weight reducing.

Clinically: Probable mechanism of anti-cancer action is thought due to the known, and most active, ingredient called "nordihydroguaiaretic acid-NDGA", which has the qualities to convert fermentation processes thought to be out of balance.

In a few words, medical science believes the processes in which Chaparral supports the system works by inhibiting the unwanted rapid growth, via the vital respiratory process throughout the body.

The magazine articles stated taking from one tablet with each meal, to as many as ten tablets every hour. The most sensible, also with results was instructions from the following Indian use.

Dose: Place 1 tablespoonful of Chaparral leaves and small twigs into a glass screw-top jar. Pour 1 pt. of boiling water over this, cover and let stand overnight. Do not refrigerate, do not remove surface settlement. Drink a quarter of the liquid $\frac{1}{2}$ hr. before each meal and at night time.

To some, the strong taste of creosote is unpleasant as a tea. Different strengths of tablets are available. Tablet form, 1 before each meal and 1 at bedtime. When using the loose tea in the above amounts, approximately 40 per cent of the available properties is extracted with total daily intake around 200–250 mg. Herbalists combine other herbs with Chaparral as case requires.

Externally: Our Indian nation of Papoga, Pimas and Maricopas of the south-western states boiled the leaves and branches for bruises and rheumatism. In some areas salt was added to the boiled herb for the above. The dry heated leaves and branches were applied as a poultice for chest and other body pain. Young branches were sharpened, placed in the fire until hot, then inserted into tooth cavities to relieve pain.

Veterinary: After the resins have been obtained for commercial use as a preservative, the leaf residue is fed to livestock. It contains as much protein as Alfalfa.

"In springtime if an old cow can pull through until the greasewood puts out tender shoots she will get fat, shed off her old rough winter coat, and be glossy and pretty in four weeks, and she will bring her calf and be able to nurse it into a fine animal. This drama of life I have witnessed year after year for the past 50 or more."—Ralph W. Davis, N.D., H-O-H, August 1971.

CHERRY BARK   Prunus virginiana, L.
(N.O.: Rosaceae)

Common Names: WILD BLACK CHERRY BARK, CHOKE CHERRY.
Features: This large fruit tree is native to North America and is found in Canada, Florida, Minnesota, Nebraska, Kansas, Louisiana, Texas.

The outside bark is blackish and rugged. The young branches are smooth, red or purplish; flowers appear after the leaves in May and

June, followed by the delicious Cherry in August. The bark has a distinct aromatic odour, resembling bitter almond when macerated in water; the taste is astringent and agreeably bitter. The young, thin bark is the best; very large or small branches should be rejected. Stem bark is collected in the autumn and carefully dried; slouching dead tissue, if present, should be removed. Will keep well in tightly closed containers in a dark place.

Solvent: Hot or cold water.

Medicinal Part: The young thin bark.

Bodily Influence: Mild tonic, Soothing astringent, Sedative, Pectoral.

Uses: Wild Cherry bark is extensively used in cough medicines as a vehicle base. This agent is useful in many other classes of disease. For diarrhoea of children it is excellent in the form of syrup and may be pleasantly combined with neutralizing cordial; lack of stomach tone causing indigestion will be greatly relieved. Cough, Bronchitis, Scrofula, Heart palpitation (should not be used in dry cough), Dyspepsia, Hectic

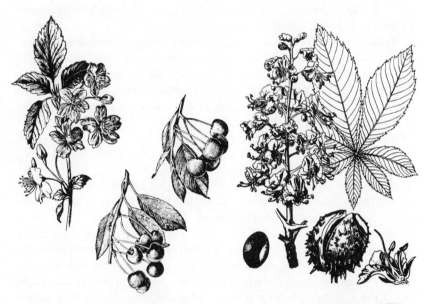

CHERRY BARK   Prunus virginiana, L.
(Department of Education,
Moscow, 1957)

CHESTNUT   Castanea dentata, Mill.
(Bello-Russ. Academy of Science,
Minsk, 1969)

fever, debility of old or protracted and enfeebled cases of congested feeling of phlegm in the throat and chest. It contains a small amount of hydrocyanic acid. The Cherry contains malic acid, and is high in life-giving properties.

85

Dose: 15 drops in water. Cherry bark will dissolve stones but should be combined with other herbs and administered carefully and over a period of several months, as when taken too fast will expel the stones abruptly without being softened.

Homoeopathic Clinical: Cold infusion or tincture of inner bark; solution of concentrated resinous extract, Prunin—Acidity, Anorexia, Dyspepsia, Heart (weakness of, hypertrophy of, irritable), Pyrosis.

CHESTNUT Castanea dentata, Mill.
(N.O.: Fagacaae)

Common Names: SPANISH CHESTNUT, HORSE-CHESTNUT, SWEET CHESTNUT.

Features: The stately Chestnut tree grows in North America, western Asia and southern Europe. The species are usually self-sterile, requiring more than one tree for the production of chestnuts. The flowers consist of long catkins, which may contain the female or fruit bearing organs at their base, or may be purely male of staminate.

If the female flowers are fertilized they develop spiny burrs, containing 1–5 one-seeded nuts. The leaves are dark green above, light beneath; slightly broken, folded or matted together, the odour is light with an astringent taste. The chestnut is low in protein, high in carbohydrates and starch, contains minerals such as phosphate of potash, magnesia, some sodium and iron.

Medicinal Parts: The leaves and inner bark.

Solvents: Boiling water, alcohol (partially).

Bodily Influence: Tonic, Mild Sedative, Astringent.

Uses: Culpeper made use of the inner skin that contains the nut: "Is of so binding a quality that a scruple of it being taken by a man or ten grains by a child, soon stops any flux whatsoever."

The green or dried leaves can be used, and it is considered a particular herb for whooping cough or nagging distressing coughs, controlling the paroxysmal; and in frequent hiccoughs and other irritable and excitable conditions of the respiratory organs. Fevers, ague respond to the soothing of the mucous surfaces and the nervous system, acting as an antispasmodic. Lobelia inflata, Blue cohosh and Caulophyllum thalictroides are most successfully combined for the above mentioned.

Dose: 1 oz. to 1 pint of boiling water, infused for 15 min. A wineglassful three times a day, children half the amount. The fluid extract is convenient: dose, 10 drops three times a day; 5 drops for children.

Homoeopathic Clinical: Tincture of leaves gathered in summer—Diarrhoea, Whooping cough.

Russian Experience: Konsky cashtan, known as Horse-chestnut, does not grow wild, but has long been cultivated in European Russia, Middle Asia and Kaukaz (Eaucasus).

Folk Medicine: Its value is recognized and is used for Arthritis, Rheumatism, Female bleeding, Haemorrhoids, and chronic inflammation of the intestines.

Clinically: Extracts used for bleeding haemorrhoids, varicose veins, arteriosclerosis.

CHICKWEED Stellaria media, Cyrill.
(N.O.: Caryophyllaceae)

Common Names: STITCHWORT, SCARWORT, SATIN FLOWER, ADDER'S MOUTH, STARWEED.

Features: There are about twenty-five species native and naturalized in the American continent. The Indians used native Chickweed for many years, but also adopted naturalized species. It is common in Europe and America, growing in fields and around dwellings, in moist shady places. The stem is weak and straggling, freely branched; there is a line of white hairs along one side only, changing direction at each pair of leaves. The very small white flowers bloom from the beginning of spring until autumn; taste, slightly salty. The seeds are eaten by poultry and birds.

Solvents: Water, alcohol.

Medicinal Part: Whole herb.

Bodily Influence: Demulcent, Emollient, Pectoral, Refrigerant.

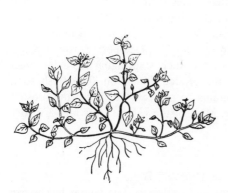

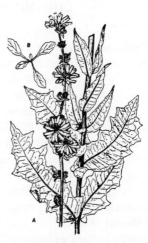

COMMON CHICKWEED Stellaria media, Cyrill.
(Ontario Department of Agriculture, Toronto, 1966)

A—CHICORY Chicorium intybus, L. B—SEEDLING
(Ontario Department of Agriculture, Toronto, Canada)

Uses: The many areas of internal inflammation are soothed and healed by this so-called troublesome garden weed. The uses are many, from salad greens, and spinach, to preparations of fresh, dried, powdered, poultice, fomentations and salves.

The awareness of this creation for bodily correction is qualified for liver ailments (internally and externally), bronchitis, pleurisy, coughs, colds, hoarseness, rheumatism, inflammation or weakness of the bowels and stomach, lungs, bronchial tubes, scurvy, kidney trouble, to ease the heat and sharpness of the blood in haemorrhoids; to release cramps and shrunken sinews, which are small vessels that transmit blood from the liver and into the hepatic veins, making them more pliable again. This so-called common plant could be included among the all-purpose herbals.

Dose: 1 oz. of Chickweed to 1½ pints of water, simmered down to 1 pint. A wineglassful every 2–3 hr. Use externally as a poultice for inflamed surfaces, boils and skin eruptions.

Externally: Effective for all swellings, redness of the face, weals, scabs, boils, burns, inflamed or sore eyes (apply on cotton pads over closed eyes), erysipelas, tumours, haemorrhoids, cancer-swollen testes, ulcerated throat and mouth. For broken or unbroken skin conditions, Chickweed is your medicine.

Homoeopathic Clinical: Gout, Liver (inflammation of), Rheumatism, Psoriasis.

CHICORY ROOT   Chicorium intybus, L.
(N.O.: Compositae)

Common Names: GARDEN CHICORY, ENDIVE, SUCCORY.

Features: Naturalized in the United States from Europe. This perennial bears a most heavenly shade with star-like petals of blue, with a violet cast that is so outstanding when in bloom it is restful to behold.

The flowers are abundant from July to October; shrub reaches heights of from 1–6 ft., with abrupt branches springing from the erect stem; leaves similar to those of the related dandelion. The fresh root, when collected in the spring, contains 36 per cent of inulin; the roasted root is mixed to adulterate coffee. Most of the U.S.A. cultivated Chicory is grown in Michigan State.

Medicinal Part: The root.

Solvent: Water.

Bodily Influence: Hepatic, Laxative, Diuretic, Tonic.

Uses: The uses are much the same as Dandelion. The tender leaves can be chopped fine and mixed with salad greens. The tea from Chicory eliminates unwanted phlegm from the stomach that interferes with absorption and secretion of the internal system—in this way aiding in superfluous gall material—purifies the liver and spleen, is effective in uratic acid conditions of gout, rheumatics and joint stiffness. Tea made from the dried root is good for sour or upset stomach.

Dose: 1 oz. of the root to 1 pint of boiling water, and infusion of the fresh root in the same proportions used for gravel in the bladder and kidneys. The bitter, milky juice flows from the rind, which is the medicinal virtues it possesses. The cold preparation taken a mouthful at a time two or three times a day.

Externally: The juice of the bruised leaves applied externally allays swelling and inflammation pain due to abundance of milk.

Homoeopathic Clinical: Tincture or trituration of dried root—Amblyopia, Constipation, Headache.

Russian Experience: Tzicory (Chicory) is very popular in Russian Folk Medicine and clinical practice. It is a food supplement alone, or with combinations of ordinary coffee and other herbal teas.

Clinically: As antiseptic and astringent alone, or combined as a sedative of the central nervous system and heart conditions. Medically as Carminative, Tonic, Astringent, Digestive, used in cases of Liver inefficiency.

CLEAVERS Galium aparine, L.
(N.O.: Rubiaceae)

Common Names: GOOSE GRASS, CATCHSTRAW, BEDSTRAW, CLEAVERS.

Features: Common to Europe and the United States, growing in cultivated grounds, moist thickets and along banks of rivers; flowering from June to September; stems rough and weak but very lengthy, with little prickly hooks and many side branches, always in pairs; leaves small and six to nine on the round stem, topped with very small white flowers of petals in arrangement of the Maltese cross. Medicinally the green herb may be used as well as the dry. The root is a permanent red dye.

Medicinal Part: The whole herb.

Solvent: Water (do not boil).

Bodily Influence: Diuretic, Tonic, Refrigerant, Alterative, Aperient.

Uses: Notably one of our best-known herbs for obstructions of the urinary organs, especially when combined with Broom, Uva ursi, Buchu and Marshmallow. It is particularly useful for stones or gravel and seems to soften and reduce the calculous and/or accumulation to where it can be eliminated, making sure the bowels are active at all times.

For children or adults suffering from scalding urine it is invaluable and the refrigerant qualities are soothing in cases of scarlet fever, measles and all acute diseases. The book "Vitalogy" (1925) by Dr. Wood and Dr. Ruddock says: "The cold infusion will remove freckles when it is drunk two or three times a day, for two or three months and the parts frequently washed with it, and has recently been used with decided success in treating children for bed wetting, it should be drunk three times a day."

Claudie V. James (1963) gives us another use: "The juice mixed with oatmeal to the consistency of a poultice and applied over an indolent tumour three times a day, keeping the bowels open and taking a teaspoonful of the juice every morning, will often drive the tumour away in a few days. It is one of the best known herbs for reducing."

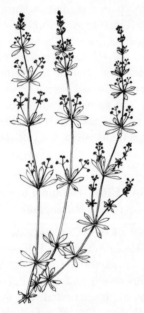

CLEAVERS   Galium aparine, L.
(U.S. Agricultural Department, Appalachia, 1971)

For reducing, $\frac{1}{4}$ cup of the fresh or dried herb in $\frac{1}{2}$ pint of boiling water, one-third of the amount taken three times a day.

Externally: Cleavers may be used in all acute diseases and deep perplexing psoriasism eczema, cancer, scrofula, ulcers and all skin trouble. An infusion is prepared by macerating $1\frac{1}{2}$ oz. of the herb in 1 pint of warm water for 2 hr.

Dose: 2–4 oz. given three or four times a day cold; may be sweetened with honey or brown sugar. Of the tincture, 20–40 drops in water three or four times a day.

COLTSFOOT Tussilago farfara, L.
(N.O.: Compositae)

Common Names: COUGH WORT, HORSE HOOF, BULL'S FOOT, FOAL'S FOOT, GINGER ROOT.

Features: Naturalized in the United States from Europe, Siberia and East Indies. Although found growing in many areas, from the sea shores to elevations of nearly 8,000 ft., our local Coltsfoot prefers certain clay soil. This low succulent perennial has smooth green leaves with a white and cottony underside that appear in March. They do not appear until the large daisy-type, bright yellow flower has withered, and are from 5–8 in. long and like a colts foot in shape.

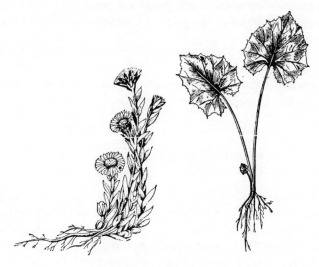

COLTSFOOT   Tussilago farfara,
(Vishaya Schkolla, Moscow, 1963)

The stem is covered with a loose cottony down. The whole plant is used, more especially the leaves, and they should be collected when they have almost reached maturity. Collect the root after the fullness of the leaves; the flowers, as soon as they open. When dried, all three have a faintly herbaceous bitter taste.

Medicinal Part: The leaves.

Solvents: Water, diluted alcohol.

Bodily Influence: Emollient, Demulcent, Expectorant, Slight Tonic, Pectoral.

Uses: For congestion of the pulmonary system, especially if inclined to consumption. For these symptoms Horehound, Ground ivy, Marshmallow and Elder flower have been successfully combined with Coltsfoot,

91

making up half of the compound. However, the juice of Coltsfoot by itself is effective in troublesome coughs. The botanical name Tussilago means "Cough Dispeller"; this includes Coughs, Asthma, Whooping cough, in short, a chest and lung expectorant.

Dose: Steep 1 teaspoonful of the leaves in 1 cup of boiling water for $\frac{1}{2}$ hour; drink $\frac{1}{2}$ cupful at bed time, hot or cold, or a mouthful three times a day, or administer according to case, up to 2 cupfuls daily. Of the tincture, 1–2 fl. drams.

Externally: The leaves, bruised or steeped in hot water, may be applied to the chest for relieving fever, feebleness and easing the heart, also for open wounds to draw out the injurious matter. Use as a poultice in scrofulous tumours. For sore feet, or when bruised externally, fevered swelling and skin irritations, apply fresh, and often.

Homoeopathic Clinical: Tincture of the whole plant—Corpulence, Plethora.

Russian Experience: "Mat i Matcheha", "Mother and step mother". is Russia's name for Coltsfoot.

Folk Medicine: The leaves and flowers are first aid home treatment for colds, acute and chronic lung infections.

COMFREY   Symphytum officinale, L.
(N.O.: Borraginaceae)

Common Names: GUM PLANT, HEALING HERB, KNIT BONE, NIPBONE.

Features: The genus includes some twenty-five species of herbs native to Europe, Asia Minor, Siberia and Iran. The common Comfrey is naturalized in much of North America. Comfrey is a perennial with a stout spreading root, brownish-black and wrinkled, the stem about 3 ft. high and large, coarsely hairy, egg to lance shaped leaves, with wavy edges.

The blue-purplish, yellow, white, or red tubular flowers, less than 1 in. long, are borne in coiled clusters. They have five stamens and the fruit consists of four shiny brown to black nutlets, which can be seen in August. It flowers in May and June and grows by riversides and in most moist places. The root contains a large amount of mucilage and is rich in easily assimilated organic calcium.

Medicinal Parts: Root and leaves.

Solvent: Water.

Bodily Influence: Demulcent, Astringent.

Use: American Indians found the value of medical Comfrey and used it with many other naturalized plants. When internal functions are weakened or injured to the degree of showing bloody discharge, whether in sputum, urine or bowels, Comfrey will prevent serious complications by healing the tissue and easing the pain of the involved areas of bones, tendons, ruptured lungs and other delicate cells.

By knowledge of the past and present, Comfrey has long been accepted as being of great value as a soothing demulcent, a general stimulant to the mucous membrane of the respiratory organs and to help increase expectoration, thus aiding the bronchial tubes.

A syrup made of equal parts of Comfrey and Elecampane roots is a most valuable agent for coughs, consumption and all affections of the lungs. In "Natures Healing Agents" S. Clymer (1963) tell us: "Numerous uncontradicted reports of lung cancer cured where all other means have failed and in which the sole treatment consisted of infusion made from the whole green plant and, even in some instances, of infusion made from the powder of entire plant."

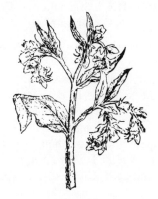

COMFREY   Symphytum officinale, L.
(Dr. A. J. Thut, Guelph, Canada)

For the purpose of cleansing the entire system of impurities and establishing a normal condition, Comfrey is useful in Arthritis, Gall-stones, Stomach conditions, Asthma, Ulcerated tonsils, in some cases of various forms of Cancer, Ulceration of the kidney, Scrofula, Anaemia, Dysentery, Diarrhoea, Leucorrhoea and Female debility.

Dose: The entire fresh or powdered plant. 1 teaspoonful to 1 cup of boiling water, steeped for $\frac{1}{2}$ hr., taken four times daily, 1 cup a day. Of the tincture, 5–20 drops fours times daily, by prescription.

Externally: A poultice of the fresh or dried leaves or powder for ruptures, sore breasts, fresh wounds, ulcers, swellings, burns or bruises.

Homoeopathic Clinical: Tincture of fresh root-stock collected before flowering and in autumn. Tincture of fresh plant. Dr. Dorothy Shepherd, J. H. Clark, M.D., and other homoeopaths highly appraised Symphytum and used it in many cases. Abscess, Backache (from sexual excess), Bone (cancer of) (injuries of), Breast (sore), Eye (pains in) (injuries of),

93

Fractures (non-union of) (nervous), Glands (enlarged), Gunshots wounds, Hernia, Menses (arrested). Peritonium (sensitive, painful), Psoas abscess, Sexual excess (effect of), Sprains, Wounds.

Russian Experience: Russian Comfrey is known as Okopnik, which is used less in Russia than abroad. In medicine they consider an excess to be poisonous. However they do admit scientific and clinical analysis is not complete.

Folk Medicine: Has a wide and varied reputation. They use the fresh or dried roots and rhizomes in decoctions and teas as an astringent. In cases of internal and external bleeding, broken bones, female complaints, ulcers, wounds and many of the above mentioned.

CORN SILK   Stigmata maydis, L.
(N.O.: Gramineae)

Common Names: SEA MAYS, INDIAN CORN, MAIZE, JUGNOG, TURKEY CORN.

Features: Corn is a member of the grass family, the genus Zea, and the species Mays. Its scientific name is Zea Mays. The common Indian corn is generally believed to have originated in the New World, where it was cultivated before Christopher Columbus discovered America. Columbus took it to Spain and many thought it was brought from Asia and it was frequently known as Turkey corn, or Turkey wheat. The silk should be taken when the corn will shed its pollen. The active principle is maizenic acid.

Solvents: Water, dilute alcohol.

Medicinal Part: The green pistils.

Bodily Influence: Diuretic, Demulcent, Alterative.

Uses: So well known and yet not recognized by most for its purpose in aiding mankind. Herbalists and naturopaths think first of Corn silk when dangerous deposits of brick dust are present in the urine and for removing the condition which is responsible for the disturbance in cystic irritation due to phosphatic and uric acid build up. Stigmata maydis will assist all inflammatory conditions of the urethra, bladder and kidney, which is the cause of much local and general malfunction of the body due to uric acid retention. So often the scanty and offensive release of urine of the aged calls for the appreciable comfort of Corn silk. Also indicated in local dropsy and heart trouble.

Children of uncontrolled, often swollen, bladder tissue will be happy to know Corn silk tea prevents bed wetting.

Dose: Tincture of Corn silk (Stigmata maydis) 15–30 drops, tincture of Agrimony (Agrimonia eupatoria) 10–30 drops, in water between meals and at bedtime. For more advanced urinary complaints combine

4 oz. Corn silk, 2 oz. Dandelion root (Leontodon taraxacum), 1 oz. Golden seal (Hydrastis canadensis). Steep 1 teaspoonful to 1 cup of boiling water. Take every three or four hours or as needed. Sweeten with honey to taste.

Homoeopathic Clinical: Albuminuria (st), Cystitis (st), Dropsy (st), Gonorrhoea (chronic) (st), Heart (failure of) (st), Malaria (chronic) (sh), Renal colic (st), Pyelitis (st), Urine (retained; suppressed) (st).

Russian Experience: Kukuruza, or Maize, is well known to Russian Folk Medicine. Lately they have found that Corn oil is prophylactic for high blood pressure, Cholesterol, Arteriosclerosis, to promote bile, activate the liver and many other benefits.

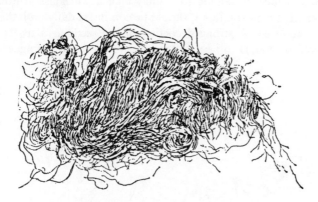

CORN SILK   Stigmate maydis, L.
(Vishaya Schkolla, Moscow, 1963)

Folk Medicine: The use of Corn silk tea, or decoctions, has material Folk Medicine history for bleeding, as it is rich in Vitamin K, bed-wetting, high blood pressure, cholesterol and arteriosclerosis.

Externally: As a Corn silk powder, or ointment, with corn oil for wounds and ulcer-like skin disturbances.

Clinically: Given medicinally in extract, powder and tablet decoctions for gall-bladder conditions, kidney and bladder stones, inflammation, slow urination, bed-wetting and all involvements of the urinary tract.

COTTON ROOT   Gossypium herbaceum, L.
(N.O.: Malvaceae)

Common Name: COTTON ROOT.

Features: There are many different species of Gossypium, a member of the Malvaceae, or Mallow, family. Economically, cotton is one of the most valuable of all plants. The biennial or triennial herb is a branching

95

shrub about 5 ft. high, with woody roots, and branches. The flower seems to open only for pollination, as it withers after one day. The boll grows to golf ball size with pointed tip. The boll cracks and splits from the tip showing locks, or 8–10 seeds with fibres attached. The open dried boll, which holds the fluffed-out cotton is called the burr. Native to Asia, but is cultivated extensively in many parts of the world. In the United States more successfully in the southern portion.

Part Used: The inner bark of the root.

Solvent: Boiling water.

Bodily Influence: Emmenagogue, Parturient, Oxytocic.

Uses: For parturient in childbirth add $\frac{1}{4}$ lb. of the bark to $1\frac{1}{2}$ quarts of water and reduce by boiling to 1 pint; take a wineglassful every $\frac{1}{2}$ hr. For obstructed menstruation it should be continued daily until the desired effect is produced. A strong decoction of the seeds as a tea is mucilaginous and is reputed to be an effective cure for fever and ague.

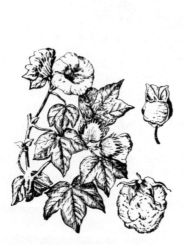

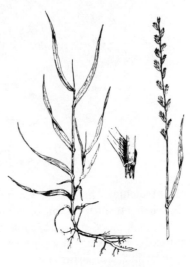

COUCH GRASS
Triticum or Agropyrum, Beav.
(Ontario Department of Agriculture,
Toronto, Canada, 1966)

COTTON ROOT
Gossypium herbaceum, L.
(Botanic Medicine, Moscow, 1951)

Homoeopathic Clinical: Tincture of fresh inner root bark—Abortion, Amenorrhoea, Dysmenorrhoea, Labia (abscess of), Ovaries (pains in), Pregnancy (vomiting of), Sterility, Tumour, Uterus (bearing down in).

Russian Experience: Time never passes without the use of absorbent Cotton in Russia, and elsewhere, for industrial, commercial, and clinical use. Known in Russia as Hlopok or Vatta.

Folk Medicine: The root is used to stop bleeding, especially internally.

Clinically: Common in the form of extract.

India and Pakistan: The many and different uses of the whole Cotton plant has long been established in India and Pakistan.

Root Bark: As an Abortifacient, in uterine disorder, and as effective Emmanenagogue. Root powder, 20–60 grain dose; its decoction, 1–2 oz. every 30 min.

Leaves: Crushed to make a fresh extract and used in Diarrhoea, Dysentery, Piles, Strangury, Gravel.

Seed: Is used as a decoction or in powder form as Laxative, Expectorant, Antidysenteric, Aphrodisiac, Demulcent, Nervine, Tonic, Galactagogue and Abortifacient.

Externally: Cotton seed oil: an application for Rheumatic disease and dressing for Freckles, Herpes, Scabies and Wounds. Local applications will act as a sedative for Neuralgia and Chronic headache.

Cotton Ash Fibres: Are effective applied to Ulcers; Sores and Wounds.

Leaves and Seeds: As a poultice for Bruises, Burns, Scalds, Sores, Swellings. For Uterine colic, a hot leaf infusion is applied.

COUCH GRASS   Triticum or Agropyrum repens, Beav.
(N.O.: Gramineae)

Common Names: DOG GRASS, QUICK GRASS, DURFA GRASS, TWITCH GRASS, TRITICUM REPENS, AGROPYRUM.

Features: Known to farmers in Europe and North America as a pest. The spikes resemble wheat or rye when in bloom, reaching heights of 1–3 ft.; the pale yellow, smooth rootstock is long and trailing, with each joint sending forth a shoot which becomes a new plant. It should be gathered in the spring and carefully cleaned and dried. Culpeper says an acre of Couch grass is worth 10 acres of carrots.

Medicinal Parts: Rootstock, rhizome.

Solvent: Water.

Bodily Influence: Diuretic, Aperient, Demulcent.

Uses: Couch grass is recommended by Dr. Thompsom for lessening the frequency and pain in cases of excessive irritation of the bladder from any cause. It is a Botanical for general catarrhal treatment, which if not eliminated advances more seriously. The troublesome plant has been used by famous Herbalists for Gout, Enlarged prostate gland (when chronic gonorrhoea), Prulent cystitis, Incipient nephritis. Some physicians trust its timely use in dissolving small calculi. This being so, it is a herb to remember for all rheumatic and jaundice sufferers. The accepted administration is in an infusion of 1 oz. of Couch grass to 1 pint of boiling water, steeped 20 min. and given in wineglassful doses every 2 hr. Or a decoction of the root made by boiling 1 oz. of the herb in 1 pint of water until reduced to $\frac{3}{4}$ pint, 10–20 drops in water two or more times a day.

Dr. Clymer, M.D., gives us the following from "Natures Healing Agents". In chronic gonorrhoea:

Tincture of Couch grass (Triticum repens), 5–20 drops
Tincture 2 Motherwort (Leonurus cardiaca), 9–15 drops
Tincture 2 Sandalwood (Santalum album), 10–20 drops
Tincture 2 Buchu (Barosma betulina), 10–20 drops

Dose: In water, three or more times a day.

For enlarged prostate (non-operative):

Tincture of Couch grass (Triticum repens), 5–15 drops
Tincture of Fringe tree (Chionanthus virginica), 3–7 drops
Tincture of Saw palmetto (Sabal serrulata), 5–20 drops

Dose: In water, three or more times a day.

In rheumatism complicated with prostatic involvement:

Tincture of Couch grass (Triticum repens), 5–20 drops
Tincture of Motherwort (Leonurus cardiaca), 9–15 drops
Tincture of Scurvy grass (Cachlearia officinalis), 7–15 drops
Tincture of Black cohosh (Cimicifuga racemosa), 1–15 drops

Dose: In water three or four times a day. Black cohosh should be used with caution.

Dose: Tincture of Couch grass alone, 10–20 drops in water, two or more times a day. Specifically, one of the most important symptoms for the prescribing of Triticum is a burning sensation and constant desire to urinate.

Homoeopathic Experience: Bladder (irritation of), Dysuria, Urine (incontinence of).

Russian Experience: Familiar Couch grass can be seen all over the country, the prevailing pattern of life has many rewards of merit. Pirey Polzutchy (Couch grass) by Russian translation means, Fire of Field. Even in Latin they call it Agros ("A field") and pyr ("Fire"), hence Agropyum. To most Couch grass has a reputation as a troublesome, persistent weed.

Professor N. B. Tzitzin, Academy of Science, may be a blessing to mankind for his awareness of this hearty plant. First he noticed how the plant could survive in any soil or weather conditions; and how it had a fantastic power to multiply. One plant produced over 10,000 seeds by crawling rhizomes. Lengths up to 1,500 ft. can be produced in an area of 9 sq. ft. This will yield over 20,000 buds ready to start at the first opportunity, meaning one plant can produce over 30,000 plants in one season, either by rhizomes in immediate area or by seeds in distant soil.

If one lonely plant settles in a cultivated field it overcomes the field in a very short time and the more you cut it the more it grows. Observing this strong power of survival, Professor Tzitzin, being a young and ambitious scientist, decided to use this characteristic for the betterment of mankind and brilliantly gave new life to wheat by this hybrid omnipotent quality. In countries where agricultural production is critical this improvement deserves attention and consideration. This much-improved academic find adapts to any soil, good or bad; resists sickness and fungus parasites; resists frost, drought and wet periods. It is perennial and very self protected, giving much improved larger and nutritious grain.

The qualities as medicine to persons aware of its possessions are openly accepted.

Folk Medicine: The tea is used in every part of the country for serious cases of uncontrollable urination, to restore poor eyesight, Tubercular lungs, Chest pain, Fever, Jaundice, Rheumatism, Lumbago, Syphilis, and as a female corrective agent.

Clinically: They find Couch grass rich in Vitamin C, Carotene, Polysaccharide, Inulin, Glucose and other nutritional elements. Used in extract form and considered the best for blood purifying, kidney and bladder, stomach stimulant, liver and spleen. The thick extract is also used as a tablet binder.

COWSLIP   Primula officinalis, Hill
(N.O.: Primulaceae)

Common Names: PAIGLES, PALSYWORT, HERB PETER.

Features: Growing in moist pastures and open places in the United States and Canada from the Atlantic coast of Nebraska, as well as in Arctic and temperate regions of the eastern hemisphere, Cowslip, a glabrous perennial commonly applied to various species of Caltha (the Marsh Marigold family) reaches a height of 2 ft. with bright yellow flowers up to 2 in. in diameter that bunch together on one stalk, each flower emerging from the same point, outer blossoms drooping, flowers in April and May followed by a cluster of many seeded pods; the brightest yellow flowers should be collected when in bloom and dried thoroughly, as they will putrefy if moisture is present.

Medicinal Parts: Flowers, leaves (less valued).

Solvent: Water.

Bodily Influence: Sedative, Antispasmodic.

Uses: The Greeks called Cowslip "Paralysis", for the embracing strength given to the brain and central nervous system. For various infirmities such as heat waves of the head, vertigo, false apprehension, frenzy, epilepsy, convulsions, cramps, trembling, palsy, articular diseases of any

99

name with violent pains, a daily drink of Cowslip tea will gradually make the symptoms disappear. Culpeper used the root to ease pains in the back and bladder, and to open the passage of the urine.

Externally: The leaves (some say both, leaves and flowers) are made into an ointment by extracting the juice and mixing with linseed oil or coconut oil, for skin conditions of scaldings, or burns by fire, water or sun. As a beauty aid the ointment will nourish the skin, softening wrinkles, lightening freckles and discolorations, if applied faithfully.

Homoeopathic Clinical: Tincture of entire fresh plant—Apoplexy (threatened), Eczema, Fevers, Migraine, Neuralgia, Vertigo, Voice, (affections of).

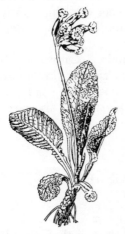

COWSLIP   Primula officinalis, Hill
(Medicina, Moscow, 1965)

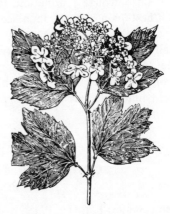

CRAMPBARK HIGH   Viburnum opulus, L.
(Bello-Russ. Academy of Science,
Minsk, 1967.)

Russian Experience: Pervo-Tzvet, First Flower of Spring, a joy in its beauty and fragrance, is one of nature's signs of the fresh and alive unfolding beauty of the countryside, with many unsuspecting treasures, some of which are yet untold. The fresh leaves are used in spring salads, giving a pleasant aroma and sweet taste. The flowers are an export item and widely used abroad. Powder for Avitaminosis (deficiency of vitamins) as it is rich in Vitamin C and carotin.

Folk Medicine: The importance as a home medicine for colds was known and employed as Diaphoretic, Expectorant, Diuretic and Antispasmodic. Used equally with Senega root (Polygala senega) for Bronchitis and respiratory trouble.

Leaves: As a vitamin source are used as tea and food.

Root and Rhizome: Medicinal for Bronchitis, etc.

100

Clinically: Used as an extract or powder with other herbs, or separately, without toxic accumulation, as a mild laxative, stomach tonic, stimulant, vitamin builder to regenerate the blood.

CRAMPBARK HIGH Viburnum opulus, L.

(N.O.: Caprifoliaceae)

Common Names: HIGH CRANBERRY, SNOWBALL TREE, GUELDER ROSE, SQUAW BUSH, CRAMP BARK.

Features: Indigenous to the northern part of the United States and Canada; a handsome shrub, growing in low rich lands, woods and borders of fields, presenting a showy appearance of flowers in June. The flowers are succeeded by red, very acid berries, resembling low cranberries, and sometimes substituted for them. They remain on the bush after the leaves have fallen and throughout the winter. The bark has no smell, but has a peculiar bitterish and astringent taste, which leaves a clean feeling in the mouth. Viburnine is the active principle found in the dried bark of the stem. The berries are a rich source of Vitamins C and K.

Medicinal Part: The bark.

Solvents: Water, diluted alcohol.

Bodily Influence: Antispasmodic, Nervine, Tonic, Astringent, Diuretic.

Uses: Known to American practitioners for the conditions of which the name implies, Cramp bark, giving relief to cramps and spasms of involuntary muscular contractions such as in asthma, hysteria; cramps of female during pregnancy, preventing the attack entirely if used daily for the last two or three months of gestation.

Steep 1 teaspoonful of the cut bark in 1 cup of boiling water for $\frac{1}{2}$ hr.; when cold, drink 1 or 2 cupfuls a day. Of the tincture, $\frac{1}{2}$ fl. dram. Spasmodic Compounds:

> Add to 2 quarts of the best sherry wine
> 2 oz. Cramp bark (Viburnum opulus),
> 1 oz. Skull cap (Scutellaria)
> 1 oz. Skunk cabbage (Symplocarpus foetidus)
> $\frac{1}{2}$ oz. Cloves (Eugenia caryophyllus)
> 2 dram. Capsicum

Combine ingredients in powder form, or coarsely bruised. Let stand in covered container at least 24 hr. shaking daily.

Dose: Half a wineglassful, two or three times a day.

Externally: Seasonal but worth remembering. The low cranberry (and probably the high cranberry will have the same results) is known to be direct medication for dangerous erysipelas. If applied early this

101

malady yields at once. Also for malignant ulcers and scarlet fever when applied to the throat. Pound the berries and spread them in a fold of old cotton cloth and apply over the entire diseased surface and the inflammation will speedily subside. Its usefulness is universally acknowledged.

Homoeopathic Clinical: Tincture of fresh bark, collected in October or November—After-pains, Cough (of pregnancy), Cramps, Dysmenorrhoea (spasmodic, neuralgia, membranous), Ears (painful), Epididymitis. Headache, Hysteria, Labour pains (false), Lumbago, Menstruation (painful), Miscarriage, Ovaries (pain in), Paralysis, Uterus (cramps in, bearing down in).

Russian Experience: If you attend a Russian concert, or listen to one on the radio you will hear a beautiful heartfelt song which is touching to people in all corners of the globe. It will be Kalina or Kalinushka, well known to North American Indians as Cramp bark.

Russians like Kalina so much they plant it in parks as well as for home garden decoration and medicinal use. They feel that the beauty and tenderness of its creation is only one of its merits, as a deeper meaning is known to them as a shrub for health. Ukraine, White Russia and Siberia supply the country commercially, but it is grown throughout the land.

Folk Medicine: White Russia especially has a very impressive list of uses. Berries are rich in vitamins, especially C and K, and minerals. They are used alone, fresh or dried, with honey for high blood pressure, heart conditions (recommended with the seeds), Cough, Cold, Tubercular lungs, Shortness of breath, Kidney; Bladder and Stomach conditions, Bleeding, Stomach ulcers. A decoction of the flowers for Coughs, Cold, Fever, Sclerosis, Lung tuberculosis, Stomach sickness (including stomach cancer).

Externally: Children and adults are bathed with a strong decoction of the flowers for Tubercular skin, Eczema and various other skin conditions. For Scrofula a decoction of both berries and flowers in 1–10 parts, used as a tea.

Clinically: Prescribed in doses of 20–30 drops, two to three times a day, in cases of female bleeding, hysteria, cramps, etc.

Industry: Supplied by commercial farms to the food industry which uses an extract and the berries for candy, fillers, pastry, marmalade and aromatics. Pharmacy uses the bark, Folk Medicine, every part of Kalina.

CRANESBILL   Geranium maculatum, L.
(N.O.: Geraniaceae)

Common Names: DOVESFOOT, CROWFOOT, ALUM ROOT, SPOTTED GERANIUM, WILD GERANIUM.

Features: Native to the United States, the Spotted Cranesbill is a very familiar species in the eastern and northern areas. Geranium grows in nearly all parts of the low grounds, open woods, etc., of North America. The dark green palmately-lobed leaves stem from up to 3 ft. high plants; with swollen joints, and freely branched. Flowers, blossoming in June, are five-lobed ovary terminated by a long thick beak (hence the common

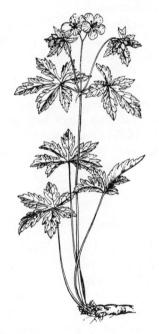

CRANESBILL   Geranium maculatum, L.
(U.S. Agricultural Department, Appalachia, 1971)

name Cranesbill) and five stigmas; coming to maturity the carpels separate from the base and become resolute or spirale. The root is the official part. Geranium is its active principle. The so-called Geranium of gardens are mostly species of Pelargonium, and are native to southern Africa.

Medicinal Part: The dried root.

Solvents: Water, alcohol.

Bodily Influence: Astringent, Tonic, Diuretic, Styptic.

Uses: The powerful astringent is used in secondary dysentery, diarrhoea, and infantile cholera: in infusion with milk. Internally and externally it may be used whenever astringents are indicated, in haemorrhages, gleet, leucorrhoea, relaxed vagina, throat, sore mouth, rectum, indolent ulcers, diabetes and excessive chronic mucus discharges. Also to alleviate the abuse of mercurial retention in the body, causing more serious conditions that the cause for which the mercury was taken. Troublesome bleeding from the nose, wounds or small vessels, and from the extraction of teeth, may be checked effectively by applying the powder to the bleeding orifice and, if possible, covering with a compress of cotton.

For Diabetes and Brights disease (disease of the kidneys) a decoction taken internally has proven effective: Unicorn root (Aletris farinosa), Cranesbill (Geranium maculatum).

For chronic mucous disease, as in gleet, leucorrhoea, ophthalmia, gastric affections, catarrh and ulceration of the bladder, a decoction of: 2 parts of Golden seal (Hydrastis), 1 part of Cranesbill (Geranium maculatum).

Dose: From 1 tablespoon to 1 wineglassful three times a day. Administered as an injection for gleet and leucorrhoea: 1 part of Blood root (Sanguinaria), 2 parts of Cranesbill (Geranium maculatum).

Homoeopathic Clinical: Tincture and triturations of root; infusion of the plant—Diarrhoea, Dysentery, Haemorrhages, Leucorrhoea, Stool (ineffective urging to), Throat (sore).

CRAWLEY Corallorhiza odontorhiza, Nutt.

Common Names: CORAL ROOT, DRAGON'S CLAW, CHICKENTOE.
Features: This singular, leafless plant has a collection of small, fleshy tubers as roots; the stalk is coral-like, of pale yellow colour, with a covering of a sort of sticky wool and scales, answering for leaves. The flowers, from ten to twenty, are of a brownish-green colour in bloom from July to October, and the fruit is a large oblong capsule. Resembles Beechdrops, growing from 10–20 in. high, and depends on roots of trees and the rich soil of the woods for survival, as does Beechdrops. The root is small, dark brown, resembling cloves, or a hen's claw; has a strong nitrous smell, and mucilaginous slightly bitter, astringent taste.

The plant is a native of the United States, found from Maine to Florida, and in Canada. The entire plant is destitute of verdure. The Herbalist, J. E. Meyers, says the entire plant is used for medical purposes. Its scarcity and high price have prevented its general use.
Medicinal Part: The root.
Solvent: Water.
Bodily Influence: Diaphoretic, Sedative, Febrifuge.
Uses: Crawley is recognized as the most powerful, prompt and certain

104

diaphoretic in the "Materia Medica"; its chief value is as a diaphoretic in fevers, especially in typhus and inflammatory low stages of diseases, and may be relied upon in all cases to bring on free perspiration without increasing the heat of the system, or accelerated action of the heart. It has proven effective in acute erysipelas, cramps, flatulence, pleurisy, and night sweats, it relieves hectic fever without debilitating the patient. Combined with Leptandra virginica (Black root) or Podophyllum peltatum (Mandrake) when it is found necessary to act upon the bowels or liver, and mixed with Dioscorea (Wild yam root) it will be found almost a specific in flatulent and bilious colic. Combined with Caulophyllum (Blue cohosh) it forms an excellent agent in amenorrhoea and dysmenorrhoea or scanty or painful menstruation and is unsurpassed in after-pains, suppression of Lochia, and the febrile symptoms which sometimes occur at the parturient period.

From 20–30 grains of the powdered root given in water as warm as the patient can drink (when in bed) and repeated every $1\frac{1}{2}$–2 hr., according to circumstances.

Steep 1 teaspoonful of the root in 1 cup of boiling water for $\frac{1}{2}$ hr. When cold (if ambulent) drink 1 or 2 cupfuls a day a good mouthful at a time. Crawley is recognized as the fever powder by some practitioners; should be kept well closed, away from light.

CROWFOOT   Ranunculus bulbosus, L.
(N.O.: Ranunculaceae)

Common Names: BUTTERCUP, CROWFOOT.

Features: Do not classify the virtues of this plant with the Geranium maculatum (Cranesbill), which is also called Crowfoot, and belonging to the genus Ranunculus, family Ranunculaceae.

The 250 species are native in cold temperate regions throughout the United States and Europe, growing in fields and pastures; the root of this herb is a perennial, solid, roundish, and depressed, sending out radicals from its undersides, with annually erect hairy stems, 6–8 in. in height.

The leaves are on long petioles, each stem supports several solitary golden yellow flowers; five petals; stamens are numerous and hairy; flowering in May, June and July. When any part of these plants are chewed, the pain and much heat in the stomach will also be expressed by inflammation and excoriation of the mouth. Do not take internally.

Solvent: Water.

Bodily Influence: External rubefacient, Epispastic.

Uses: This plant is too acrid to be used internally, especially when fresh. When applied externally it is powerfully rubefacient and epispastic. It is

105

employed in its recent state in rheumatic neuralgia and other diseases where vestication and counter-irritation are indicated. Its action, however, is generally so violent that it is seldom used. The beggars used to use it to produce and keep open sores to excite sympathy.

Homoeopathic Clinical: Tincture of the whole plant—Alcoholism, Breast (pain below), Chest (pains in), Chilblains, Corns, Delirium tremens, Diarrhoea, Dropsy, Dyspnoea, Eczema, Epilepsy, Feet (pains in), Gastralgia, Hay-fever, Herpes zoster, Hiccough, Hydrocele, Jaundice, Liver (pain in), Neuralgia, Nyctalopia, Ovaries (neuralgia of), Pemphigus, Pleuritic adhesion, Pleurodynia, Rheumatism, Spinal irritation, Warts, Writer's cramp.

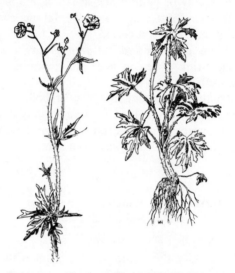

CROWFOOT   Buttercup, Ranunculus bulbosus, L.
(Weeds, Canadian Agricultural Department, Ottawa, 1967)

CYPRESS   Cupressus, L.
(N.O.: Coniferous Cupressaceae)

Common Names: MONTEREY CYPRESS, GOPHER WOOD.

Features: The best-known species is probably the European or Italian Cypress (Cisemper virens). It is indigenous to the Mediterranean area and is believed by some authors to be the "gopher" wood and cypress referred to in the Bible. Cupressus is represented by twenty or more species ranging from Asia to the Mediterranean, and from southern Oregon to Costa Rica. The habit varies from trees 150 ft. or more in height to small shrubs. The leaves are small (seldom used) triangular, scale-like, closely appressed to the branches, and generally in opposite arrange-

106

ment. The small ovulate cones are globular, consist of a few knobbed, peltate scales, and require two years to mature. The fruit is ripe about the beginning of winter. Much used in landscapes.

Part Used: Cones or nuts.

Solvent: Water.

Bodily Influence: Astringent.

Uses: The cones or nuts are very drying and binding and will stop bleeding of all kinds, as spitting of blood, bleeding or haemorrhages of the lungs and stomach, useful in diarrhoea, dysentery, bleeding haemorrhoids, immoderate flux of monthly periods (the tea at body temperature may be inserted, also taken internally). If the gums are spongy in pyorrhoea, and bleeding gums where the teeth feel loose, rinse the mouth with the tea several times a day for results. Place a few of the cones, with water, in a covered container and simmer for 10 min.

Dose: Internally, 2 tablespoons every 2 hr.

Homoeopathic Clinical: Tincture of berries and leaves—Keloed, Tumours, Warts.

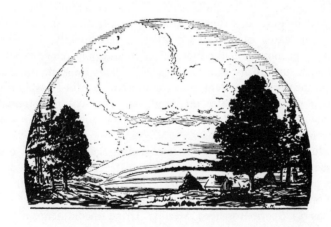

DAMIANA   Turnera aphrodisiaca, UrB.
(N.O.: Turneraceae)

Features: Indigenous to Texas, and found in lower California (Mexico), South America and West Indies. The small yellow-flowered shrub has long, broad, obovate, light-green leaves, with few hairs on the rib; frequented by reddish twigs. The plant has an aromatic odour and contains a volatile oil (0.51 per cent) with a warm, bitter, camphor-like taste, two resins, a bitter principle (Damianin) tannin, sugar and albuminoids.

Medicinal Part: The leaves.

Solvent: Diluted alcohol.

Bodily Influence: Aphrodisiac, Tonic, Stimulant, Laxative.

Uses: Damiana has strong claims as a great sexual rejuvenator, in lethargy of the sexual organs, whether the result of abuse or senility. The use, or administration, should be with care, as the claims are justified by many who know of its influence. In this case, for those who ever will, please remember that when the system is run down, overworked, subject to nervous tensions, etc., Damiana often stimulates beyond the limit of our safe and healthy resources, and encouragement beyond our natural energy level may have ill effect on the heart.

W. H. Myers, M.D., of Philadelphia, writes concerning Damiana: "I have given it quite an extensive trial in my practice, and as a result I find that in cases of partial or other sexual debility, its success is universal. I pronounce it the most effective and only remedy that in my hands had a successful result in all cases." There are some objections to its use on the digestive system but by combining it with Phosphorus, Nux vomica, it partially obviates this tendency. The required strength will not be noticed immediately; usually one portion once a day for ten days. Also given in nervous diseases.

Dose: Fluid extract, 15–30 drops once a day. Solid extract, 3–6 grains. Also used in pill form.

Homoeopathic Clinical: Tincture of fresh part—Amenorrhoea, Dysmenorrhoea, Fatigue impotence, Leucorrhoea, Migraine, Prostate (affections of), Spermatorrhoea, Sterility, Urine (incontinence of).

DANDELION Leontodon taraxacum, Wigers
(N.O.: Compositae)

Common Names: BLOW BALL, CANKERWORT, LION'S TOOTH, WILD ENDIVE, ETC.

Features: This plant is a native of Greece but can now be found in most parts of the world, almost all the year round. Taraxacum is a genus of less than one hundred species of biennial or perennial herbs belonging to the sunflower family (Compositae).

Dandelions are characterized by shiny green rosette of leaves, nearly entirely or variously tooth-edged in a slightly backward direction. The flower stem is longer than the leaves, 5–6 in. in height, and bearing a single yellow flower. The root and stem yield a milky fluid when cut. The root is the official part and should be collected when the plant is in flower.

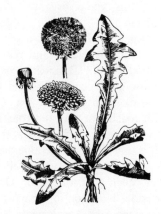

DANDELION   Leontodon taraxacum
(Wigers. "Med," Moscow, 1969)

The spring leaves are used in salads and possess some slight narcotic properties. Can be found outside of most doors throughout the United States, in bloom from April to November. Dry some of your once thought of as worthless Dandelion roots for winter use, they will aid you in many ways.

Medicinal Part: The root.

Solvents: Boiling water, alcohol.

Bodily Influence: Diuretic, Tonic, Stomachic, Aperient, Deobstruent. Native Aborigines of North America realized the great value of dandelion and used it as food and medicine by their experience and knowledge.

Uses: The common Dandelion has had intelligent use as a medical plant before science strikingly opened our eyes to some of the contents of the shiny green leaves: They contain 7,000 units of Vitamin A per oz. and are an excellent source of Vitamins B, C and G. As a comparison, Vitamin A content in lettuce is 1,200 per oz. and carrot 1,275 per oz. A wise and easy addition to our diet.

The root is the official part of the plant and is a constituent of many prescriptions for dropsical and urinary complaints, and is indicated for impostumes and inward ulcers in the urinary passage; atonic dyspepsia and rheumatism. It is of an opening and cleansing quality and therefore very effective for obstructions of the liver, gall and spleen and the diseases that arise from the biliary organs. It is a splendid agent for skin diseases, scurvy, scrofula and eczema; has a beneficial effect on the female organs. Herbalists use Dandelion more generally than any other herb as it combines well with other herbal preparations for the liver and is so mild, wholesome and safe. Its prolonged use can only be beneficial in all rheumatic complaints. The natural nutritive salt in Dandelion is twenty-eight parts sodium; this type of organic sodium purifies the blood and destroys the acids therein.

J. Kloss tells us in "Back to Eden": "Anaemia is caused by the deficiency of nutritive salts in the blood, and really has nothing to do with the quality of the good blood." Dandelion root cut up and dried is used for coffee by health-minded people. From a health point of view, it is more desirable to drink than coffee or tea. For this purpose it is frequently combined with roasted acorns and roasted rye in equal parts, or according to taste. As a vegetable for salads it has no equal, being rich in many minerals. It is a medicinal vegetable plant.

Dose: Of the tincture 5–40 drops. For infusions, fill a cup with the green leaves, add boiling water, steep $\frac{1}{2}$ hr. or longer. Drink when cold, three or four times a day. Or add 1 teaspoon of the cut or powdered root to 1 cup of boiling water and steep $\frac{1}{2}$ hr. Drink when cold three times a day.

Homoeopathic Clinical: Tincture of whole plant just before the perfection of the flower—Ague, Bilious attacks, Debility, Diabetes, Gall-stones, Headaches (gastric), Jaundice, Liver (affections of), Neuralgia, Night-sweats, Rheumatism, Tongue (mapped), Typhoid fever.

Russian Experience: Dandelion is known as Oduvanchik or Pushki in Russia. Taraxacum, part of the official name, comes from Greece, and in ancient time Taraxacum was used for yellow spots (liver spots) of the skin and freckles.

It is recorded that in Germany the roots were used as a sedative as early as the sixteenth century. Arabian knowledge is much the same as other nations. The French people use the fresh young leaves for salads. To remove the bitter taste they soak them in salt water for 30 min. and use as a spicy addition to mixed vegetables, at the same time getting natural protein, iron, calcium, phosphorus, and inulin, which are all part of our human formula.

Uses: In Russia the root is the most popular, prepared as an extract with vodka, as a tea, or coffee. Ancient home medicine calls it Life Elixir, and it has acceptance for blood purifying, liver treatment, jaundice, gall-bladder, skin conditions, digestive disturbance and as an expectorant, sedative and calming.

Clinically: In the form of extracts, tinctures, powders; loose and in tablets, for the long-established conditions above.

DOGWOOD, AMERICAN   Cornus florida, L.
(N.O.: Cornaceae)

Common Names: BORWOOD, FLOWERING CORNEL, GREEN OZIER.

Features: Dogwood, the common name of many of the larger of the forty or so species frequently cultivated, of hardy shrubs, trees and herbs that comprise the genus Cornus (family Cornaceae). The above specie grows from 12–30 ft. high in Canada and the United States. The slow growing and compact wood is covered with a rough and brownish bark used for many purposes. The leaves are smooth ovate, dark green above and pale beneath; the flowers are in bloom April to May, and are of a greenish-yellow colour and constitute the chief beauty of the tree in the springtime. The action of the Dogwood flowers are close to Chamomile for their soothing, tonic, and adaptability to weakened and debilitated conditions of the stomach. The fruit is an oval drupe of a glossy scarlet colour, containing a nut with two cells and two seeds, which the birds are very fond of. The chemical quality of the bark is tannic, and gallic acids, resin, gum, oil, wax, lignin, lime potash and iron, cornine is its active principle.

Medicinal Part: The dried bark.

Bodily Influence: Tonic, Astringent and slightly Stimulant.

Solvents: Water, alcohol.

Uses: It is much used as substitute for Peruvian bark (Cinchona), from which quinine is made, and may be used when the foreign remedy is not to be had, or when it fails, or when it cannot be administered. By some, Dogwood is prized for ague, but it is better adapted to the diseases caused by weakness of the stomach and bowels, by inducing circulation of healthy blood to the parts, removing effete matter, vitalizing the tissues and speedily removing pain from the diseased parts. To over-come water brash and other stomach weaknesses, capsules combined with Golden seal (Hydrastis canadensis) and Ginger (Zingiber) in powder form can be taken after meals. "Dogwood, or Green ozier, exerts its best virtues in the shape of an ointment"—Dr. O. P. Brown (1875). Both are effective. Internally, 1 teaspoonful of the bark in 1 cup of boiling water, steeped for $\frac{1}{2}$ hr. Drink $\frac{1}{2}$ cupful upon retiring at night, hot or warm, or take a mouthful three times a day. 1 or 2 cupfuls may be taken. Of the tincture, ½–1 fl. dram.

Homoeopathic Clinical: Tincture of fresh bark—Dyspepsia, Intermittent fever, Pneumonia.

DRAGON ROOT   Arum triphyllum, L.

(N.O.: Araceae)

Common Names: WAKE ROBIN, JACK IN THE PULPIT, DRAGON'S ROOT.
Features: Found in damp localities of North and South America; the whole plant is acrid, but the root is the only part employed. It is of various sizes, turnip-shaped, dark and corrugated externally, and milk white and mealy within, seldom exceeding 2½ in. in diameter; the leaves are generally one or two, standing on long, sheathing footstalks; oval and pale on the inside. The flower looks much like the funnel-shaped lily, except the Jack in the pulpit has straight veins coming from the base of the flower, extending through to the tip end. The root when first dug is too fiercely acrid for internal use; it will leave a burning impression on the tongue, lips and fauces, like a severe scalding, followed by inflammation and tenderness, which, however, may be somewhat mollified by milk. The root dispenses its biting reputation with age, and should always be used when partially dried. Contains volatile acrid principle, starch, fat, gum, resin, calcium oxalate. When the acrid matter is driven off by heat, the root yields a pure delicate, amylaceous matter resembling arrowroot, very white and nutritious.
Medicinal Part: The dry root.
Bodily Influence: Stimulant, Expectorant, Diaphoretic.
Uses: Due to the aggressive influence on the mucous cells Dragon root should only be employed by persons understanding both patient and medication. If there is no excess of mucus, your unqualified deed could endanger the life of alimentation (the act of giving or receiving nutritional material into the body). Helpful in certain asthma complaints, whooping cough, chronic bronchitis, chronic rheumatism, pains in the chest, colic, low stage of typhus, and general debility.
Amount: 10 grains of grated root in syrup or mucilage, three or four times a day.
Homoeopathic Clinical: Tincture of fresh tuber or corn—Brain (inflammation of), Clergyman's sore throat, Delirium, Diphtheria, Glandular swellings, Headache, Jaw joint (painful), Mouth (sore), Scarlatina, Tongue (cracked), Typhoid fever, Voice (hoarse).

112

ECHINACEA   Echinacea angustifolia, L.
(N.O.: Compositae)

Common Names: WILD NIGGERHEAD, PURPLE CONEFLOWER, BLACK SAMPSON, KANSAS NIGGERHEAD.

Features: Native to the prairie regions of America, west of Ohio. This native herbaceous perennial belongs to the Aster family. The plant grows 2–3 ft. high, with single, stout, bristly, hairy stems. Leaves are thick, rough, hairy, broadly landscaped, 3–8 in. long, narrowed at the end and strongly three nerved. The single, large flower head appears from July to October, the colour varying from whitish rose to pale purple. Taste is sweetish, then tingling, as in aconite, but without its persistent benumbing effect, when administered wrongly. Faint odour, aromatic, and should not be used after it has lost its characteristic odour and taste. Contains inulin-bearing parenchyma tissue.

Medicinal Parts: Dried rhizome, root.

Solvent: Alcohol.

Bodily Influence: Diaphoretic, Sialagogue, Alterative.

Uses: Useful in all diseases due to impurities in the blood. Thompsonian, Physio-medical and Naturo-physicians have always maintained that Echinacea is a natural herbal antitoxin. Orthodox physicians have not generally been willing to accept it as such, though many do. Controversy being permitted, falsehood will appear more false, and truth more true.

"Echinacea is a corrector of the deprivations of the body fluids", was Dr. Niederkorn's opinion, and this whether the morbific changes of the fluid of the body are internal, or caused by external introductions.

Echinacea has an honoured place for septic infections, septicaemia in its various forms, blood poisoning, adynamia fever, typhoid fever, cellular abscesses, salpingitis, carbuncles, cancerous cachexia, and in fevers or conditions where there is a bluish discoloration of the mucous membranes, of any condition which points to sepsis, internal or external.

The Sioux Indians used fresh scraped root for hydrophobia, snake bites, septicaemia.

Dose: Steep 1 teaspoonful of the granulated root in 1 cup of boiling water for ½ hr., strain, take 1 tablespoonful three to six times a day. Of the tincture, 5–10 min.

Externally: Steep as above and apply, or bathe parts concerned.

Homoeopathic Clinical: Tincture of whole fresh plant—Appendicitis, Bites of rabid animals, Blood poisoning, Carbuncles, Diphtheria, Enteric fever, Gangrene, Poisoned wounds, Pyoemia, Rhus poisoning, Scarlatina,

Septicaemia, Snake bites, Struma, Syphilis, Typhoid, Ulcers, Vaccination (effects of).

Russian Experience: Echinacea is not native to Russia. Careful study, research and experiment has given many opportunities for cultivation in Ukraine, Kaukaz and other places. They use the Latin name Echinacea for identification, pronounced with a Russian influence. Another species, Echinacea angustifolia, or narrow leaf Echinacea, grows on the North American plains and is used for the same purpose.

Uses: According to experiments it is not toxic in large amounts but has been known to cause salivation. They use it as an antiseptic, internally and externally. Internally it is healing by reducing pain; improves the quality of blood to resist infection, or further spread of disease.

Externally: Antiseptic and healing for skin conditions of carbuncles, boils, wounds, ulcers, burns and bed sores.

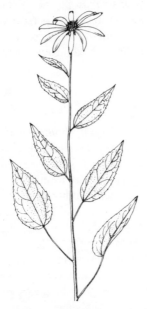

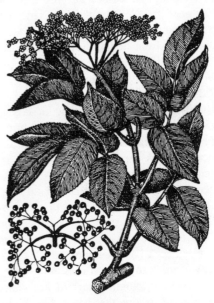

ECHINACEA
Echinacea angustifolia, L.
(U.S. Agricultural Department,
Appalachia, 1971)

ELDER or ELDERBERRY
Sambucus canadensis, L.
(L. Y. Skliarevsky, Lekarstevennye Rastenia,
Moscow, 1968)

ELDER OR ELDERBERRY   Sambucus canadensis, L.
(N.O.: Caprifoliaceae)

Common Names: SAMBUCUS, AMERICAN ELDER, SWEET ELDER.

Features: An indigenous shrub growing in all parts of the United States

114

and Canada, in low, damp grounds, thickets and waste places. Elders are frequently cultivated for their ornamental foliage. They grow from 5–12 ft. high, blooming in June and July, with star-shaped fragrant flowers $\frac{1}{4}$ in. across, grouped in flat flower clusters about 8 in. across. Purple black berries containing three or four round seeds, maturing in September and October. The fruit is often made into jellies, pies and wine. The branching stems are covered with a rough, pitted grey bark; large central stems are smooth. The odour is faintly sweet, aromatic; taste slightly bitter. The European Elder, though larger than the American, is in general characteristics and properties similar.

Medicinal Parts: The roots, inner bark, leaves, berries and flowers are all recognized as natural medical treatment.

Solvent: Water.

Bodily Influence: Emetic, Hydragogue, Cathartic; Flowers: Diaphoretic, Diuretic, Alterative, Emollient, Discutient, Gentle Stimulant.

Uses: No education is required as to which part may be used. From the tree top to root's end is a symbol of medical properties. Often all that is needed is the virtue of necessity as a teacher. The flowers, berries, leaves, inner bark and roots have expressed gratitude for many in conditions of headache due to colds, palsy, rheumatism, scrofula, syphilis, jaundice, kidney and epilepsy.

Dr. Brown (1875) gives us the following: "The inner bark of Elder is hydragogue, emetic and cathartic. Has been successfully used in epilepsy by taking it from branches 1 or 2 years old, scraping off the grey outer bark, and steeping 2 ounces of it in 5 ounces of boiling water for 48 hours. Strain and give a wineglassful every 15 minutes when the fit is threatening, have the patient fast. Resume it every 6 to 8 days." The tea of the flowers is quieting to twitching and inflammation of the eyes, taken internally. The tea simmered for 10 min. longer and cotton soaked in the solution provides an eye application over closed lids. The berries are rich in organic iron and therefore an excellent addition to the autumn menu, especially if anaemic. Combine Elderberry and Black-berry juice, 1 oz. three times a day.

The inner green bark is cathartic; an infusion of it in wine, or the expressed juice, in doses from $\frac{1}{2}$ fl. oz. to 1 fl. oz. will purge moderately. A large dose produces vomiting. In small doses it produces an efficacious deobstruent, promoting all the fluid secretion, and is much used in dropsy, to expel the water from the engourged organism. It is scarcely excelled by any other medication. Can be used for children's diseases, such as liver derangements, erysipelas, etc., decreasing the amount according to age.

Externally: The Elder may be called the Herbalist's cosmetic tree, as every part will aid in complexion beauty, removing spots, allaying

115

irritation, removing freckles and preserving and softening the skin if applied faithfully, internally and externally.

For various swellings, tumours, joints, etc., simmer any or all parts of the elder; apply as a poultice, or bathe when skin is broken. Also excellent mixed with coconut oil for a discutient ointment, used for burns and scalds. Any part is advisable to keep in its dried form for out-of-season use.

Homoeopathic Clinical: Tincture of fresh leaf and flower—Albuminuria. Angina pectoris, Asthma, Larynx (dry), Lumbago.

Russian Experience: The decorative and medical yellow, red and black Elder grows in many parts of Russia and has been used as home medicine from the time of their early history. However they consider the North American white Elder superior. In the Middle Ages it was considered a Holy Tree, capable of restoring good health, keeping good health, and, it is reasonable to say, as an aid to longevity, as this, too, was one of its contributions.

Uses: The roots, bark, twigs, leaves and berries are used alone or in combinations for every type of infection or inflammation.

Flowers: contain oil, rutin, vitamins and minerals extensively for treatment of dropsy, rheumatism, appendix inflammation, bladder and kidney infections, intestinal conditions, eyes, and external skin trouble.

Berries: Diuretic, Astringent, Diaphoretic, much used as a gargle.

Leaves: The young spring leaves boiled in honey are excellent in chronic constipation; boiled in milk for inflammation of burns of the skin and piles.

Clinical: Used for conditions of above, in extracts, tinctures and powders.

Food: Home and hospital foods are made from the flowers and berries, including vitamin- and mineral-rich jam, and marmalade used in many dietetic preparations. Elderberry wine, with its pleasant aroma and taste, is a familiar in the wine industry.

Externally: Leaves, flowers, bark and twigs are excellent as a hot poultice, mixed equally with Chamomile (Matricaria chamomilla), for soreness, inflammations, joint stiffness, etc.

In a seventeenth-century Botanic book is a story about a king and a small hunting party. Most of the day had passed away when they realized they were lost in the thick timber brush. Wandering in various directions they happily found a lonely farmhouse of prosperous condition. As they approached closer they saw an old gentleman, who had been crying, sitting on the porch. When the king asked why, he explained he slipped and fell while carrying his grandfather from one room to another, and his father was angry for such misbehaviour and beat him.

The king listened suspiciously and then entered the house. To his surprise he observed elders of advanced generations peacefully talking and going about their daily routine. After talking, and observing the family, he inquired how they kept in such good health to advancing years. They told the king that for as long as they could remember they had only eaten simple food, salt, home-prepared bread, milk and cheese, with emphasis on Elderberries.

As in name, legend and story, grateful people of all continents and in all times admire and appreciate virtues of herbs. The same herb in different countries and used, of course, by different people have come to the same objective, whether it be useful or dangerous. Many such simple things will not be accepted by stories, or experience alone. It seems when tested scientifically and given allopathic approval, only then will thoughts be changed.

ELECAMPANE   Inula helenium, L.
(N.O.: Compositae)

Common Names: ELF DOCK, SCABWORT, VELVET DOCK, AUNEE.

Features: Native of Europe and north Asia, and now naturalized over much of eastern North America. This stout perennial herb, of the sunflower family (Compositae), thrives in moist, sandy, mountainous areas. The stems are vigorous, 3–4 ft. high, downy above, and branched. The leaves are large, ovate and toothed, the upper ones clasping the stem, the lower ones stalked. The flower heads are golden yellow, large, solitary, and with narrow rays, blooming in July and August. The root is slightly grey, hard, horny and cylindrical, and should be dug in the autumn of the second year, usually split into longitudinal, oblique pieces having one or more roots. The whole plant is similar in appearance to the horseradish.

The main component of the root is a carbohydrate, inulin, which in the autumn may comprise as much as 45 per cent of its weight; its taste is bitter and acrid and the odour reminiscent of camphor.

Medicinal Part: The root.

Solvents: Alcohol, water (partially).

Bodily Influence: Stimulant, Diaphoretic, Diuretic, Expectorant, Emmenagogue, Tonic.

Uses: Elecampane is a constitutional treatment for general catarrhal conditions such as chronic pulmonary affections that have symptoms of cough, shortness of breath, wheezing in the lungs, a specific for whooping cough in children, diseases of the breast and malignant fevers, hepatic torpor, dyspepsia, and the feeling of stitches in the side caused by the spleen. This well-known root strengthens, cleanses and tones up the pulmonary and gastric membranes, encouraging a more harmonious metabolism by assisting the pancreas with the large amount of natural inulin contained in the root, and valued in incipient tuberculosis.

117

Culpeper also used Elecampane for intestinal worms, retention of water, to lessen tooth decay, and for firming the gums. A personal opinion but one which we believe to be true, is that inulin decreases excessive sugar in the blood—and sugar causes tooth decay. Hurray for Culpeper!

Dose: Of the powder, from 1 scruple to 1 dram; the decoction, 1 oz. to 1 pint of boiling water taken in wineglassful doses. Mixes well with other herbs.

Homoeopathic Clinical: Tincture of fresh root dug in autumn of the second year—Back ache, Cough, Cramp, Dysmenorrhoea, Erysipelas, Leucorrhoea, Rectum (pain in), Sciatica, Toothache.

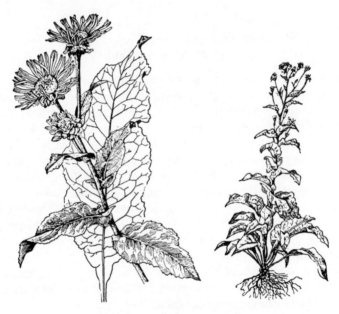

ELECAMPANE   Inula helenium, L.
(Moscow University, Moscow, 1965)

Russian Experience: There are many names for this gracious flower, but in 1804 inulin was discovered as being a large part of the plant's make-up. Since then Inula is the official name.

In Russia they call it De-via-sil, or Deviat Sil, which means nine powers. Also Di-vasil, which means fair or magic power. This is how the Russian people apprize Elecampane as a medicine.

At one time Elecampane in Russia was almost forgotten, but lately interest has been renewed and the Government now encourages the collection and growth of this flower. In Ancient Greece and Rome, Elecampane had prominent recognition in medical botanics, and in the

Middle Ages it had the same strong reputation. Europe and Britain cultivate this flower for medical purposes. In the Far East, and isolated Tibet, Elecampane is extensively used by their own independent experience.

Uses: In Russia today Elecampane grows in many gardens. They preserve the fresh root in vodka and keep this for winter use when in need of restoring health after sickness, or for stomach trouble. Other preparations consist of tea, or powder for colds, chest colds, inflammations, female trouble, skin conditions, especially itching, and wounds, catarrh, indigestion, kidney and bladder trouble, weak pancreas; in all a general blood builder.

Bodily Influence: Diaphoretic, Diuretic, Antiseptic, Blood builder.

Clinical: Directly or in combinations as drops, powder or tablets.

Externally: Poultice or a strong tea is made and used for itching, skin rash and wounds.

Food: In confectionery to give better aroma, colour and nutrition.

ERYNGO Eryngium aquaticum, L.
(N.O.: Umbelliferae)

Common Names: BUTTON SNAKEROOT, RATTLESNAKE MASTER.

Features: There are about 220 species in the genus, of which about twenty-two are found in America. E. aquaticum grows in wet soil and in the pine barrens, from New Jersey south to Florida; and west to Texas, Missouri and Minnesota.

The white flowers bloom in August and a number of species are cultivated for the steel blue colour of the stem and branches, and unusual manner of growth. The root is tuberous, aromatic and of a sweet acrid taste, resembling the parsnip.

Medicinal Part: The root.

Solvents: Water, alcohol.

Bodily Influence: Diaphoretic, Expectorant, Sialagogue. In large doses Emetic.

Uses: Very useful in dropsy, nephritic and calculus affections, also in scrofula and syphilis. It is valuable as a diaphoretic and expectorant in pulmonary affections and used when Senega (Polygala senega) is not available. The British and American Physio-Medical associations relay the following: "For sluggishness of the liver with uric acid accumulation as follows: Boil 1 ounce each of Eryngo (Eryngium aquaticum) and Wild carrot (Daucus carota) in 1½ pints of water, reduced to 1 pint, strain, and take a wineglassful 4 times a day. In case of Jaundice take 1 ounce of Eryngo (Eryngium aquaticum), ½ ounce Barberry bark (Berberis vulgaris), boil in 1 quart of new milk for 10 minutes, strain and take

2 wineglassfuls every 3 hours. Most obstinate cases have been known to yield to this remedy in from 7 to 14 days."

The pulverized root, in doses of 2–3 grains, is very effective in haemorrhoids and prolapsus, and 2 oz. of the pulverized root, added to 1 pint of good Holland gin, is effective in obstinate cases of gonorrhoea, and gleet; to be administered in doses of 1–2 fl. drams three or four times a day. By some practitioners the root is employed as a specific in gonorrhoea, gleet and leucorrhoea, used internally in syrup, decoctions, or tinctures, and the decoction applied locally by injection. Used externally and internally, it cures the bite of snakes and insects. Dose

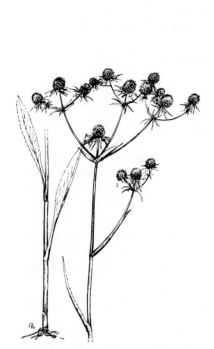

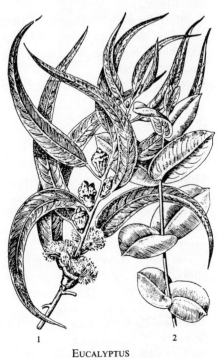

1   2

ERYNGO   Eryngium aquaticum, L.
(U.S. Agricultural Department,
Appalachia, 1971)

EUCALYPTUS
Eucalyptus globulus, Labill.
1—Old branch with flowers.
2—New branch
(Vishaya Schkolla, Mosow, 1963)

of the powder, from 20–40 grains; of the decoction, which is principally used, from 2–4 oz. several times a day.

Homoeopathic Clinical: Tincture of fresh root—Anus (prolapsus of), Conjunctivitis, Constipation, Cough, Diarrhoea, Dropsy, Gleet, Gonorrhoea, Haemorrhoids, Influenza, Laryngitis, Leucorrhoea, Renal colic, Sclerotitis, Sexual weakness, Strabismus, Spermatorrhoea, Urine (incontinence of), Wounds.

EUCALYPTUS   Eucalyptus globulus, Labill
(N.O.: Myrtaceae)

Common Name: BLUE GUM TREE.

Features: Approximately 600 species belong to the family "Myrtaceae". Although the majority are trees, some forms, like the "mallees", are shrub-like. They are largely confined to Australia, however about ninety species grown in California and a few can be seen in Florida. They are widely planted for ornamental purposes.

The violet-brown trunk peels off in long thin strips, exposing the smooth underlayer. The simple leaves are without teeth, smooth, and frequently have a waxy sheen. Depending on species, white, yellow or red flowers adorn the Eucalyptus, and attract honey-bees from which a distinctive Eucalyptus honey is enjoyed. The sepals are small or absent, and the petals stick together to form a cap which falls when the flower opens. Looks much like an acorn cap.

The tallest known living specimen is 322 ft., found in 1956 in the Styx Valley, Tasmania.

As children we remember coming home with the tree's gum on hands and clothing after having played around the large Eucalyptus.

The peppermint-lemon fragrance is most agreeable.

Medicinal Parts: Oil, leaves, bark.

Solvents: Alcohol, water.

Bodily Influence: Astringent, Tonic, Antiseptic, Antispasmodic.

Uses: A reliable medical journal of Europe gives credit to the power of the Eucalyptus tree for destroying miasmatic influence in fever-stricken districts, entirely abating the pestilent fever in areas where the trees grow.

Among the diseases in which it is employed are: croup, diphtheria, bronchitis, asthma, piles, neuralgia, malarial diseases, catarrh, in subacute or chronic inflammation of the genetic urinary organs, ulcers and sores. It has been proven an effective remedy in some cases of rheumatism. For some, the mode of using it in asthma is to smoke the dried leaves.

In Britain the oil is the preparation best known and most widely used. It may be inhaled for asthma, diphtheria, sore throat, etc.

For haemorrhoids, the area is washed with a decoction of the leaves. As an agent for suspicious leucorrhoea and discharges, 1–2 drams in 1½ pints of tepid water, injecting it slowly. For toning up weakened and prolapsed uterus, Buchu leaves and bark is also effective combined with the above, for strengthening, quick healing, and diminishing offensive odours. Its efficiency depends chiefly upon its antiseptic properties, which are extremely potent, though quite safe.

Dose: 15–30 drops of the fluid extract three times a day; 3–10 grains of the solid extract three times a day. The leaves crushed and steeped can be used in tea form.

Externally: As a local antiseptic, stimulant and corrective when applied to ulcers and wounds; 1 oz. of the extract to 1 pint of lukewarm water.

Homoeopathic Clinical: Tincture of fresh leaves, essential oil Eucalyptol —Aneurism, Acritis, Asthma, Bladder (affections of), Bronchitis Diarrhoea, Dysentery, Dyspepsia, Dysuria, Fistulae, Gonorrhoea, Gout, Intermittent fever, Kidney (diseases of), Quinine cachexia, Rheumatism, Spleen (affections of), Strychnine poisoning, Syphilis, Tumours, Typhoid, Urethra (stricture of), Urethral carbuncle, Varicose ulcers, Worms.

Russian Experience: Two species of Eucalyptus are cultivated for medical and decorative purposes, known by the same name, pronounced in their own way, Eucalyptus globulus, Labill and Eucalyptus cinera.

Dr. Ramel introduced Eucalyptus to Europe in 1856 and Southern France soon followed with cultivation of this medical tree. Dr. Muller has written a valuable monography about Australian Eucalyptus which has stimulated interest in this valuable plant. About eighty years ago Russia started to cultivate Eucalyptus for decorative reasons; later its interest was of a deeper meaning. Today the Black Sea area has active plantations. About 15,000–18,000 seedlings are obtained from 1 kg. of seeds, which are then transplanted. The young trees yield leaves for oil extract, or are cut and used as a tea.

Uses: The tea, decoctions, oil or Nastoika with Russian vodka is on hand for all conditions of respiratory malfunctions: colds, bronchitis, chest tightness, catarrh, etc.

Externally: Skin conditions of carbuncles, boils, wounds, ulcers.

EVENING PRIMROSE   Oenothera biennis, L.
(N.O.: Onagraceae)

Common Names: TREE PRIMROSE, SUN DROP.

Features: The English name for the species of the genus Primula; also applied to a number of other unrelated flowering plants as evening primrose (Oenothera biennis). This is not to be confused with the Butter rose (Primula veris).

Evening primrose can be found in the United States. The 500 species of Primula are mostly perennial herbs, spring flowering, native in the north temperate zone, especially at high altitudes. Only six or eight are known from North America. The leaves all grow from a short underground stem; the flowers are borne usually in umbels on a leafless stem. The petals form a tube which flares at its summit. They are of many colours, from white to purple.

Medicinal Parts: Leaves, bark.

Solvent: Water.

Bodily Influence: Astringent, Nervine, Sedative.

122

Uses: To quiet nervous sensibility, this agent acts on the alimentary toxins due to combined faulty diet, and nervous tensions of long standing which create toxic waste, causing depression of the solar plexus and the central nervous system.

Evening primrose stimulates the vital actions of the stomach, which has a direct association on the liver and spleen. Rendering renewed success in the treatment of gastro-intestinal disorders such as neuralgia, affection of the lungs, dyspepsia, hepatic torpor, heart, spasmodic asthma, cough of a nervous or spasmodic character, whooping cough, fullness of the bowels, and in female disorders associated with pelvic fullness.

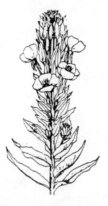

EVENING PRIMROSE   Oenothera biennis, L.
(Ontario Department of Agriculture, Toronto, Canada, 1966)

Dose: From ½–1 teaspoonful of the fluid extract every 4–6 hr., or more frequently as required. Dose of tincture of Evening primrose alone: 5–40 drops according to symptoms. Especially favourable combined with 15–30 drops of Cone flower (Echinacea angustifolia).

Homoeopathic Clinical: Tincture of fresh plants—Cholera infantum, Diarrhoea, Hydrocephaloid.

FEMALE FERN   Polypodium vulgare, L.
(N.O.: Polypodiaceae)

Common Names: ROCK POLYPOD, BRAKE ROOT, COMMON POLYPODY, FERN ROOT.

Features: The fern family is common throughout the United States in shady woods and on mountains. This perennial has a creeping, irregular brown root which has a peculiar and rather unpleasant odour and somewhat sickening taste. The lush green and decorative fronds are from 6–12 in. high, smooth and deeply pinnatified. The fruit on the lower surface of the frond is in large golden dots or capsules. Should be gathered from June to September.

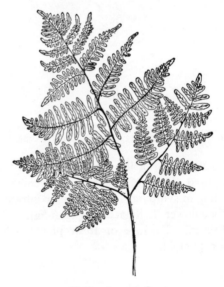

BRACKEN FERN, L.

Medicinal Parts: Root and tops.

Solvent: Water.

Bodily Influence: Pectoral, Demulcent, Purgative, Anthelmintic.

Uses: The starchy root stocks were boiled and eaten by the Indians, and they knew of their effect as a worm medicine. Our pioneers soaked them in water and wood ashes for 24 hr. and cooked the young leaves like pot herbs.

The many species of ferns were also used in decoction as a cure for rickets in children. The strong decoction is purgative. A specific in expelling tape worms, by influencing their muscle release. The presence of worms causes serious anaemia, undermining various organs of the body. The syrup as a decoction has been found very valuable in pulmonary and hepatic diseases.

The ancients used the roots and the whole plant in decoctions and diet drinks for the spleen and other disorders. The Japanese use it in soup. Combined with liverwort it is said to have restored patients severely affected with disease of the lungs. Do not use extensively.

Dose: 1–4 drams of the powdered plant, 4 fl. oz. of the syrup decoction, three or four times a day.

FEVERFEW   Pyrethrum parthenium, Sm.
(N.O.: Compositae)

Common Names: FEATHER FEW, FEBRIFUGE PLANT, FEATHERFOIL, PYRETHRUM.

Features: The plant is native to Europe but common in the United States. Found occasionally in a wild state, but generally cultivated in gardens. The tapering root, with dark brown, furrowed bark, contains a large percentage of inulin. The yellowish, porous wood has a distinct odour; sweetish taste, very pungent acrid, tingling, with a sialagogue effect. The flower resembles Chamomile with its yellow disc, and white petals, one to a stalk; flowering in June and July. The centre stem grows to about 2 ft. high with serrated-edge alternate leaves; very short hairs.

Bees are said to dislike this plant very much, and a handful of the flower heads carried, where they are, will cause them to keep their distance.

Medicinal Part: The whole herb.

Solvents: Alcohol, boiling water (partially).

Bodily Influence: Aperient, Carminative, Tonic Emmenagogue, Vermifuge, Stimulant.

Uses: The warming infusion of Feverfew upon the circulation influences the skin, nervous system and the genito urinary organs and relieves the head of dizziness, brain and nerve pressure, and tensions of over-excitement.

Culpeper recommends it as "a special remedy against opium when taken too liberally".

The relieving assistance of hyperemic conditions of the mucous membrane have a trustworthy regard for this garden herb in conditions of colic, flatulence, general indigestion, colds, suppressed urine, expelling worms, hysteria, and in some febrile diseases. It is largely used in female correction of scanty or delayed monthly periods. Dr. G. P. Wood,

M.D., and Dr. E. H. Ruddock, M.D., in the book "Vitalogy", say that it is "An admirable remedy for St. Vitus dance". Dr. Clymer. M.D., dealing with Natures healing agents, administers the following for fevers:

Tincture of Feverfew (Pyrethrum parthenium), 10–30 drops
Tincture of Cone flower (Echinacea angustifolia), 10–20 drops
Tincture of Cayenne pepper (Capiscum), 10–20 drops.

Taken every 2–3 hr., depending on symptoms. The cold infusion or extract makes a valuable tonic. The warm infusion is nervine and very useful for hysteria and promoting perspiration in fevers.

Dose of Feverfew alone: 10–30 drops in water every 2–3 hr., or as indicated by condition. Can be used as tea, 1 teaspoonful to 1 cup of boiling water steeped for $\frac{1}{2}$ hr.; 2 cups a day in small mouthful doses.

Externally: The leaves boiled for hot compresses for pain of congestion, or inflammation of the lungs, stomach and abdomen is beneficial.

Homoeopathic Clinical: Tincture of fresh plant—Convulsions, Delirium, Dysentery, Fevers, Loquacity, Rheumatism.

FEVER WEED   Gerardia pedicularis, L.
(N.O.: Scrophulariaceae)

Common Names: FEVER WEED, AMERICAN FOXGLOVE, LOUSEWORT.

Features: A most elegant plant grown in dry copses, pine ridges, barren woods and mountains from Canada to Georgia. The plant reaches the

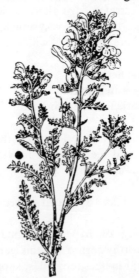

FEVER WEED (Mitnik, Bolotny)   Pedicularis palustris, L.
(Bello-Russ. Academy of Science, Minsk, 1965)

126

height of 2-3 ft., with busy stems supporting numerous leaves opposite, ovate and lanceolate in form. The large yellow flowers are trumpet-shaped and show themselves in August and September, followed by a two-celled fruit capsule.

Medicinal Part: The whole herb.

Solvents: Water, alcohol.

Bodily Influence: Diaphoretic, Sedative, Antiseptic.

Uses: Used principally in febrile and inflammatory diseases. A warm infusion produces a free and copious perspiration in a very short time. Very valuable in ephemeral (short duration) fever.

Dose: Of the infusion, from 1-3 fl. oz. Cut the herb small or granulate. Of the tincture, 5-20 min.

Russian Experience: One species of Feverwood, Mitnik (Pedicularis palustris, L.) is found growing wild in Central and Northern Russia and Siberia.

Folk Medicine: Use it as diuretic for Haemorrhage of the bladder and excessive female bleeding.

Externally: Healing to wounds.

FIRE WEED   Erechthites hieracifolia, Raf.
(N.O.: Compositae)

Common Names: PILE WORT, VARIOUS LEAVED FLEABANE.

Features: This so-called annual weed naturalized in the United States of America; especially thrives where areas have been cleared by burning, also in moist woods. Height from 1-6 ft., with thick, rough, fleshy, branching stems. The white flowers bloom from July to October, some-what resembling the Sowthistle. The fruit, an achenium, oblong and hairy. The plant has a strong unpleasant odour and bitter, disagreeable taste.

Medicinal Parts: Root, herb.

Solvents: Water, alcohol.

Bodily Influence: Emetic, Cathartic, Tonic, Astringent, Alterative.

Uses: As a prompt botanical in purifying the system in diseases of the blood, and discharges of bloody flux. Administered either in a strong decoction, or the alcoholic extract. It is unrivalled in accumulation of excess mucus and the many progressive disease symptoms this condition brings on. To mention a few: the common cold, allergies, hay fever, tonsilitis, cholera, dysentery, haemorrhoids, etc. It is strongly astringent and will quickly relieve pain due to its influence in arresting the dis-charges and effectively diminishing unwanted accumulation. It is invariably successful in summer complaints of children, even in cases where other means have failed.

Dose: Steep 1 heaped teaspoonful of the root and herb in 1 cup of boiling water for ½ hr. Prompt relief will follow when taken hot in small amounts, often. Of the tincture, ½–1 fl. dram as called for.

Homoeopathic Clinical: Tincture of whole fresh plant—Diarrhoea, Gonorrhoea, Haemorrhage, Metrorrhagia, Orchitis.

FIVE FINGER GRASS   Potentilla tormentilla, Neck.
(Potentilla (L.) Rausch.), (Tormentilla erecta, L.).
(N.O.: Rosaceae)

Common Names: FIVE LEAVES GRASS, CINQUEFOIL, ROUGH-FRUITED, SILVERY CINQUEFOIL.

Features: Five finger is common to the United States, growing by roadsides, on meadow banks and waste ground. The herb grows like the strawberry, rooting at joints; the leaflets have five parts, scattered hairs, veins prominent below. The bright yellow flowers bloom from June to September, extending on long stalks from the stem. The root has a bitterish, styptic taste.

Medicinal Part: The root.

Solvents: Water-milk, vinegar.

Bodily Influence: Astringent, Tonic.

Uses: The long established, hidden talent of Cinquefoil has many uses. Culpeper states: "Let no man despise it because it is plain and easy, the ways of God are all such." He gives us a preparation for epilepsy, or as it used to be called, falling sickness: "The juice here of drunk, about 4 ounces at a time for certain days together cureth the quinsey, and yellow jaundice; and taken for 30 days together, cureth the falling sickness."

It is a specific in all inflammations and fevers of infections, or mixed with other herbs to cool and temper the blood and humours in the body. The root boiled in milk is effective for male and female complaints to the extent of haemorrhage. The juice or decoction taken with a little honey clears hoarseness of the throat and cough of the lungs, makes an excellent gargle for spongy, bleeding gums and ulcerated mouth and throat.

Externally: The root boiled in vinegar and applied to all kernels and hard swellings growing in any part of the flesh will soften them, and is quietening to shingles and all sorts of running and foul scabs, sores, itch and bruises. At the same time, drink the tea of Five fingers.

Dose: 20 grains in white wine, milk or water in wineglass amounts.

Russian Experience: Kalgan, Lapchatka, Kurinye Lapke (Chicken Foot) and many other names are given to this small but potentially useful plant. Used in Russia for medical and industrial purposes.

128

Folk Medicine: Use the rhizome, which is collected late in the spring before the leaves are overgrown, or in late autumn. The decoction as a very strong astringent for inflammation of the mouth or stomach, colitis, loose bowels, dyspepsia to stop bleeding of the stomach or female disorders. Mostly used in Folk Medicine (Saratov University, 1965).

In some parts of Russia the home medicine is given as a tonic for heart conditions, pains in the chest, inflammation (internal and external), amenorrhoea, coughs (Bello-Russ. Academy of Science, 1965).

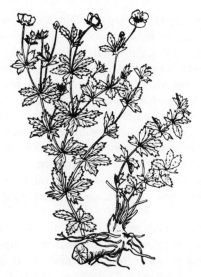

FIVE FINGER GRASS   Potentilla tormentilla Neck.
(Potentilla (L.) Rausch.); Tormentilla erecta, L.
(Bello-Russ. Academy of Science, Minsk, 1967)

Dose: 1 tablespoonful of the crushed rhizome to 1 cup of boiling water; drink from 3–5 tablespoonfuls a day, 1 or $1\frac{1}{2}$ tablespoonfuls before each meal.

Industrial: Used to process leather; also in the textile industry for dying in red colour.

FRINGE TREE   Chionanthus virginica, L.
(N.O.: Oleaceae)

Common Names: OLD MAN'S BEARD, SNOWDROP TREE, WHITE FRINGE, POISON ASH.

Features: The species is native in the eastern United States, from Pennsylvania to the Gulf of Mexico. A shrub or small tree of the Oleaceae, or

129

olive, family. The plants are 10–30 ft. high, possess oval, smooth, entire leaves, and bear snow-white flowers which hang down like a fringe, hence the common name and synonyms. Fruit fleshy, purple, ovid drupe. They form an attractive feature in garden shrubbery, growing well on river banks and on elevated places, presenting clusters of snow-white flowers in May and June. Root about ⅛ in. thick, dull brown with irregular concave scales on outer surface, inside smooth, yellowish brown. The inner layer shows projecting bundles of stone cells. Very bitter taste.

Medicinal Part: Root bark.

Solvent: Water.

Bodily Influence: Alterative, Hepatic, Diuretic, Tonic.

Uses: Generally useful in stomach and liver disorders and in poor digestive functions, by slightly influencing all the organs engaged in digestion and blood making. A specific in spleen malfunction, and for congestion of the liver when failure to excrete the residue from food, thus resulting in constipation (one of the reasons for gall-stone, jaundice and stomach inefficiency). In some, the involuntary muscles of the heart will also be impaired by the inactivity of the above mentioned.

In pregnancy, when indications of yellow skin, the white of the eyes are of a yellow colour, bilious colic, heartburn, etc., 5–10 drops in water before meals is indicated. Useful in malignant tumours of the stomach or bowels, and in uterine tumours, also in most chronic conditions of the liver and spleen.

Combine: Tincture of Golden seal (Hydrastis canadensis), 7–10 drops.
   Tincture of Fringe tree (Chionanthus virginica), 3–7 drops.

Dose: 10–20 drops in water before meals and at bedtime has proven effective.

In bilious colic it is best to first evacuate the stomach by giving an emetic dose of Lobelia and then to administer the above. The powdered root bark is used professionally; however, the cut root bark can be infused in hot water for ½ hr. and taken in small amounts throughout the day. Pulsatilla (Anemone) is also used in conjunction with Fringe tree.

Externally: The skin will respond to the application of an infusion of 1 oz. to 1 pint of water, when other attempts have failed. Also as an injection.

Homoeopathic Clinical: Tincture of the bark (which is the part employed and which contains saponin)—Constipation, Debility, Emaciation with liver disorder, Gall-stone colic, Headache, Jaundice, Liver (disease of, hypertrophy of), Malaria, Neurasthenia, Nursing women (complaints of).

FROSTWORT   Helianthemum canadense, Michx.
(N.O.: Cistaceae)

Common Names: ROCK ROSE, FROST PLANT, FROSTWEED, SUN ROSE, SCROFULA PLANT.

Features: This flowering plant, with its large, bright yellow face, is indigenous to all parts of the United States, growing in dry, sandy soils and blossoming from May to July. The flowers open in sunshine and cast their petals the next day. When seen growing you will notice some with petals and some without. The Rock rose is a perennial herb, simple, ascending downy stems about 1 ft. high. The leaves are alternate, from ½–1 in. long, and about a quarter as wide. The leaves, as well as the stem, are covered with a white down, hence its name.

The whole plant is official, having slight aromatic odour; and astringent and bitter taste.

Professor Eaton, in his work on Botany, records this curious fact of the plant: "In November and December of 1816, I saw hundreds of these plants sending out broad, thin covered ice crystals, about an inch in breadth from near the roots. These were melted away by day, and renewed every morning for more than twenty-five days in succession."

Medicinal Part: The herb.

Solvents: Dilute alcohol, water.

Bodily Influence: Tonic, Astringent, Alterative, in large dose Emetic.

Uses: Has been used for cancerous degenerations, especially the oil procured from the plant. In scrofula, its valuable contents have performed with astonishing admiration.

It can be used with advantage in diarrhoea, as a gargle in scarlatina and aphthous ulcers (small white ulcers on the tongue, and in the mouth) and as a wash in scrofulous ophthalmia. Effective in venereal treatment, obviating the many side-effects of the popular treatment.

It is used in the form of decoction, syrup, or fluid extract, but is advised to be used with Dicentra canadensis (Corydalis) and Stillingia.

Dose: Steep 1 teaspoonful of the granulated herb in 1 cup of boiling water for ½ hr., strain, take 1 tablespoonful three to six times a day. Of the tincture, 5–10 min.

Externally: The leaves made into a poultice are effective in treating scrofulous tumours, and ulcers.

Surely there is something in the unruffled calm of nature that exceeds our anxieties and doubts, and is in control by obeying her.

GARDEN NIGHTSHADE   Solanum nigrum, L.
(N.O.: Solonaceae)

Features: Often thought of as the Deadly Nightshade, but should not be confused with Belladonna. The Solanum nigrum is the rarer of the many species.

In comparison with Belladonna it has smaller, smoother stems; a purple colour; it is more erect; 1–3 ft. high, and it has dull, instead of shining black berries. It is found along walls and fences, and in gardens, in various parts of the United States of America.

The small white or pale violet flowers can be seen in July and August; in some areas the ripe berries, green berries and the flowers are seen on the plant together. The berries are poisonous, but boiling destroys the toxic properties in the ripe, black berries, and they are often made into pies.

Medicinal Part: The leaves.

Solvents: Water, alcohol.

Bodily Influence: Narcotic, Sedative.

Uses: The Indians used a decoction as an eye wash. It is said that the young leaves and stems can be boiled as pot herbs.

Parkinson wrote: "The root boiled in wine and a little thereof held in the mouth eases the pain of toothache."

It can be used to tighten the gums when teeth are loose. In consequence of its peculiar power over the nerve centres, it is an appropriate remedy for epilepsy, spasms and cramps of the extremities.

Dr. G. P. Wood, M.D., and Dr. E. H. Ruddock, M.D.: "In angina pectoris (one form of heart disease) it is said it often acts admirably, and likewise in inflammation of the eyes. In small doses it relieves headache of a nervous, congective character.

The leaves have been freely used in cancer, scurvy and scrofulous affection, in the form of an ointment. For home use it is best to use the plant in the ointment preparation, as in internal, large amounts it will produce sickness and vertigo, and in most cases should be prescribed by persons knowing both patient and medication.

Dose: 1 teaspoonful of the leaves cut small to 1 cup of boiling water, taken a teaspoonful at a time. Of the tincture, ½–1 min.

Homoeopathic Clinical: Tincture of fresh plant—Amaurosis, Chorea, Headache, Heartburn, Hydrocephalus, Mania, Meningitis, Night-terrors, Parotitis, Peritonitis, Puerperal convulsions, Scarlatina, Smallpox, Stammering, Tetanus, Tympanites, Typhoid fever, Varicosis, Vertigo, Ulcers.

India and Pakistan: Black nightshade is Makoy, or Kakmachi, to the people of India and Pakistan. The detailed knowledge of the plant, leaves and berries elaborate our study. Accordingly a valuable Heart tonic, Alterative, Diuretic, Sedative, Expectorant, Diaphoretic, Cathartic Hydragogue, Anodyne.

The berries contain the toxic alkaloid, solanine. They are alterative, diuretic and tonic, used in fever, diarrhoea, anasarca and heart disease. Also used to dilate the pupil. The plant juice in doses of 6–7 oz. in chronic enlargement of the liver, chronic skin diseases, spitting of blood and haemorrhoids. The leaf juice for inflammation of the kidneys and

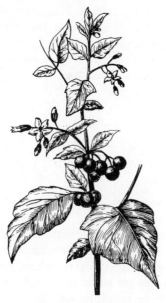

GARDEN NIGHTSHADE
Solanum nigrum, L.
(N. E. Kovaleva, Lecheye Rasteniamy
Medicina, Moscow, 1971)

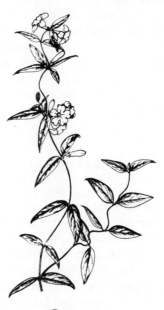

GELSEMIUM
Gelsemium sempervirens (L.) Ait.
(U.S. Agricultural Department,
Appalachia, 1971)

bladder, gonorrhoea, chronic enlargement of the liver and spleen. A hot infusion is a strong diaphoretic, 1–2 grains only. As a diuretic and depurative a decoction of the leaves is used for dropsy, chronic enlargement of liver and jaundice. Syrup of the herb is used as expectorant, diaphoretic, in cooling drinks for fevers.

Externally: A paste of the plant is a useful application for corroding ulcers, chancre, severe burns, herpes and rheumatic joints. The hot leaves applied in poultice form will relieve swollen and painful scrotum and testicles, also rheumatic gout, eruptions of the skin, corroding ulcers, tumours, whitlow and burns. A decoction of the leaves is used for bathing

133

tumours, inflamed, irritated and painful parts of the body. This diluted decoction is effectively added to the syringe for vaginal discomfort.

Russian Experience: Of all the medical literature available it is only in Bello-Russian (White Russia) literature that any reference can be found of Solanum nigrum (Garden nightshade) or Russian paslen cherry.

From days of long ago, Werenko (1896) used the berries for expelling tapeworms, as a gargle and as a poultice for inflamed boils. Cholovski (1882) found the contents of use for rheumatism. More recently it has been used as a tea for stomach pain and for baby's eczema (Nikolaeva, 1964). They also referred to French literature (Hoppe, 1958).

Industrial: Another species, Paslen dolchaty (Solanum lacimiatum) has better attention for industrial and commercial cultivation. Plantations in Ukraine, Moldavia, South Kazakhstan and elsewhere have had professional Agro-Technic assistance. For approximately 1 acre, $3\frac{1}{2}$–4 lb. of seed is needed. In South Kazakhstan they cut three times a season. The raw material is delivered to State chemical factories in 50 kg. bundles. With this a cortisone and other hormone preparations are processed.

GELSEMIUM   Gelsemium sempervirens (L.), Ait.
(N.O.: Loganiaceae)

Common Names: YELLOW JASMINE, WILD WOODBINE, GELSEMIUM.

Features: Abounding throughout North America, from Vancouver to Florida. The beautifully woody climber with its yellow flowers in March through May has an agreeable odour, and is cultivated as an ornamental vine. The plant has a twining stem with perennial leaves, which are dark green above and pale beneath. The roots are numerous, tough and splintery, containing Gelsemium as its active principle, also fixed oil, acrid resin, yellow colouring matter, a heavy volatile oil, a crystalline substance, and salts of potassium, lime, magnesia, iron and silica.

Medicinal Part: The root.

Solvents: Water, alcohol.

Bodily Influence: Nervine, Sedative, Mydriatic, Antispasmodic, Antiperiodic.

Uses: Has been used for many purposes by former generations, and still seems to be credited, but with careful administration. Close resemblance to Hemlock (Tsuga canadensis) in action.

It is an unrivalled febrifuge, possessing relaxing and antispasmodic properties. It is efficacious in nervous and bilious headache, colds, pneumonia, haemorrhage, leucorrhoea, ague-cake, but especially in all kinds of fevers, quietening all nervous irritability and excitement, equalizing the circulation, promoting perspiration, and rectifying the various

134

secretions, without causing nausea, vomiting and purging, and is adapted to any stage of the disease. Useful in inflammation of bowels, diarrhoea, dysentery, but with great success in neuralgia, toothache, insomnia, wherever a sedative is called for.

In pelvic disorders of women it is a favourite herb. It is also of great service in various cardiac diseases, spermatorrhoea and other genital diseases, but its use should be confined to persons understanding the pathology.

Dose: The tincture is the form in which it is employed, the dose being from 10–15 drops in a wineglass half full of water; to be repeated every 2 hr. as long as required. In large doses it depresses the nervous system and gives rise to convulsions and toxic symptoms such as clouded vision, double-sightedness, or complete prostration, and inability to open the eyes. This, however, completely wears off in a few hours, leaving the patient refreshed and completely restored. When the effects are induced no more of the remedy is required.

Homoeopathic Clinical: Tincture of the bark of the root—Amaurosis, Anterior crural neuralgia, Aphonia, Astigmatism, Bilious fever, Brain (affections of), Cerebro spinal meningitis, Choroiditis, Colds, Constipation, Convulsions, Deafness, Dengue fever, Diarrhoea, Diphtheria, Dupuytren's contraction, Dysentery, Dysmenia, Emotions (affects of), Epilepsy, Eyes (affections of), Fever, Fright, Gonorrhoea, Hay-fever, Headache, Heat (effects of), Heart (diseases of), Hydro-Salpingitis, Hysteria, Influenza, Intermittent fever, Jaundice, Labour, Liver (affections of), Locomotor ataxia, Mania, Measles, Meningitis, Menstruation (painful; suppressed), Metrorrhagia, Myalgia, Neuralgia, Nystagmus, Oesophagus (stricture of), Paralysis, Paralysis agitans, Paraplegia, Pregnancy (albuminuria of), Ptosis, Puerperal convulsions, Remittent fever, Retina (detachment of), Rheumatism, Sexual excess (effects of), Sleep (disordered), Spasms, Sun headache, Sunstroke, Teething, Tic-douloureux, Tobacco (effects of), Tongue (affections of), Toothache, Tremors, Uterus (affections of), Vertigo, Voice (loss of), Writer's cramp.

GILLENIA   Gillenia trifoliata, Moench.
(N.O.: Rosaceae)

Common Names: INDIAN PHYSIC, AMERICAN IPECAC, WESTERN DROP-WORT.

Features: This indigenous shrub can be found scattered in North America: Canada to Florida, on the eastern side of the Alleghenies. Does well in open hilly woods, in light gravelly soil.

The root is quite thick with thin bark and many fissured rootlets, of bitter taste. The several erect, slender and smooth stems are 2–3 ft. high, and of a reddish or brownish colour. The leaves are alternate. Flowers are of white and pinkish colour, and can be seen in May. Matured fruit of two-valved, one-celled capsule, seeds are oblong, brown and bitter.

Medicinal Part: The bark of the root.

Solvents: Boiling water, alcohol.

Bodily Influence: Purgative, Tonic, Emetic, Cathartic, Expectorant.

Uses: Very popular with the North American Indians for amenorrhoea (absence or abnormal interruption of the menstrual flow), rheumatism, dropsy, costiveness, dyspepsia, worms and intermittent fever. It may be used in all fevers where emetics are required.

Dose: As an emetic, 20–35 grains of the powder, as often as required; as a tonic, 2–4 grains. As a diaphoretic, 6 grains in cold water, and repeated at intervals of 2–3 hr.

GINGER—WILD Asarum canadense, L.
(N.O.: Aristoloch)

Common Names: CANADA SNAKE ROOT, INDIAN GINGER, VERMONT SNAKE ROOT.

Features: Ginger, being of many species, differs in appearance according to habitat; Africa, Calcutta, India, Pakistan, China, Jamaica, Japan, etc., have their own special native herb.

Our native Ginger is a beautiful little plant found growing in rich woods during April and May, from Maine to Michigan, and southwards. The root of the plant is round and fleshy, with dividing stem supporting a heart-shaped, deep green above and light below, soft, woolly, and handsomely veined leaf, there being two to a plant. The flower is one to a plant, small and of a brownish-purple colour, growing only a few inches high and sometimes becoming covered by the dead leaves that carpet the woods. Odour: ginger-like, or recalling serpentaria; taste: pungent, bitter.

Medicinal Part: The root.

Solvent: Boiling water.

Bodily Influence: Stimulant, Carminative, Tonic, Diaphoretic, Diuretic.

Uses: As a carminative it is useful in all painful spasms of the bowels and stomach, also to promote perspiration, in all cases of colds, female obstructions, whooping cough, and fevers. Practitioners of the American Physic Medical School hold that this root exerts a direct influence upon the uterus, and prescribe it as a parturient when nervous fatigue is observed. It can be made into a tea and administered in small doses. frequently repeated, as large doses are apt to nauseate the stomach.

Dose: As a cordial made with a tincture and syrup of molasses it is most agreeable. 1 teaspoonful of the granulated root to 1 pint of boiling water, 2 tablespoonfuls at a time as often as required. Of the tincture, 2–5 min. Powder may be taken dry, 20–30 grains.

Homoeopathic Clinical: Tincture of root and whole fresh plant (Asarum europeum)—Alcoholism, Anus (prolapse of), Catarrh, Cholerine, Diarrhoea, Dysmenorrhoea, Eyes (affections of; operations of), Fidgets, Headache, Hysteria, Levitation (sensation of), Typhus.

Russian Experience: Kopiten (Ginger) grows wild in the European and West Siberia of Russia, and the Far East. There is a special time for collecting the different sections of the well-known plant. Leaves in the early spring, rhizomes when the flower begins to form, roots in the fall.

Folk Medicine: The different parts of the plant play an important specific as to their use, or perhaps in combinations of ailments and use. In Bello-Russia (White Russia) the properties of the rhizome are used as an expectorant, for jaundice, dropsy, to promote milk for the nursing mother, heart trouble, lung tuberculosis, nerve excitement, migraine headache, and laxative. The rhizome as Nastoika (with vodka) for scrofula (Cholousky, 1882; Antonov, 1888), heart palpitation, weakness and lack of stamina of children (Werenko, 1896), poisoning with mushrooms, stomachic (Federevski, 1897), migraine headache, alcoholism, scrofula (Nikolaeva, 1964). The leaves are used for malaria.

Clinically: Of late use as tea from leaves for heart trouble, and decoction of rhizome as expectorant for vomiting.

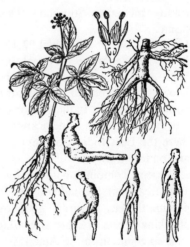

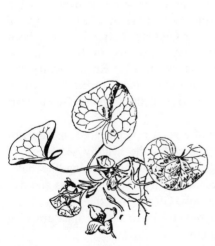

GINGER—WILD   Asarum canadense, L.
(Zdorovie, Kiev, U.S.S.R., 1964)

GINSENG   Panax quinquefolium, L.
1—Flowering plant   2—Cross section
of flower   3–7—Different forms of the
roots (Medicine Encyclopedia, Moscow,
1961)

137

GINSENG   Panax quinquefolium, L.
(N.O.: Ararliaceae)

Common Names: FIVE FINGER ROOT, AMERICAN GINSENG, SANG, NINSIN, PANAX, PANNAG, RED BERRY.

Features: Indigenous to China, North America; East Asia, American ginseng grows naturally on the slopes of ravines and other shady but well-drained places in hardwood forests, in varying abundance, from eastern Canada to Maine and Minnesota and southwards into the mountain regions of Georgia and Carolina. In its wild state it grows from 8–20 in. high, bearing three large leaflets at the top and two smaller ones beneath.

Yellowish green clusters of flowers are produced in midsummer, followed by as many bright crimson berries, which can be seen until the frost. They are edible and taste much like the ginseng root. The berries contain from one to three flattish wrinkled seeds the size of a small pea. The root is thick, spindle shaped, 2–4 in. long and $\frac{1}{2}$–1 in. or more in thickness. The older specimens usually have branched protrusions somewhat resembling a human form. It usually takes at least six years for the root to reach marketable size. Can be cultivated from cracked or partly germinated seed. Ginseng is very shy and must be protected from the sun. The roots should be dug in the autumn when they are not so full of sap.

Medicinal Part: The dried root.

Solvent: Water.

Bodily Influence: Stimulant, Demulcent, Stomachic, Nervine, Aphrodisiac.

Uses: If we look in Ezekiel 27:17, we find Ginseng was known to Judah in the market place of Israel. Trading was done in wheat, honey, oil balm and "Pannag", or the all-healing Ginseng. Certainly it has been known and respected for centuries. Father Jartoux, in 1679, after he noticed American Indians from the Ozarks and Blue Ridge country employing Ginseng as a medication, started exporting it to England. From there the East India Company sent it around the Cape of Good Hope and on to the Orient.

Ginseng, combined with the juice of a good ripe pineapple, is superior as a treatment for indigestion. It stimulates the healthy secretions of pepsin, thereby ensuring good digestion without increasing the habit of taking pepsin or other after-dinner pills to relieve the fullness and distress so common to the American people. Ginseng has the known ability to penetrate the delicate tissue our blood fails to oblige, thus arousing the malfunction of the lymphatic glands.

It is a powerful antispasmodic and suggests its use in other spasmodic and reflex nervous diseases, such as whooping cough and asthma. For

138

many people Ginseng has had beneficial results in the home for general strengthening and appetite, as well as to relieve eructations from the stomach, neuralgia, rheumatism, gout, irritation of bronchi or lungs from cold, gastroenteric indigestion, weak heart, spinal and nervous affection.

Ellingwood, speaking of the medical properties of Ginseng, says: "It is a mild sedative to the nerve centres, improving their tone, and if persisted in, increases the capillary circulation of the brain." Dr. Raymond Bernard A.B.M.A., Ph.D., says: "The term 'aphrodisiac' should not be misunderstood, and we must differentiate between aphrodisiacal drugs which produce their effects by irritation of the sexual centres and herbs like Ginseng which regenerate and rebuild the vitality but do not act by mere stimulation or irritation." A modern Chinese herbalist avows that it is "most energy giving, and is distinguished by the slowness and the gentleness of its actions." Ginseng is known to give off organic radioactive rays resembling the Gartwitch rays of onions which stimulate vital processes in living cells. It is adaptable to the treatment of young children as well as the aged.

Dose: To make a tea, take 3 oz. of powder (Ginseng 6–7 years old), add 1 oz. of honey and 60 drops of wintergreen, and blend. Use 1 teaspoonful to 1 cup of boiling water, let it stay a little short of the boiling point for 10 min., drink as hot as you can before each meal. To make tea from the dried leaves, steep as you would for ordinary teas. Excellent for nervous indigestion.

Homoeopathic Clinical: Trituration and tincture of the root—Appendicitis, Debility, Headache, Lumbago, Rheumatism, Sciatica, Sexual excitement.

Russian Experience: The history of Ginseng has come through periods of belief and disbelief in many continents when laboratory technicians could not give explanations to its unalterable physiological and psychological accomplishment of centuries of belief. For the latest information on Ginseng you must go abroad. Up to 1964–5, Anglo-American literature did not pay too much attention to the long-held belief in the useful properties of Ginseng.

China has always been a good market for Ginseng, the highest prices being paid for old roots. About seventy years ago a Chinese Emperor sent a present of the best selected roots to a Russian Tzar. Being unaware and suspicious, the Russian official understandably though it best to have the root analysed to see why so much importance was given to this man-like root. The Military Academy of Medicine was elected for this purpose, as the international diplomat was a military figure. The top staff, heads of wisdom, could not find any health-giving properties after long and careful research. So at this time Ginseng was thought of as a Chinaman's prejudice, and was once again rejected because of insufficient evidence for further scientific research. (This gift object was sent to St.

139

Petersburg botanic museum, where it can be seen today.) This did not dampen the original thought of the Chinese, as they still came to the Russian Far East to collect and buy Russian and Manchurian Ginseng, which they considered the best. The price did not restrict their demands, as they would pay ten to twenty times more than gold, or the traditional oriental silver. Time and experience has led to plantations of Ginseng in Korea, China, Manchuria and Japan.

In 1675 is the first record of Ginseng in Russia, experienced by Boyarin N. G. Sapfary; 300 years later we consider their acceptance ahead in world research. Twenty-five years ago, team after team was sent to neighbouring countries to study, on the spot, established plantations. The highly protected secret of this culture is not given charitably. Today all information from observation and study leads us to Russia's own army of Ginseng specialists in all parts of Russia, but more especially in the Far East. All work and research is directed and co-ordinated by the Committee for Ginseng Research, which includes universities, institutes, laboratories, Agro-Technical methods, field work, plantations, publications, etc.

There are plantations of Ginseng in the Russian Far East, Moscow regions, Bello-Russia (White Russia) and the Caucasus (Bello-Russ. Acad, 1965). In the past, Russian Ginseng was always exported from a wild source but today the cultivated plant is exported, being collected in August.

Lengthy study and research of Chinese belief in the Folk Medicine of Ginseng, not only confirms fundamental impressions but has opened new horizons to its proven value beyond reality ("Vishaya Scholla", Moscow, 1963).

We wish to mention two monographs we have on hand of the Siberian branch of the Academy of Science. One work was published in 1960, with 1,500 copies printed (usually Herbal book publications run to 100,000–200,000). It contains 248 pages, and a few hundred authors contributed 5–10 pages each, as a collective work of 5–8 different teams.

Another work, compiled by one author, is a 342-page book dealing with the biological aspect of Ginseng. Here the author refers to the bibliographies of all available languages, but mostly original works and research of Russian experience.

In North America we think of Ginseng as the slow-growing herb, as it takes from five to seven years before the root is considered usable. To find a plant fifty years old is considered sensational, as collectors usually find the plants before they reach this age. The age is told by the rings around the plant.

The older roots in North America are uncommon, but theoretically the older the root the smaller should be the dose.

In the Far East there are plants that have reached the age of 100, 200 and even 400. Some Hong Kong roots sell for 500 dollars per ounce. A five- to ten-year-old root will weigh only a few ounces but a 200–300-year-old one will weigh nearly 1 lb. The young Ginseng is used in large amounts, 1 teaspoonful to each cup. The old Ginseng requires careful use, starting with 1 drop a day and adding extra drops day by day. If one drop too much is taken, bleeding will start, as the old root is very strong.

There are many beautiful common names for Ginseng: Root of life, Root of man, Santa root, Seed of earth, Panax, Panacea, Life for ever lasting, etc. (Moscow University, 1963).

After having had the history, research data and facts, we are sure you will be interested in its uses. In short, it prolongs life (Saraton University, 1962).

In Russia they recommend to all people over forty to have six weeks (forty-two days) of consecutive daily intake of Ginseng twice a year. This will regenerate the glands and invigorate the blood, thus bringing the properties of Ginseng to the endocrine system. This activates metabolism, improves blood circulation and positively activates the kidney, bladder, liver etc. In general, an over-all tonic.

Ginseng increases vitality by carefully improving the condition. The activating process improves the mental, physical and spiritual efficiencies of the brain, so inducing better feeling, sleep, appetite and well-being. Ginseng has a long list of accomplishments when other means have failed.

It is not only used as a physical restorative, but acts psyschologically for tiredness of heart and blood circulation, sugar diabetes, depressions, neurasthenia, neurosis, psychasthenia. You may be interested in the properties of this plant as a special study, but the above mentioned is impressive as it is.

In Russia, Ginseng is used, of course, as Nastoika (with vodka) and as tea and powder. Clinically, in the form of extracts, pills, tablets, capsules.

GOLDEN ROD   Solidago canadensis and Solidago juncea, L.
(N.O.: Compositae)

Common Names: SWEET SCENTED GOLDEN ROD, BLUE MOUNTAIN TEA.
Features: Nearly 100 members of the species of Solidago are centred in North America, especially the eastern United States. These are fibrous, creeping-rooted, perennial herbs; they have erect stems which are sometimes rather woody at the base. The leaves are alternate, simple, entire, or toothed; they have a fragrant odour and a warm, aromatic, agreeable taste. The golden yellow flowers are rather small, arranged in terminal, panicled racemes.

Golden Rod blooms in the summer and autumn, forming in the eastern United States a conspicuous part of the autumnal scene. Different species may be found in a great variety of habitats, from brackish coastal swamps to meadows, woods, fields, prairies, cliffs and alpine fields. The species are difficult to identify and many hybridize in nature, as is shown in the illustrations.

Medical Parts: The leaves and tops.

Solvent: Water.

Bodily Influence: Aromatic, Carminative, Stimulant, Astringent, Diaphoretic.

Uses: For sickness due to weakness of the stomach, Golden rod has been proven effective. It promotes perspiration and is often used to dissolve stones in the bladder.

A good herb to remember for the unsuspecting, repeated colds of tuberculosis and hay fever. Mixes well with other unpleasant medicinal tasting herbs to improve the flavour. Golden rod is aromatic, moderately

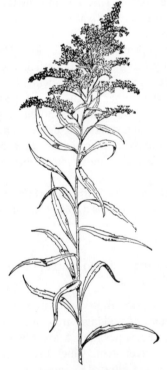

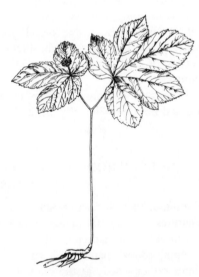

CANADIAN GOLDENROD
Solidago canadensis, L.
(Weeds, Canadian Agricultural
Department, Ottawa, 1967)

GOLDEN SEAL
Hydrastis canadensis, L.
(U.S. Agricultural Department,
Appalachia, 1971)

142

stimulant and carminative when cold. Diaphoretic as a warm infusion. **Dose:** 1 teaspoonful of the leaves to 1 cupful of boiling water.

Externally: The Indians used the solution from boiled leaves as an external lotion for wounds and ulcers, sprinkling the affected parts with the powdered leaves as a protective dressing. The same was used for saddle sores on horses. The Spanish Americans used the fresh plant mixed with soap for a plaster to bind on sore throats. Missouri golden rod (S. missouriensis), recognized by its unusually long stemmed and fluted leaves, was eaten as salad greens.

Homoeopathic Clinical: Tincture of flowers, infusion of dry leaves and flowers—Albuminuria, Calculus, Croup, Deafness, Dysuria, Eruptions, Gout, Leucorrhoea, Ophthalmia (scrofulous), Phosphaturia, Prostate (enlarged), Rheumatism, Sciatica, Scrofula, Urine (scanty, suppressed).

Russian Experience: Only in one book can information on Solidago be found, which in Russia is Zolotarnik obiknovenny (from Zoloto—Goldsmith vulgaris).

Uses: The flowers and leaves have long been used in Bello-Russia as a tea for diarrhoea, inflammation of the bladder and amenorrhoea (Federowske, 1897).

Externally: Powdered flowers have a reputation for treating unhealed wounds of long standing (Uladzimirau, 1927). Floral powder is mixed with fresh cream for skin sickness, especially TB of the skin (Nikolaiva, 1964) (Bello-Russ. Academy of Science, 1966).

GOLDEN SEAL Hydrastis canadensis, L.
(N.O.: Ranunculaceae)

Common Names: YELLOW PUCCOON, GROUND RASPBERRY, TUMERIC ROOT, YELLOW ROOT, ORANGE ROOT.

Features: A perennial herb native to the moist woods and damp meadows of eastern North America.

The rough, wrinkled yellow root contains several alkaloids; odour is distinct, with a bitter taste. When fresh it is juicy and is used by the Indians to colour their clothing, etc. The plant sends up a simple hairy stem 8–20 in. tall with three to five lobed, dark green leaves that in the summer may become 4–10 in. broad. The May and June flower is a solitary one, small, white or rose coloured, appearing in early spring proceeded by a crimson head or small berries resembling raspberry, and consists of many two-seeded drupes. The wild plant is scarce today and is cultivated for medicinal purposes.

Medicinal Part: The root.

Solvent: Alcohol, diluted alcohol, boiling water.

Bodily Influence: Tonic, Alterative, Laxative.

Uses: The Cherokee Indians introduced Golden seal as an agent for treating ulcers and arrow wounds. Since then it has gained a title of being one of the most powerful agents in the entire herb kingdom.

Its recognition for usefulness is in congested conditions, sustaining the circulation of blood in the veins, and this attribute is valuable in heart affections where the extremities are usually cold and lips bluish. To strengthen the weakened condition, it is best to combine 1 part each Capsicum, Skull cap to 4 parts Golden seal.

For debilitated conditions of mucous membrane of the stomach (the harbour of much injustice, usually self-administered), Golden seal pulls rank. Can be used in a wide range of illnesses ranging from the common cold to complicated advancements, La grippe, ulcerated stomach, dyspepsia, enlarged tonsils, diphtheria, chronic catarrh of the intestines, skin eruptions, scarlet fever and smallpox.

Combine 1 part Golden seal, $\frac{1}{4}$ part Myrrh gum for a strong decoction which is very valuable in gleet, chronic gonorrhoea, leucorrhoea, incipient stricture, spermatorrhoea, and inflammation and ulceration of the internal coat of the bladder. The latter may be treated by Golden seal alone. It must be injected into the bladder and held there as long as the patient can conveniently retain it. To be repeated three or four times a day immediately after emptying the bladder. Should be injected by experienced persons.

It is a specific in passive haemorrhages from the pelvic tissue. For this 2 parts Golden seal to 1 part Geranium or Cranesbill, simmer covered for 20 min. Golden seal combined with Scullcap and Hops is a very fine tonic for spinal nerves, including spinal meningitis. As a mouth medication for pyorrhoea or sore gums, make a solution and gently brush or massage teeth and gums. Golden seal can be given alone in weak proportions, but is most effective combined with other suitable medications.

Dose: Of the powder, from 10–30 grains; of the tincture, 1–2 fl. drams. Roots: place 1 teaspoonful of the powdered root into 1 pint of boiling water, let stand until cold, drink 1–2 tablespoonfuls three to six times a day.

Externally: Externally it is used as a lotion in treatment of skin eruptions and eye affections, and as a general cleansing application. Tired, irritated eyes will be relieved by saturating cotton with a weak solution and applying to closed eyes.

Homoeopathic Clinical: Tincture of fresh root—Alcoholism, Asthma, Cancer, Catarrh, Chancroids, Constipation, Corus, Dyspepsia, Eczema impetiginoids, Ears (affections of), Faintness, Fistula, Gastric catarrh, Gonorrhoea, Haemorrhoids, Jaundice, Leucorrhoea, Lip (cancer of), Liver (affections of), Lumbago, Lupus, Menorrhagia, Metrorrhagia, Mouth (sore), Nails (affections of), Nipples (sore), Noises in the head,

144

Nursing women (sore mouth of), Ozaena, Placenta (adherent), Postnasal catarrh, Rectum (affections of), Sciatica, Seborrhoea, Stomach (affections of), Syphilis, Taste (disordered), Throat deafness, Throat (sore), Tongue (affections of), Typhus, Ulcers, Uterus (affections of).

Russian Experience: Golden seal does not grow in Russia or any other known place except North America. However, the value of this wonder plant is known to them medicinally. They use the Latin name with Russian dialect—Hydrastis Kanadsky. Their studies and experiments are seriously in favour of the possible cultivation in Russia.

Clinically: Not a home medicine in Russia. Only the extract is used, prescribed clinically in hospitals. At the present time it is limited to female conditions of excess bleeding, disturbance and pain of monthly periods, etc. (Atlas, Moscow, 1965).

GOLD THREAD   Coptis groenlandica, Salisb.
(N.O.: Ranunculaceae)

Common Names: MOUTH ROOT, YELLOW ROOT, CANKER ROOT, VEGETABLE GOLD.

Features: Gold thread is found growing in dark swamps and mossy woods in northern parts of the United States, and Canada, Iceland, Siberia and India.

The plant has a small, creeping perennial root of many fibres, and a bright yellow colour, faint odour, and bitter taste without stringency. The leaves are evergreen, on long, slender 1 ft. long stalks, growing three together. The white and yellow star-like flowers grow on a separate stem, rising to the same height as the leaves. They flower early in the spring to July, proceeded by oblong capsules containing many small black seeds. Autumn is the proper season for collecting this creation from above.

Medicinal Part: The root.

Solvents: Boiling water, dilute alcohol.

Bodily Influence: Tonic.

Uses: Exactingly helpful as a mouth wash for canker sores, gargle for sore throat, and ulcers of both stomach and throat. It may be beneficially used in all cases where a bitter tonic is required, such as dyspepsia and chronic inflammation of the stomach. It is a good herb to give to children occasionally as a tonic; it invigorates the stomach and is a preventive of pin worms. It may be given alone or in combination with other suitable medicines; it promotes digestion, improves the appetite and acts as a general stimulant to the system. In convalescence it is highly beneficial. Made into a decoction, Gold thread (Coptis trifolia) and Golden seal (Hydrastis canadensis), it will often release the driving desire for alcoholic beverages.

145

Dose: The tincture, made by adding 1 oz. of the powdered root to 1 pint of diluted alcohol, is preferable to the powder. The dose is from 20 drops to 1 teaspoonful, three times a day. As a tea, steep 1 teaspoonful of the granulated root in 1 cup of boiling water for ½ hr., strain, take 1 tablespoonful three to six times a day.

GRAVEL ROOT   Eupatorium purpureum, L.
(N.O.: Compositae)

Common Names: QUEEN OF THE MEADOW, KIDNEY ROOT, JOE-PYE WEED, TRUMPET WEED, PURPLE BONESET.

Features: Found in low places, dry woods or meadows in northern, western and middle regions of North America and in Canada.

Gravel root is distinguishable by the purple band about 1 in. broad around the leaf joint. The perennial plant reaches heights of 5–6 ft., with pale purple to white tubular flowers that bloom in August and September. The leaves, from three to five at a joint, are broad, rough and jagged. The root is the official part, with a fragrance resembling that of old hay, and slightly bitter, aromatic taste which is faintly astringent but not unpleasant.

Medicinal Parts: The root; floral decoctions are diuretic and tonic.

Solvent: Water.

Bodily Influence: Diuretic, Stimulant, Tonic, Astringent, Relaxant.

Uses: The strong decoction of the root is esteemed almost an infallible remedy for gravel and accumulations of the associated bladder, kidney and the urinary system. To mention a few: dropsy, neuralgia, lumbago, gout, rheumatism and joint stiffness caused by uric acid deposits. It has also been recognized as being an agent for sterility, threatened abortion, as well as incontinence of urine. Queen of the meadow is also used in nerve fibres, which once destroyed can never be replaced.

Homoeopathic Clinical: Tincture of the root—Albuminuria, Calculi, Cystitis, Diabetes, Dropsy, Enuresis, Gravel, Headache, Home-sickness, Hysteria, Impotence, Indigestion, Intermittent fever, Renal colic, Rheumatism, Sciatica, Strangury, Throat (sore), Urine (retention of), Vomiting.

GUM PLANT   Grindelia squarrosa (Pursh)
(N.O.: Compositae)

Common Names: GUMWEED, TARWEED, STICKY HEADS.

Features: A genus of the family compositae, of coarse, resinous herbs. Found chiefly in North America, west of the Rocky Mountains.

146

Of the four species, Robusta has the following identification: a perennial herb 1–3 ft. high, growing in silt marshes and along mountain ranges. Leaves are 2in. long, pale green, broadly spatulate, smooth and finely dotted; sometimes flexous and coated with resin terminating in resinous flower heads. Flowers, yellow, of aromatic taste and balsamic odour. Should be collected as soon as in full bloom.

Medicinal Parts: Dried leaves and flowering tops.

Solvents: Alcohol, boiling water.

Bodily Influence: Expectorant, Antispasmodic, Diuretic.

Uses: Antidote for the affliction of poison oak or ivy. Much used in indolent ulcers, impetigo, eczema and allergic dermatitis. For this, Dr. Clymer, M.D., in "Natures Healing Agents" informs us: "1 ounce of fluid extract of Gum Plant (Grindelia), 1 ounce of 90° proof alcohol, and 1 or 2 ounces of water, and applied as frequently as the itch demands. At night, a compress made with it may be applied to the affected portions of the body."

The tincture of grindelia, 5–20 drops in water, should be given internally in conjunction with the external application three to four times a day, according to age and condition.

Gum plant is also effective in asthma, bronchial or allergic cases, and respiratory conditions which include harsh dry cough and wheezing. Caution: of no value to asthma where the heart is involved, as in this condition it slows heart action.

The Indians boiled the root and drank the tea for the liver; buds on the plant were dried for use with smallpox and measles; a ½ cupful, hot, was said to be good for pneumonia. A decoction of leaves was made for running sores. Spring collection of the flowering tops were used as a blood purifier and to relieve throat and lung trouble. For toothache a small quantity was held in the mouth, but never swallowed. For rheumatism the fresh plant was crushed and applied to the troublesome part of the body.

Dose: Tincture of Grindelia alone, 5–30 drops according to age or condition. 1 teaspoonful of the leaves and flowering tops, cut small or granulated, to 1 cup of boiling water. Drink cold 1 cupful during the day, a large mouthful at a time.

Homoeopathic Clinical: A tincture is made of the leaves and unexpanded flowers. Bundy's proving of Grindelia squarrosa was made with a tincture of the dried plant (J. H. Clarke, 1962)—Asthma, Bites, Bronchitis, Cheyne Stoke's breathing, Conjunctivitis, Emphysema, Erythema, Eyes (pain in), Glaucoma, Heart (affection of), Iritis, Itching, Liver (pain in), Pruritus vulvae, Pruritus vaginae, Rhus poisoning, Spleen (pain in), Ulcers.

HAIRCAP MOSS Polytrichum juniperium, Wild.
(N.O.: Polytrichaceae)

Common Names: ROBIN'S RYE, GROUND MOSS, BEAR'S MOSS.

Features: Indigenous, perennial plant found in high, dry places along the margins of dry woods, mostly on poor sandy soil. The evergreen plant, with slender stem, is of a reddish colour and from 4–7 in. high Leaves are lanceolate and somewhat spreading, much darker green than the mosses in general. The fruit is a four-sided oblong capsule. Taste and smell are slight. It is said that this moss is found growing on human skulls, thus the origination of Haircap moss.

Medicinal Part: The whole plant.

Solvent: Boiling water.

Bodily Influence: Diuretic.

Uses: As a remedial agent this plant has been unnoticed but is nevertheless valuable. Professor King, of Cincinnati, says: "A strong infusion of this plant taken in doses of four tablespoonfuls every $\frac{1}{2}$ hour, has removed from dropsical patients from 20 to 40 pounds of water in the space of twenty-four hours."

Very useful in urinary obstruction and suppression, fevers and inflamations. Can be used for the most sensitive conditions, as the acceptability is met without stomach rebellion. Can be used with other hydragogue cathartics with decided advantage.

Dose: 1 teaspoonful to 1 cup of boiling water. Drink 1–2 cupfuls a day, a few swallows at a time. Of the tincture, $\frac{1}{2}$–1 fl. dram.

HELLEBORE AMERICAN Veratrum viride, Ait.
(N.O.: Liliaceae)

Common Names: HELLEBORE, INDIAN POKE, ITCH WEED, GREEN HELLEBORE.

Features: American helebore is native to North America and Canada, growing perennially in swamps, low grounds and moist meadows.

The thick and fleshy rhizome sends off a multitude of large whitish roots. The stem is from 3–5 ft. high: lower leaves from 6 in. to 1 ft. long, decreasing in size alternately up the stem. June and July find the numerous yellowish-green flowers in bloom. The roots should be gathered in autumn, and as it rapidly loses its virtues it should be gathered

148

annually and kept in a well-closed container. Has a very strong, unpleasant odour when fresh, diminishing when dry.

Medicinal Part: The rhizome.

Solvent: Alcohol.

Bodily Influence: Sedative, Emetic, Diaphoretic, Sternutatory.

Uses: It is unsurpassed by any article as an expectorant. As an arterial sedative it stands unparalleled and unequalled. In small doses it creates and promotes appetite beyond any agent known to medical men. As a diaphoretic it is one of the most certain of the whole materia medica, often exciting great coolness and coldness of the surface, sometimes rendering the skin moist and soft and in other cases producing free and abundant perspiration. In suitable doses it can be relied upon to bring the pulse down from 150 beats per min. to forty or even thirty.

The contents of Protoveratrine, being the most active heart content, slows the pulse by its powerful stimulating influence upon the vagus nerve, while Nervine, constituting more than half of the total alkaloids, plays an important part in lowering arterial tension by depressing powerfully the heart and vaso-motor centre. In fevers, in some diseases of the heart, acute and inflammatory rheumatism, and in many other conditions which involve an excited state of the circulation, it is of exceeding great value. Dr. Brown, M.D., informs us: "As a deobstruent or alterative it far surpasses iodine, and therefore used with great advantage in the treatment of cancer, scrofula, and consumption."

It is nervine and never narcotic, which property renders it of great value in all painful diseases, or such as are accompanied by spasmodic action, convulsions, morbid irritability and irritative mobility, as in cholera, epilepsy of fits, pneumonia (should never be given in the latter stages of pneumonia as it lowers blood pressure, and is relaxant to the muscles in this already weakened condition), puerperal fever, neuralgia, etc., producing these effects without stupefying and torpefying the system, as opium is known to do.

As an emetic it is slow, but certain and efficient, rousing the liver to action like other emetics, without being cathartic. It is peculiarly adapted as an emetic in whooping cough, croup, asthma, scarlet fever and in all cases where there is much febrile or inflammatory action.

Dose: Veratrum is usually given in the form of a tincture, the formula being: dried root 8–16 oz., diluted (83.5 per cent alcohol), macerating for two weeks, then expressed and filtered.

To an adult eight drops are given, which should be repeated every 3 hr., increasing the dose 1–2 drops every time until nausea or vomiting, or reduction of the pulse to 65 or 70, ensue, then reducing to half in all cases. Females and young people between fourteen and eighteen should commence with 6 drops and increase as above. For children from two to five years, begin with 2 drops and increase 1 drop only. Below two years of age, 1 drop is sufficient. If taken in so large a dose as to produce vomiting or too much depression, a full dose of morphine or opium, in a little brandy or ginger, is a complete antidote.

In pneumonia, typhoid fever and many other diseases, it must be continued for three to seven days after the symptoms have subsided. Administration of this medicine should be closely watched and when the pulse begins to recede, or if nausea or vomiting occurs, it is a signal of alarm and the administration should be stopped. In typhoid fever, while using the verartrum, quinia is absolutely inadmissible.

Homoeopathic Clinical: Tincture of fresh root, gathered in autumn— Amaurosis, Amenorrhoea, Apoplexy, Asthma, Bunions, Caecum

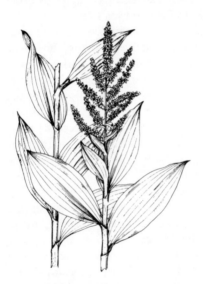 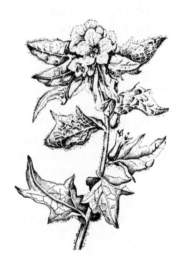

HELLEBORE AMERICAN
Veratrum viride, Ait.
(U.S. Agricultural Department,
Appalachia, 1971)

HENBANE
Hyoscyamus niger, L.
(P. T. Kondratenko, Zagotovky,
Medicina, Moscow, 1967)

(inflammation of), Chilblains, Chorea, Congestion, Convulsions, Diplopia, Diaphragmitis, Dysmenorrhoea, Erysipelas, Headache (nervous; sick), Heart (affections of), Hiccough, Hyperpyrexia, Influenza, Malarial fever, Measles, Meningitic menses (suppressed), Myalgia, Oesophagus (spasm of), Orchitis, Pneumonia, Proctalgia, Puerperal convulsions, Puerperal mania, Sleep (dreamful), Spine (congestion of), Spleen (congested), Sunstroke, Typhoid fever, Uterus (congestion of).

Russian Experience: Chemeritza Lobelia is among the several kinds of Hellebore growing in Russia. American Hellebore is valued highly and cultivation is possible.

Folk Medicine: Decoctions or Nastoika (vodka and Hellebore) and preparations of ointments are used in painful rheumatic conditions, especially in sciatica. A word of caution should be observed as it is poisonous in wrong amounts.

Clinically: Used very carefully and only under prescription.

Veterinary: The agent is strong and effective if mixed with Agrimony (Agrimonia eupatoria) for parasites and pests. It is toxic and personal protection should be taken when preparing or spraying solution; a wet mask is advised.

HENBANE   Hyoscyamus niger, L.
(N.O.: Solanaceae)

Common Names: DEVIL'S EYE, HOG'S BEAN, HENBELL, JUPITER'S BEAN.

Features: Hyoscyamus niger is the most common species of the eleven biennial or perennial nightshade or potato family, solanaceae. Native to the eastern hemisphere from Europe to India. Has been naturalized, particularly in the eastern United States from New England to Michigan.

The root is a long, tapering, fleshy, corrugated growth, which is of a brown colour externally and whitish internally, with an ill-smelling odour (could be mistakenly eaten as parsnips with fatal results). The stems are 1–4 ft. high, thickly clothed with coarsely toothed or pinnatifid, viscid, hairy, alternate leaves; collected in second year when the plant is in bloom. Flowers from July to September, in pendant, long, one-sided, leafy spikes, pale or dingy yellow in colour, with purple veins or orifice. The seeds are many, small, obovate and brownish, and are gathered when perfectly ripe. Found growing in the waste grounds of old settlements, in graveyards and around the foundations of ruined houses.

If bruised the new leaves emit a strong narcotic odour, like tobacco; when dried they have little smell or taste.

Medical Parts: Leaves, seeds.

Solvents: Alcohol, boiling water.

Bodily Influence: Anodyne, Narcotic, Mydriatic.

Uses: Henbane is powerfully narcotic. If used under the guidance of a good herbal physician, it is calmative, hypnotic, anodyne and antispasmodic. Dr. Brown, M.D., informs us: "It is much better than opium, as it does not produce constipation, and is always given where opium does not agree."

Its use is principally to cause sleep and remove irregular nervous action. Also combined with other herbal medications for gout, rheumatism, asthma, chronic cough, neuralgia, irritations of the urinary organs, etc.

All narcotics are dangerously poisonous if carelessly administered.

151

Nature grows wild her most potent medicinal herbs, and those which, if used by persons who understand them, are curative of the very worst affection of the human race, are also destructive to a small extent if applied and administered by parties who have not thoroughly studied their properties.

Externally: Gerard writes: "To wash the feet in a decoction of Henbane causeth sleep, or given in a clyster it doth the same, also the smelling of the flowers. The roots are frequently hung about childrens neck to prevent fits, and cause an easy breeding of the teeth." The leaves make a fine external preparation for glandular swelling or ulcers, etc. It is best never to use Henbane under any circumstances without the advice of a good herbal physician.

Homoeopathic Clinical: Tincture of fresh plant—Amaurosis, Angina pectoris, Bladder (paralysis of), Bronchitis, Chorea, Coma vigil, Cough, Delirium tremens, Diarrhoea, Dysmenorrhoea, Enteric fever, Epilepsy, Epistaxis, Erotomania, Eyes (affections of), Haemoptysis, Haemorrhages, Hiccough, Hydrophobia, Hypochondriasis, Lochia (suppressed), Mania, Meningitis, Mind (affections of), Neuralgia, Night blindness, Nymphomania, Paralysis, Paralysis agitans, Parotitis, Pneumonia, Rage, Sleep (disorders of).

Russian Experience: When Russians say "Beleni obelsia", it is very bad, meaning persons have lost all common sense, are unreasonable and irresponsible. They express Henbane and its effect this way. Henbane is known as Belena Vonuchaya—Henbane Sticnky, or Belena Chernaya (Black Henbane), which does not have too much approval.

A Greek physician, Dioscorides Pedanius (AD 41–68), gave the name to this herb. All literature impresses upon us that Henbane is dangerous and poisonous. Can be used clinically by prescription and under close observation by medical personnel.

Folk Medicine: Use the burned seeds and smoke to help toothache; boiled herb is added to a hot bath for swollen legs and hands; also the herb is applied when one is bitten by mad dogs or other animals; Nastoika (Henbane and vodka) as rheumatic liniment pain killer (Bello-Russ. Academy of Science, 1965).

Medicinal Use: The leaves and herb are prescribed for stomach ulcers, bronchial asthma, bronchitis, midriasis (enlargement of the pupil), nervine, rheumatic and neuralgic pain (Atlas, Moscow, 1962). A leaf preparation of Henbane, Datura and Sage is made into special anti-asthmatic cigarettes for smokers troubled with bronchial asthma (Saratov University, 1962).

Industrial: Belena grows everywhere in Russia, soil and climate being no deterrent to its livelihood; the seeds can withstand any temperature, low or high, and can be dormant for long periods and life will emerge when seed and soil meet with the vitality of water and sun. Although prevalent everywhere in Russia, and although dangerous when wrongly administered, the wild collection does not meet the supply and demand. Agro-Technics have detailed information on plantations in Ukraine, South Russia. One plant averages 10,000 seeds; some literature claims nearly one million (950,000) seeds from one single plant. For 1 acre sow 4–5 lb. of seed; 65–70 per cent will germinate. In the autumn the seed is sown, without ploughing; in this case they use 5–6 lb. for each acre. As it is a biennial, the first year they harvest only at the end of the summer, but the next year they can harvest two or three times. One acre can produce 1,000 to 1,200 lb. of the dried herbs.

HOPS   Humulus lupulus, L.
(N.O.: Moraceae)

Features: The Hop plant is a long-lived dioecious perennial and is propagated commercially from rhizome sections or "root cuttings". The Hop is one of the few crop plant species in which male and female flowers are borne on different plants. Introduced and cultivated in the United States for its cones and strobiles, which are used medicinally and in the manufacture of beer, ale and porter.

Lupulin is preferred to the Hops itself and is procured by beating or rubbing the strobiles and then sifting out the grains, which form about one-seventh part of the Hops. Lupulin is a globose, kidney-shaped grain, golden yellow and somewhat transparent. This substance is the bitter principle of Hops, and is used in aqueous solutions of Lupulin.

The stem is rough, very long and will twist around any adjacent support. Leaves in pairs, stalked, serrated, cordate. Three- or five-lobed flowers or strobiles, consisting of membranous scales, yellowish-green, round, reticulate; veined, nearly $\frac{1}{2}$ in. long. Odour is peculiar and somewhat agreeable; taste slightly astringent and exceedingly bitter.

Medicinal Parts: The strobiles or cones.

Solvents: Boiling water, dilute alcohol.

Bodily Influence: Tonic, Diuretic, Nervine, Anodyne, Hypnotic, Anthelmintic, Sedative, Febrifuge.

Uses: This old-time plant is an excellent agent for many conditions. The fluid extract of 10 drops is often used in cough syrups where there is nervousness, and in heart palpitation.

The decoction of the Hops cleanses the blood, making it useful in venereal diseases and all kinds of skin abnormalities such as itch, ringworm, spreading sores, tetters and discolorations. It will tone up the liver, assist a sluggish gall-bladder, and will increase the flow of urine. Principally used for sedative or hypnotic action, producing sleep, removing restlessness and alleviating pain, especially so if combined with chamomile flowers. Use both internally and externally.

The Lupulin tincture is used in delirium tremens, nervous exhaustion, anxiety, worms, and does not disorder the stomach or cause constipation. Also useful in after-pains and to mitigate the pain attending gonorrhoea.

A pillow made of the dried Hops, sprinkled with alcohol to bring out the active principle, is used for wakefulness and generally induces sleep.

Dose: 1 teaspoonful of the flowers, cut small or granulated, to 1 cupful of boiling water. Drink cold 1 cupful during the day, a large mouthful at a time. Of the tincture, 5–20 min.

Externally: An ointment made by boiling 2 parts of Stramonium (Jimson weed) and 1 part of Hops, in lard, is an excellent application in skin irritation and itching skin.

Homoeopathic Clinical: Tincture of the seeded spikes—Trituration. Tincture of Cupuline—Dyspepsia, Dysuria, Gonorrhoea.

Russian Experience: Hmel is the Russian name for Hops, which to them (and us) is an expression for persons that are slightly drunk. This plant grows wild in many parts of the Russian territory and is cultivated for industrial breweries.

Folk Medicine: The medical properties have long been appreciated for success as Diuretic, Sedative and Calming. Used for inflammation of the bladder, tuberculosis, and as a hair tonic. The root decoction for jaundice and dandruff.

Dose: 1–20 min., or decoction of 2 tablespoonfuls to 1 pint of water, a mouthful three times a day; as a tea, $\frac{1}{2}$ cup three times a day.

Clinically: Used as extracts and compound tablets for the purposes already mentioned.

HOREHOUND   Marrubium vulgare, L.
(N.O.: Labiatae)

Common Names: HOREHOUND, WHITE HOREHOUND.

Features: The most common of the species of plants in the mint family (Labiatae). Horehound is native to Europe, but has escaped to waste places in temperate zones of North America, especially from Maine, southward of Texas and westward to California and Oregon. It grows on dry, sandy fields, waste grounds and roadsides. The most common horehound is Marrubium vulgare, originating from the Hebrew, "marrob", meaning "a bitter juice".

The entire plant is clothed in white, downy hairs, giving it a hoary appearance. Its stems are stout, four-angled and mainly erect, with opposite, ovate, rugose, crenately-toothed and softly white hairy leaves. The white flowers are small, strongly two-lipped and densely crowded in

154

the uppermost axils of the stems. The whole herb is medicinal. The flowers appear in June to September and should be gathered before the opening of the flowers. The plant yields a bitter juice of distinct odour and aromatically agreeable taste. The extract is used by the candy houses for an old-time prescription as a cough candy. Can be used fresh or dry.

Medicinal Part: The herb.

Solvents: Boiling water, diluted alcohol.

Bodily Influence: Stimulant, Tonic, Bitter Stomachic, Expectorant, Resolvent, Anthelmintic (large doses), Diuretic, Diaphoretic, Laxative.

Uses: Perhaps the most popular of herbal pectoral remedies for congestion of coughs, colds and pulmonary affections associated with unwanted phlegm from the chest. The warm infusion will produce perspiration and flow of urine, and is used with great benefit in jaundice, asthma, hoarseness, amenorrhoea and hysteria.

Taken in large doses it is laxative and will expel worms. The cold infusion is an excellent tonic for some forms of dyspepsia. Some herbalists have found it of use for mercurial salivation. Culpeper used Horehound in various other ways: "To repel the afterbirth, as an antidote to poisons and for the bites of venomous serpents." Others used it for running sores. The hot infusion of tincture is more effective when combined with other agents for the purpose intended.

Tincture of Skull cap (Scutellaria lateriflora), 2–15 drops.
Tincture of Pleurisy root (Asclepias tuberosa), 20–45 drops.
Tincture of Horehound (Marrubium vulgare), 5–40 drops.

In warm water every 2–3 hr., according to symptoms. Tincture alone,

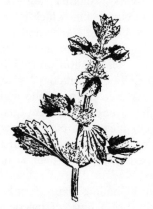

WHITE HOREHOUND
Marrubium vulgare, L.
(Dr. A. J. Thut, Guelph, Canada)

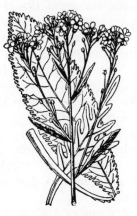

HORSE RADISH
Armoracia rusticana, Lam.
(Bello-Russ. Academy of Science,
Minsk, 1966)

155

20–30 min., as indicated by age and condition, every 2–3 hr. For children with coughs or croups, steep 1 heaped tablespoonful in 1 pint of boiling water for 20 min., strain, add honey. Should be drunk freely.

HORSE RADISH   Cochlearia armoracia, Lam.
(N.O.: Cruciferae)

Features: Originally Horse radish came to North America from eastern Europe. It has naturalized in the United States and Canada, and throughout most of the world.

The perennial root sends up numerous smooth, erect, branch stems, growing 2–3 ft. high. The large leaves are lanceolate, waved, scalloped on the edges and stand up on 1 ft. long stalks. The flowers are numerous and white, followed by seed pods divided into two cells, each containing four to six seeds. The hot, biting root is tapering, conical at the top; fleshy, whitish externally. The fresh root is much more powerful than the dried.

Medicinal Part: The root.

Bodily Influence: Stimulant, Diaphoretic, Diuretic, Digestive.

Uses: Effective for promoting stomach secretions and is used as a digestive agent. It has been used by Herbalists of the past as a most worthy diuretic. Dr. Coffin used a preparation of: 1 oz. fresh Horse radish root, sliced; $\frac{1}{2}$ oz. Mustard seed, bruised; 1 pint boiling water. Let it stand in a covered vessel for 4 hrs., then strain. Dose: 3 table-spoonfuls three times a day. This preparation is especially useful for retention of water when the body hoards water in abnormal amounts. Dr. Coffin also states that the above formula is "especially useful for dropsy occurring after fevers and intermittents". Another cause of this fearful disease is the retention of sulphur in our system, which interferes with the absorption and secretion of the endocrine glands and central nervous system. A syrup made of grated Horse radish, honey and water will control ordinary cases of hoarseness; 1 teaspoonful every 1–2 hr. Dr. Wood and Dr. Ruddock, M.D. in their book "Vitalogy" gives us more assurance of Horse radish as an agent in dropsy abnormalities "A warm infusion of the fresh root in cider, drunk in sufficient quantity to produce perspiration and repeated every night, has cured dropsy in two or three weeks." It also has merit in rheumatism, neuralgia, paralysis and in weak digestive organs, particularly the function of the pancreas.

Dose: 1 teaspoonful of the root to 1 cup of boiling water. Drink cold or hot, 1–2 cupfuls a day, a large mouthful at a time; of the tincture, $\frac{1}{2}$–1 fl. dram.

Homoeopathic Clinical: Tincture of the root—Albuminuria, Aphonia,

156

Asthma, Cataract, Colic, Cornea (spots on), Eruptions, Eyes (affections of), Gonorrhoea, Gravel, Headache, Leucorrhoea, Lungs (oedema of), Rheumatism, Scurvy, Strangury, Toothache, Ulcers, Urinary disorders. **Russian Experience:** Hren (Horse radish) is a bitter spice found growing in most gardens for home use as a food accompaniment, and Folk Medicine. This is a rich source of Vitamin C and is given in cases of scrofula, as a stomachic and diuretic. The juice of the root mixed with honey aids a sluggish liver. The whole root boiled in beer with Juniper berries is used for dropsy. Precaution: the beer should be from the old-time, naturally aged process, not artificial, fast-cured beer (Bello-Russ. Academy of Science, 1965).

HORSE TAIL   Equisetum arvense, L.
(N.O.: Equisetaceae)

Common Names: SHAVE GRASS, BOTTLEBRUSH, PEWTERWORT.

Features: Horse tail, Equisetum arvense, is among the many species of Horsetail. A perennial plant rising from creeping-root stocks, the numerous stems are furrowed, many-jointed; fruitication in terminal cone-like spikes. The spikes are the first to appear in the spring (can be prepared like asparagus) but they die after a few weeks and are followed by a clump of stems of which the outer layer contains a quality of silica. The plant grows in sand and gravel, along roadsides and railway tracks and in wet places.

The Indians and Mexicans used the stems for scouring pots; can also be used for polishing hardwood, ivory and brass (hence the common name Pewterwort).

Medicinal Part: The plant.

Solvent: Boiling water.

Bodily Influence: Diuretic, Astringent.

Uses: The Indians and early settlers used the stems as a stimulating diuretic in kidney and dropsical disorders. Horse tail is very much used today by Herbalists for eye and skin treatment because of the considerable amount of silica. Homoeopathic tablets of silica are used for catarrhal conditions with offensive, pus-like discharges of ear, nose, throat, glandular discharge, skin disorders, offensive perspiration, especially of the feet. It is also found beneficial in dropsy, gravel and all kinds of kidney affections. It strengthens the heart and lungs and is an excellent tonic when the whole system is enfeebled. For discomfort and difficulty in discharging urine, it is not to be replaced. A specific in bleeding of all kinds, taken internally, but should be discontinued when taken alone for bleeding when cessation takes place.

Internally in all indicated conditions the following is used:

157

Tincture of Shave grass (Equisetum arvense), 5–20 drops
Tincture of Couch Grass (Triticum repens), 20–40 drops
Tincture of Corn Silk (Stigma maydis), 10–20 drops.

In water three or more times a day as required by condition. As a herbal tea by itself, or combined with the above, steep 1 teaspoonful in 1 cup of boiling water for 45 min., in covered container. Cool, take a mouthful four times a day.

Externally: As a compress or sponge bath for old injuries, putrid wounds, gangrenous ulcers or external bleeding. Simmer covered for ½ hr., cool and administer; make fresh daily.

Homoeopathic Clinical: Tincture of fresh plant chopped and pounded to a pulp—Cystitis, Dropsy, Enuresis, General paralysis, Gleet, Gonorrhoea, Gravel, Haematuria, Urine (retention of).

Russian Experience: Distinction of Hvosh Polevoy (Horsetail) is given medical recognition; many others are similar, but not valued as the same.

Folk Medicine: Use Horsetail as a tea, Nastoika (with vodka), and as a powder, in many cases. Known as a Diuretic in heart conditions due to dropsy (excess of water) and deficiency of blood circulation. Is of use in kidney stones, but should not be used when the kidneys are inflamed. When bleeding from the stomach or intestinal tract, Horsetail is your medicine; also useful in excessive female bleeding. Folk Medicine has also found the properties valuable for blood purifying and liver

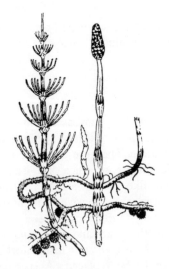

HORSETAIL
Equisetum arvense, L.
(Bello-Russ. Academy of Science,
Minsk, 1966)

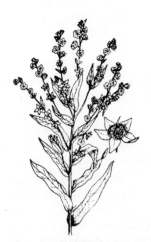

A—HOUND'S-TONGUE   B—Fruit
(Ontario Department of
Agriculture, Toronto, Canada,
1966)

158

conditions. Experimentally, an important agent to cleanse the system of lead poisoning and as a diuretic (Medical Literature, Moscow, 1962).

Clinically: In use as an extract, tincture, tablets and powder.

Externally: A powder for bleeding wounds and ulcers; also for veterinary use of the same conditions.

HOUND'S-TONGUE   Cynoglossum, L.
(N.O.: Boraginaceae)

Common Names: GYPSY FLOWER, DOG'S TONGUE.

Features: Hound's-tongue grows on the roadsides and waste places in both Europe and America. A biennial herb of medium size, 2–3 ft. high. The leaves are tongue-shaped, hoary with soft down on both sides. Flowers are blue to lavender, funnel form on terminal panicles, growing in clusters. The fruit, like Burdock, when dry sticks to livestock and hunting dogs. The leaves are bitter, and the root when fresh has an unpleasant heavy odour, diminishing when dry. It can be used in both fresh and dry stages, if when gathered it is properly dried and stored. Internally should be used by persons of professional experience.

Medicinal Parts: The leaves and root.

Solvent: Water.

Bodily Influence: Anodyne, Demulcent, Astringent.

Uses: The Indian's knowledge of Hound's-tongue was to cook the root for relief in colic, and as a poultice for scalds and burns. It is chiefly valuable for coughs, catarrh, bleeding from the lungs and other disorders of the respiratory apparatus, the action of the root being cooling, drying and binding. It is very soothing to the digestive organs in diarrhoea, dysentery and relief of piles.

Externally: According to Herbalists of long experience, bruised Hound's-tongue leaves applied to the lesion of a bite from a mad dog is the only medication needed. They also state that loss of hair from high fevers is controlled by bruising the leaves and making a salve with swine's grease and massaging over the scalp.

The leaves and root are both applied with great benefit as a poultice to old ulcers, scrofulous tumours, burns, goitres and recent bruises and abrasions.

Russian Experience: If the Russian name, Sobachyi Yazik, were translated it would be the same as our common name, Dog's tongue, but in literature it is used as Chernyi Koren—Black Root. Old Folk Medicine found many uses for Hound's-tongue: to reduce pain, swelling of boils, cramps, coughs, tuberculosis and stomach aches. The leaves were collected when in flower, May to June; roots in late summer and early autumn.

Recent literature usually warns against unexperienced use as it has a toxic effect if improperly administered.

Externally: It is used as a poultice for boils, wounds, ulcers and the bite of snakes or mad dogs. The powder mixed with grease, oil or lard as an ointment for rheumatic pains, and as Nastoika (with vodka) for wounds.

Insecticide: It is not unusual to find organic material poisonous to troublesome creatures such as insects and rodents. It has been proven that these creatures cannot stand the smell of Dog's-tongue, and will leave the premises as soon as the aroma reaches them. It is said they will abandon ship and jump into the sea if there is a trace of this used as an insecticide.

HYDRANGEA   Hydrangea arborescens, L.
(N.O.: Saxifragaceae)

Common Names: WILD HYDRANGEA, SEVEN BARKS (due to the seven separate layers of different coloured bark).

Features: Indigenous to North America and native to woodlands of rich, moist and some shady soil. There are twenty-three species of arborescens related to the well-known cultivated Hydrangea, widely distributed in eastern Asia, eastern, north central, and South America. The flowers are mostly white, often tinged with pink or purple, and in a few are entirely coloured depending on the acidity or alkalinity of the soil. Because the flowers appear from July through September (later in milder climates), the plants are highly valued for garden beauty and readily grown from cuttings or layering.

Medicinal Parts: The dried root (J. Kloss used the leaves as Tonic, Diuretic, Sialagogue).

Solvent: Water.

Bodily Influence: Cathartic, Diuretic, Nephritic (relieving kidney disorders).

Uses: An old and admirable remedy for gravel, and is best known for relieving the excruciating pain experienced when the gravelly formations pass through the ureters from the kidneys to the bladder. Also recognized for inflamed tissue of the kidney and urinary organs. Will relieve backache caused by kidney trouble, chronic rheumatism, parallelism scurvy and dropsy.

Dose: A syrup or decoction of the root may be taken in teaspoonful doses several times a day.

Homoeopathic Clinical: Tincture of fresh leaves and young shoots, fluid extract—Bladder (catarrh of; stone in), Diabetes, Gravel, Prostatic affections, Urine (incontinence of).

160

HYSSOP   Hyssopus officinalis, L.
(N.O.: Labiatae)

Common Name: HYSSOP.

Features: Native to southern Europe, sparsely naturalized in the United States. The common Hyssop, of the mint family (H. officinalis), is a perennial shrubby plant with square stems, woody at the base with rod-like branches reaching 2 ft. in height. The leaves stand in pairs without petioles. They have an agreeable aromatic odour; hot, spicy and somewhat bitter taste. The flowers are bluish-purple, growing chiefly on one side of short verticillate spikes, flowering in July.

Hyssop is spoken of in the Bible (Psalms 51:7) in connection with cleansing and purifying the body. There seems to be some controversy as to the particular plant. The Hebrew name "ezeb" has been translated "hyssop", and this is said to have grown out of the walls. It is quite possible the name is applied to several plants of similar properties.

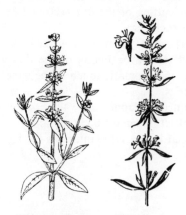

HYSSOP   Hyssopus officinalis, L.
1—Top part.   2—Flower
(Naukova Dumka, Kiev, USSR, 1965)

Medicinal Parts: Tops and leaves.

Solvents: Water, alcohol.

Bodily Influence: Stimulant, Aromatic, Carminative, Tonic, Expectorant.

Uses: Generally used in quinsy and other sore throats as a gargle with sage. Valuable in asthma, colds, la grippe and all chest affections, and shortness of breath. Excellent as a blood regulator, both increasing the circulation of the blood and reducing blood pressure. Is a fine tonic for the mucous tissue of both respiratory and gastro-intestinal tract in all weakened conditions. Serviceable in connection with hygienic herbs, scrofula, gravel, various stomach complaints, jaundice, dropsy, spleen malfunction. Has been used in Herbal preparations for epilepsy.

161

Culpeper says: "Mixed with honey will kill worms of the belly". The hot vapours of the decoction will ease inflammation and singing noise of the ear if a funnel relays the vapours of simmering Hyssop to this area.

Dose: 1 oz. to 1 pint infusion is given in wineglass doses throughout the day according to age.

Externally: The fresh leaves are valuable when bruised to relieve the pain and discoloration of the bruise. Healing to fresh wounds and old ulcers.

Russian Experience: Take the first letter "H" from Hyssop and it will be a Russian name, "Yssop". It is not considered a wild growing plant in Russia, but cultivation is profitable for medical, industrial and commercial uses.

Folk Medicine: Has known of its use as Expectorant and Stimulant for asthma and chronic bronchitis.

Externally: For healing wounds and ulcers.

Industrial: From the second year after planting Hyssop, you can harvest for the next ten years, with each yield growing stronger and more plentiful. Every year cutting of the dry herb and flowers can yield from 1,500 to 3,000 lb. for each acre.

For medical purpose Hyssop is collected before flowering. For industrial oil extract, at the beginning of the flowering season. Hyssop is used for its strong and aromatic touch in the wine, food, confectionery and cosmetic industries.

Bees like Hyssop nectar; from 1 acre they can easily, even in a short Russian summer, collect pollen for 60 lb. of honey.

Hungary has special industrial plantations for Hyssop oil extract.

INDIGO—WILD   Baptisia tinctoria, R, Rr.
(N.O.: Leguminosae)

Common Names: RATTLE BUSH, HORSEFLY BUSH, WILD INDIGO, YELLOW INDIGO.

Features: The wild Indigo of the United States is many of several species of closely related genus, Baptisia, of the pea family, which flourishes especially in the southern and eastern states of U.S.A. The blackish and woody root of this perennial plant sends up a stem which is very much branched, round, smooth and from 2–3 ft. high. The leaves are rounded at their extremity, small and alternate. The bright yellow flowers appear in July and August. The fruit is a bluish-black colour in the form of an oblong pod, and contains indigo, tannin, acid and baptisia. Any portion of the plant, when dried, yields a blue dye which is, however, not equal in value to indigo. If the shoots are used after they acquire a green colour they will cause dramatic purgation. The virtues of the root reside chiefly in the bark.

Medicinal Part: Bark of the root and leaves.

Solvents: Alcohol, boiling water.

Bodily Influence: Antiseptic, Stimulant, Purgative, Emmenagogue.

Uses: Medicinally this plant seems to have served the desert tribes for the same type of "all round" herb as did the Yerba Santa of the more western areas. A stem decoction was thought of most highly for pneumonia, tuberculosis and influenza. The tips of Indigo combined and boiled with chopped twigs of Utah Juniper (Juniperus osteosperma) was used as a kidney medication. The tea from Indigo was used in cases of smallpox, given internally in small doses and externally as a cleansing wash.

The Flower Hospital in New York made extensive experiments with this herb and found that the Indians knew their medicine. It is of great importance in all septic and degenerative conditions manifesting themselves in various forms of ulceration, and importance in serious eruptive diseases. Dependably reliable in ulceration and mucous colitis and amoebic dysentery, both of which are persistently difficult to treat. In follicular tonsilitis and quinsy it is indicated as internal medication and as a gargle.

The action of Baptisia exerts a vital influence, aiding in metabolism by stimulating the elimination of accumulated waste in the body and encourages normal organic activity. Dr. Clymer recommends the following. In all morbid, internal conditions a dependable formula is:

163

Tincture of Wild Indigo (Baptisia tinctoria), 2–20 drops
Tincture of Rhatany (Krameria triandra), 10–20 drops
Tincture of Cone flower (Echinacea angustifolia), 2–20 drops.

In water every 2–4 hr., depending on symptoms. Dosage: tincture alone, Baptisia 2–20 drops. (Keep out of children's reach.)

Generally of great importance to all septic conditions of the blood, serious forms of prostration, muscular soreness, rheumatic and arthritic pains, and constriction of the chest. Advisable to combine with other remedies when there are chills with fever.

Homoeopathic Clinical: Tincture of fresh root and its bark—Abortion (threatened), Apoplexy, Appendicitis, Biliousness, Brain softening, Cancer, Consumption, Diphtheria, Dysentery, Enteric fever, Eye (affections of), Gall-bladder (affections of), Gastric fever, Headache (bilious), Hectic fever, Hysteria, Influenza, Mumps, Oesophagus (stricture of), Plague, Tinea capitis Tongue (ulcerated), Typhus, Variola, Worms.

Indian and Pakistani Experience: Some of the local names are Guli, Nil-Nilika—Common and Indian Indigo.

Uses: The plant has Deobstruent and Alterative properties. Decoction or powder for Whooping cough, Bronchitis, Heart conditions, Dropsy, Kidney and Bladder, Lung disease, Liver and Spleen enlargement, Nervous disorders, Epilepsy.

Externally: To promote urination, applications of leaf poultice or a paste of Indigo and warm water is placed over the bladder area; also in skin conditions and haemorrhoids. Indigo dye for burns, scalds, insect sting, animal bites; Indigo dust for ulcers, boils. ("Medical Plants of India and Pakistan", J. D. Dastur, Bombay, 1962.)

IRON WEED   Vernonia, Schreb.
(N.O.: Compositae)

Common Name: IRON WEED.

Features: This is an indigenous perennial; several species grow abundantly in woods, along roadsides, prairies, beside rivers and streams throughout the eastern and southern parts of the country as far west as Kansas and Texas. The purplish-green, coarse, composite plant has stems from 3–10 ft. high. The leaves are from 4–8 in. long, dark purple and showy. They bear heads of magenta-coloured flowers from July to September somewhat like miniature thistles. The root is bitter.

Medicinal Parts: The root and leaves.

Solvents: Water, alcohol.

Bodily Influence: Tonic, Deobstruent, Alterative.

Uses: This plant is particularly useful in female complaints, amenorrhoea, dysmenorrhoea, leucorrhoea and menorrhagia. Considered a certain remedy for chills and intermittent and bilious fevers, and also valuable in scrofula, diseases of the skin and in constitutional syphilis. Some physicians employed it in the treatment of dyspepsia.

Dose: Of the decoction, ½ wineglassful or more. Of the tincture, 20–30 teaspoonfuls several times a day. A decoction of the leaves is esteemed a good gargle in sore throat.

IVY AMERICAN   Vitis quinquefolia, Lam.
(N.O.: Vitaceae)

Common Names: WOODBINE, VIRGINIA CREEPER, FIVE LEAVES, FALSE GRAPE, WILD WOOD VINE.

Features: The American Ivy is a common, familiar shrubby vine of the grape family. Ascending to the height of 50–100 ft., extensively by means of its radiating tendrils, supporting itself firmly on trees, stone walls, churches, etc. This is a woody vine, with smooth digitate leaves and many leaflets. The greenish or white flowers are inconspicuous. The bark and twigs should be collected after the small dark berries have ripened. Its taste is acrid and persistent, though not unpleasant; the decoction is mucilaginous.

Medicinal Parts: The bark and twigs.

Solvent: Boiling water.

Bodily Influence: Tonic, Astringent, Expectorant.

Uses: It is used principally in the form of syrup, in scrofula, and is a reputed remedy for dropsy, bronchitis and other pulmonary complaints.

From the herbalist, J. E. Meyers (1939), and those who have gone before us: "There is great antipathy between Wine and Ivy, and therefore it is a remedy to preserve against drunkenness, and to relieve or cure intoxication by drinking a draught of wine in which a handful of bruised Ivy leaves have been boiled."

Dose: 1 teaspoonful of the bark or twigs cut small or granulated to 1 cup of boiling water. Drink cold during the day, a large mouthful at a time. Of the decoction of syrup, from 1–4 tablespoonfuls three times a day. The common Ivy of Europe (Hedera helex) is used as a poultice or fomentation in glandular enlargements, indolent ulcers, abscesses, etc. Potter (1956): "The berries are found of use in febrile disorders and a vinegar of this was extensively used during the London plague."

Homoeopathic Clinical: Tincture of plant; Decoction of chopped inner bark—Cholera, Dropsy, Hoarseness, Hydrocele.

JIMSON WEED   Datura stramonium, L.
(N.O.: Solanaceae)

Common Names: THORN APPLE, STINKWEED, APPLE PERU, JAMESTOWN
WEED.

Features: Datura, a small genus of about fifteen species of annual, shrub
and small trees, belonging to the nightshade family (Solanaceae). "Jamestown Weed" is the name given by colonists who found the plant growing
on ship rubbish near Jamestown, Virginia. It has migrated, especially to
Michigan, and almost every part of the United States. Can be found
growing in roadsides and waste ground (never in mountains or woods).

Stramonium is an annual, over 4 ft. tall, with ovate, unevenly toothed
glabrous, strong-scented leaves; white or purplish funnel-form flowers,
and hard, prickly, many-seeded capsule splitting in four valves. Seeds
are small, roughish, dark brown or black when ripe, greyish brown when
unripe. They yield what is called "Datura". The name Stinkweed refers
to the unpleasant narcotic odour, especially of the bruised leaves, which
diminishes as it dries. Almost every part of the plant is possessed of
medicinal properties, but the official parts are leaves and seeds. The
leaves should be gathered when the flowers are full grown, and carefully dried in the shade.

Medicinal Parts: The leaves and seeds.

Solvents: Alcohol, hot water (partially).

Bodily Influence: Anodyne, Antispasmodic.

Uses: D. stramonium is seldom used by Herbalists. In four and a half
years of study with N. G. Tretchikoff we have never seen the agent in
use. In large doses it is an energetic narcotic poison, inflicting intense
agony on the victim and death by maniacal delirium. The Indians used
a preparation of the plant in various ways. The main reason being to
induce fanciful dreams. They dried the leaves and smoked them as a
cure for asthma, if the patient had a sound heart. We prefer other plants
that have mutual effect without the possibility of uncertain tolerance.
Medicinally it is often used as a substitute for opium. It has fairly good
effect in cases of mania, epilepsy, gastritis, delirium tremens and enteritis.
Also neuralgia, rheumatism and all periodic pains.

The information regarding this herb is only for identification, as in this
case, what is not fully understood should not be in possession.

Externally: The Indians sometimes crushed the plant and bound it on
bruises and swellings and there is record of its use in extreme cases of
saddle sores on horses and also a cure for rattlesnake and tarantula bites.

Its medicinal qualities are quite important if its use is entrusted to proper and educated persons.

Homoeopathic Clinical: Tincture of fresh plant in flower and fruits— Anasarca (after Scarlatina), Aphasia, Apoplexy, Burns, Catalepsy, Chordee, Chorea, Delirium tremens, Diaphragmitis, Ecstasy, Enuresis, Epilepsy, Erotomania, Eyes (affections of), Headache (from sun), Hiccough, Hydrophobia, Hysteria, Lochia (offensive), Locomotor ataxia, Mania, Meningitis, Nymphomania, Oesophagus (spasm of), Scarlatina, Stammering (starting), Strabismus, Sunstroke, Tetanus, Thirst, Tremors Trismus, Typhus.

Russian Experience: Durman Vonuchyi, Durman Indyisky is Russia's name for Datura stramonium. The plant was first introduced as a botanical garden specimen, now it invades nearly all of the Russian territory. The Datura implies that the brain and nerves are so affected that persons no longer are in control of themselves, or are deadly poisoned.

Folk Medicine: Use is made of Stramonium in many assorted ways. The amount of seeds in vodka (Nastoika), depending on the child's age, for treatment when paralysis due to a severe scare; decoction for epilepsy, stenocordid (Angina Pectoris); leaves were shredded and rolled to smoke for bronchial Asthma (Bello-Russ. Academy of Science, 1965).

Externally: A liniment of Nastoika (vodka and Jamestown weed) is

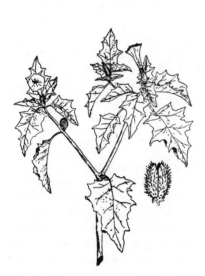

A—Jimson weed
Datura stramonium, L.   B—Pod
(Ontario Department of Agriculture,
Toronto, Canada, 1966)

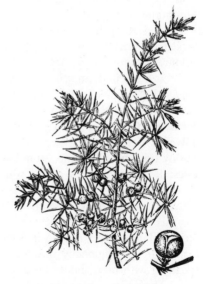

Juniper   Juniperus communis, L.
A—Branch   B—Berry
(Vishaya Schkolla, Moscow, 1963)

167

applied to rheumatic and radiculitis (inflamation of the nerve root) pain (Bello-Russ. Academy of Science, 1965).

Clinically: Prescribed mainly for Asthma, Angina Pectoris, Bronchitis; all possible caution should be taken when administering Datura stramonium, even by medical personnel.

Industrial: Soon after introduction, distribution was felt throughout the land. The wild collection soon led to successful special cultivated plantations in South Russia, Ukranie, Don river regions (Krasnodar).

Dose: To plant 1 acre, 1–1¼ lb. of seed are required, if planted by the "nest" system; 5 lb. if planted in "row" system (Atlas, Moscow, 1963). As this plant is poisonous, gloves should be worn when collecting the leaves and plant. Jamestown Weed is poisonous to horses, cattle and geese; fresh, or portions of the dry herb, is in hay, even in the minimum dose.

JUNIPER   Juniperus communis, L.
(N.O.: Pinaceae)

Common Names: JUNIPER BUSH, JUNIPER BERRIES.

Features: An ornamental evergreen of the pine family with trees and shrubs of about forty species. The common Juniper (J. communis) is a smaller species, usually less than 25 ft. tall, and many of its numerous varieties are less than 10 ft. This shrub is common on dry, sterile hills from Canada south to New Jersey, west to Nebraska, and in the Rocky Mountains of New Mexico.

The leaves open in whorls of three, are glaucous and concave above, keeled underneath. Flowers in May, with fleshy fruit of dark-purplish colour, ripening in the second year after the flower. Every part of the shrub is medicinal, and the French peasantry prepare a sort of tar which they call "huile-de-cade" from the interior reddish wood of the trunk and branches. This is our popular Juniper tar.

Medicinal Part: The ripe dry berries.

Solvents: Boiling water, alcohol.

Bodily Influence: Diuretic, Stimulant, Carminative.

Uses: If we may speak of the conditions of internal accumulative filth we would suggest Juniper berries as an agent used for fumigating the system to ward off contagion. S. Kneip, of "My Water Cure" (1897), has this to say about the berries: "Those who are nursing patients with serious illness as Scarlet fever, small pox, typhus, cholera, etc. and are exposed to contagion by raising, carrying, or serving the patient, or by speaking with him, should always chew a few juniper-berries (6 to 10 a day). They give a pleasant taste in the mouth and are of good service to the digestion, they burn up as it were, the harmful miasms, exhalations, when these seek to enter through the mouth or nostrils."

168

Persons with weak stomach should chew five softened berries a few days in succession, increasing the amount one a day until fifteen berries a day are taken. Then decrease the amount by one berry a day for five more days. Obstinate stomach troubles have been relieved by releasing pressures that cause stomach tissue weakness, indigestion, in general poor assimilation. For sluggish conditions of the kidneys, Juniper berries will be found most serviceable; they increase the flow of urine, but should not be used alone in sensitive conditions. Small doses reduce irritation, while large doses may increase it, so it is best to combine with Peach leaves (Amygdalus persica), a little Marshmallow root (Althea officinalis), Uva ursi (Arctostaphylos), Parsley (Petroselinum sativum), Alfalfa (Medicago sativa), etc.

A useful agent for many ailments: expels wind and strengthens the stomach, for coughs and shortness of breath, consumption, rupture, cramps, convulsions, gout, sciatica, dropsy and ague. It will strengthen the nerves and is an agent used for epilepsy; some causes are aggravated due to stomach, intestinal and nerve vibratory interference. Kills worms in children and adults. Dr. Coffin tells us: "If Juniper boughs are burnt to ashes and the ashes put into water, a medicine will be obtained that has cured the dropsy in an advanced stage."

For fumigating a room which has been used by a patient with an infectious disease, a solution used as a spray destroys all fungi.

Dose: To make an infusion, several tablespoonfuls of the berries are generally prepared by macerating (softening by soaking), then adding them to 1 pint of boiling water for $\frac{1}{2}$ hr. or more. Cool and divide the mixture into four portions, which is then taken morning, noon, afternoon and evening. Dose of the tincture, 10–30 drops.

Homoeopathic Clinical: Tincture of fresh ripe berries—Dropsy, Dysmenorrhoea, Haemorrhage.

Russian Experience: Mozshevelnik Obiknovennyi, or Juniper vulgaris, grows in many parts of Russia. The berries and twigs are used for medical purpose with Nastoika (in vodka) as Diuretic, Expectorant, Disinfectant, Digestive, Antiseptic (Atlas, Moscow, 1962).

Junipers are direct in affect and the doses should be kept very small; steep 1 teaspoonful in 1 cup of boiling water for 15 min., strain, take 1 tablespoonful three times a day. Warning: cannot be used when kidneys are inflamed. Used successfully in Colpatitis (vaginal inflammation) (Saratov University, 1962). The raw berries for stomach ulcers, decoction of berries and twigs for menstrual restoration and diatheses (uric acid) retention throughout, or specific parts of the body.

169

KIDNEY LIVER LEAF   Hepatica americana, Schreb.
(N.O.: Ranunculaceae)

Common Names: NOBLE LIVERWORT, LIVER LEAF, CHOISY, LICHEN CANINUS.

Features: One of our earliest harbingers of spring. The purplish-white flowers appear almost as soon as the snow leaves the ground. The leaves are all radical, on hairy evergreen stems. Fruit an ovate achenium. The Liverworts include some 8,500 species in approximately 237 genera. Most of them are small, leafy plants, easily and commonly mistaken for mosses. More common are Round-lobed Hepatica (Americana) and Sharp-lobed (H. acutiloba). They are common to both the U.S.A. and Canada and are found in warm, moist tropical conditions, along stream banks and in damp shaded forests; some occur in drier situations, however.

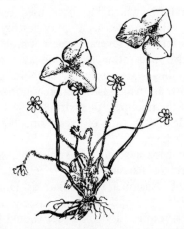

KIDNEY LIVER LEAF   Hepatica nobilis, Schreb.
(Bello-Russ. Academy of Science, Minsk, 1967)

Medicinal Part: The whole plant.
Solvent: Water.
Bodily Influence: Tonic, Demulcent, Deobstruent, Mild Mucilaginous, Astringent.
Uses: An innocent herb which may be taken for all diseases of the liver, which in sickness or health influences so many functions of our system. Recommended in lung affections, coughs, bleeding of the lungs and the

170

early stages of consumption, by cooling and cleansing the inflamed areas. Usually combined with other herbal plants, but can be taken as infusion of 1 oz. to 1 pint of boiling water in wineglassful doses, repeated frequently. Of the tincture, $\frac{1}{2}$–1 fl. dram.

Homoeopathic Clinical: Tincture of full-grown leaves—Bronchitis, Catarrh, Dyspepsia, Epistaxis, Throat (sore).

Russian Experience: Hepatic Noble, or in Russian, Pereleska blagorodnaya, grows plentifully in Russia.

Folk Medicine: From earliest historical use for jaundice, fever, cough, chronic bronchitis, headache, eye-wash. As medication for cattle of mouth sickness (Sibirskaya Yazva) Bello-Russ. Academy of Science, 1965).

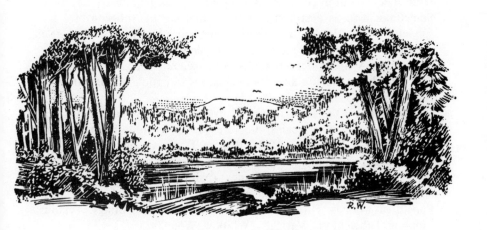

LABRADOR TEA   Ledum latifolium, Jacq.

(N.O.: Ericaceae)

Common Names: JAMES TEA, MARSH TEA, WILD ROSEMARY, CONTINENTAL TEA.

Features: An evergreen shrub common to North America and is found as far south as Wisconsin and Pennsylvania. They are low ornamental plants from 1–6 ft. high, having narrow, dark leaves lined underneath with rust-coloured wooly hairs and bearing white, bell-shaped flowers in the early spring. During the American Revolution the leaves are said to have been used as a substitute for commercial tea.

Medicinal Part: The leaves.

Solvent: Boiling water.

Bodily Influence: Pectoral, Expectorant, Diuretic.

Uses: Very useful in coughs, colds, bronchial and pulmonary affections. Sometimes used as a table tea. For internal use the infusion of 1 teaspoonful of dried leaves to 1 cup of boiling water in wineglassful doses as needed for the control of the above mentioned.

Externally: A strong decoction has been recommended for external use as a remedy for itching and exanthematous (eruptions accompanied by fever) skin diseases.

Homoeopathic Clinical: Tincture of dried small twigs and leaves collected after flowering begins; tincture of whole fresh plant—Ascites, Asthma, Bites, Black eye, Boils, Bruises, Deafness, Ear (inflammation of), Eczema, Erythema nodosum, Face (pimples on), Feet (pains in, tender), Gout, Haemoptysis, Hands (pains in), Intoxication, Joints (affections of, cracking in Menier's disease), Pediculosis, Prickly heat, Punctured wounds, Rheumatism, Skin (eruption on), Stings, Tetanus, Tinnitus, Tuberculosis, Varicella, Whitlow, Wounds.

Russian Experience: The common Russian name is Bogulnik but literature gives it another, Herba Ledu, which is very close to Canadian Ledum palustra, or Ledum marshland. Bogulnik sometimes covers miles of marshland in European Russia, Siberia and the Far East, making it impossible for other plants to invade this strong shrub abode.

The young leaves and twigs are collected in August and September. Care must be observed when drying as one of the various volatile ether oils it contains is $7\frac{1}{2}$ per cent Ledum; the strong aroma from which could seriously affect the heart if one is in too close confinement during this plant drying stage (Moscow University, 1963).

Folk Medicine: Medical literature gives full credit to Folk Medicine

172

though it is not fully experimented clinically. Leaves and twigs are officially collected for state institutes and sold to pharmacies and dispensaries (Atlas, Moscow, 1962).

Uses: Accommodates Coughs, Bronchitis, Bronchial asthma, Tubercular lungs, Stomach sickness, Headache, Kidney and weak Bladder, Rickets, Diarrhoea, Rheumatism (internally, and as a liniment or ointment), Pains in the chest, Scrofula, Scaby dandruff (blanketed on the scalp, or in patches). Additional: fertility, infections, tightness of breath (Bello-Russ. Academy of Science). Can cure Bronchitis in two weeks. Recommended as a tea decoction of 1 oz. tea to 2 pints boiling water; drink as required, a mouthful at a time (Medicina, Moscow, 1965).

Externally: Russian Homoeopaths boil the flowers in fresh butter making an ointment for skin diseases, bruises, wounds, bleeding and rheumatism (Moscow University, 1963).

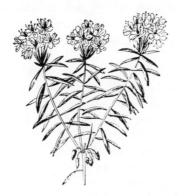

LABRADOR TEA   Ledum latifolium, Jacq.
(Medicina, Moscow, 1965)

LADY'S SLIPPER—Cypripedium pubescens, Willd.
(N.O.: Orchidaceae)

Common Names: NERVE ROOT, NOAH'S ARK, YELLOW LADY'S SLIPPER, AMERICAN VALERIAN, YELLOW MOCCASIN FLOWER.

Features: Lady's slippers are among the primitive members of the family Orchidaceae and are among the most beautiful and best known orchids. Some fifty species comprise the genus cypripedium, found in Europe, Asia and North America and as far south as the tropics. There are eleven species found in North America. Professor Rainesque, in "Medical Botany", of the University of Pennslyvania, says: "All species are equally remedial."

The plant grows in North America in rich woods and meadows and flowers in May and June. The two or more folded and prominently ribbed

173

leaves are sheathed, located near the base of the plant or on the stem. The usually showy flowers (numbering one to twelve) are characterized by the sessile, inflated or pouch-shaped, variously coloured lip, from which the plant received its general name, Aphrodite's shoe. The Indians called the beautiful plant "Mocassin Flower", its use being known to them for generations. The empyrics of new England, particularly Samuel Thompson, had much respect for mutual evidence. The fibrous roots are the parts used in medicine and they should be gathered and carefully cleaned in August or September.

Medicinal Part: The root.

Solvents: Boiling water, diluted alcohol.

Bodily Influence: Antiperiodic, Nervine, Tonic.

Uses: This medicine is an excellent nervine and acts as a tonic to the exhausted nervous system, improving by circulation and nutrition of the nerve centres. It relieves pain (if present) and produces a calm and tranquil condition of body and mind. From the quick response and high attributions many suppose it possesses narcotic properties, but to this the answer is "none present".

It is of special value in reflex functional disorders or chorea, hysteria, nervous headache, insomnia, low fevers, nervous unrest, hypochondria and nervous depression accompanying stomach disorders. During fevers its use is indicated for restlessness and during the early fever stages of pneumonia, combined with a little lobelia (Lobelia inflata) and Ginger (Zingiber), it will often cut short the trouble. Combine with Skull cap (Scutellaria) in various nervous affections such as hysteria, headache, St. Vitus dance or other diseases of this nature. For the feeling of depression due to stomach disorders, Lady's slipper (Cypripedium) and Chamomile (Anthemis nobilis) is your preparation, before meals, and on retiring. As a home remedy the root is best roughly ground, 5 tablespoonfuls in 1 pint of boiling water; steep for an hour, 1 tablespoonful every hour, as needed. Of the tincture of Cypripedium alone, 5–30 drops, according to age and severity of condition.

Homoeopathic Clinical: Tincture and infusion of fresh root gathered in autumn—Brain affections, Chorea, Convulsions, Debility and sleeplessness, Delirium tremens, Ecstasy, Epilepsy, Mental despondency, Nervous debility, Neuralgia, Post-influenza debility, Sleeplessness, Spermatorrhoea, Stye.

LARKSPUR Delphinium consolida, L.
(N.O.: Ranunculaceae)

Common Names: LARK'S CLAW, LARK'S HEEL, KNIGHT'S SPUR.

Features: An annual herb native to Europe, but has become naturalized

174

in the northern states of the U.S.A. The American species are known either as Tall larkspurs, which are 3–7 ft. in height and grow in moist places of higher altitudes and bloom in summer; or Low larkspur, which are found in open or exposed places to an elevation of 3,000 ft. Only four species of the seventy-nine native to North America occur east of the Mississippi, the majority being western in distribution, often in small areas.

The leaves are palmate and variously cut or divided. The flowers are mostly blue, but some are scarlet, red, bluish, white, or even yellow, in cultivated forms. The corolla consists of two sets of two petals each, the lower bearing a slender claw extending into the large calyx spur. The root is simple and slender; capsule—fruit or seed. Odour faint; taste bitter, then biting, acrid.

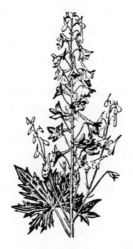

LARKSPUR Delphinium consolida, L.
(Medicina, Moscow, 1965)

Medicinal Parts: The root and seeds.
Solvent: Dilute alcohol.
Bodily Influence: Emetic, Cathartic, Narcotic, Parasiticide.
Uses: The Hopi tribes used the pollen of S. Scaposum, by grinding the flowers with corn to make blue meal (blue pollen). Seldom used internally and only when prescribed by physicians of experience.

The flowers and leaves were extensively used in the United States army during the rebellion to kill lice and it is pretty well authenticated that the same substance forms the basis of many preparations offered for the destruction of all noxious insects whose room is better than their company. Dr. Brown (1875): "A tincture of the seeds, it is said, will cure Asthma and Dropsy, also a specific for cholera morbus."

Dose: 1 oz. of the seeds added to 1 quart of diluted alcohol makes the tincture, of which 10 drops may be given three times a day. This, however, should be used only in extreme cases, and with the approval of persons of knowledge on the subject.

Russian Experience: Szivokost, or Alive Bone, is Russia's Larkspur. They use the herb and flower, but with caution, as Delphinium is very poisonous. However, it has its useful place in Herbal practice if the "how and when" are observed.

Folk Medicine: As a poultice and wash, but very carefully given. For enlarged liver, stomach and intestinal trouble, urinary system, and venereal diseases. Decoction of Delphinium for inflammation of the lungs, pleurisy, headaches, tapeworm, female sickness, chronic coughs, toothaches, and when frightened.

Dose: 20 grams to 4 cups of boiling water; do not drink more than 3 cups a day, a mouthful at a time. Decoction of the flower as a poultice when eyes are inflamed with pus. The same decoction as a tea for cramps, convulsions, amenorrhoea (Bello-Russ. Academy of Science, 1965).

Clinically: As tablets, ampoules and powder in compounds when muscle tension, or excitement, after operations when the brain and central nerve system has expended involuntary vital energy, Parkinson's disease, spreading sclerosis, paralysis. Also used in surgery combined with narcotics (Atlas, 1962).

Industrial: A dye of especially beautiful blue colour for silks and woollens is made for the textile industry; also blue writing ink (Moscow University, 1963).

LEVERWOOD   Ostria virginiana (Mill) K. Koch
(N.O.: Betulaceae)

Common Names: IRONWOOD, HOP HORN BEAM, DEERWOOD.

Features: Probably the best-known species in America is Ostria virginiana, Leverwood, a popular name for many trees whose timber is very hard and heavy. Indigenous from Nova Scotia to Florida and westward to Minnesota and Texas. This medium-sized tree (25–30 ft.) has fine, narrowly furrowed, brownish bark, protecting the white, hard and strong underneath structure. A Birch-like foliage appears with the pistillate flowers in April and May, resembling the female flowers of hop, hence its popular name, hophornbeam. The bark should be gathered in August and September.

Medicinal Part: The inner wood and bark.

176

Solvent: Boiling water.

Bodily Influence: Antiperiodic, Tonic, Alterative.

Uses: It is very good for intermittent fever, neuralgia, nervous debility, scrofula and dyspepsia. Sometimes administered with fair success as a remedy for fever and ague.

Dose: 1 teaspoonful of the inner wood cut small or granulated to 1 cup of boiling water; drink cold 1 cupful during the day a large mouthful at a time. Of the tincture, 5–20 drops.

Homoeopathic Clinical: Tincture of hardwood—Headache (dull), Head, (numb), Intermittent fever, Liver (affections of), Lumbago, Malarial anaemia.

LICORICE   Glycyrrhiza glabra, L.
(N.O.: Leguminosae)

Common Name: SWEETWOOD.

Features: A perennial species introduced into various countries from southern Europe and western Asia. It grows 3–5 ft. tall, bears imparipinnate dark green leaves in pairs of 4–7, ovate and smooth. The yellowish-white, pale blue or purplish spike-shaped flowers are followed by one to six seeded 1 in. long, brown ovate, flat fruit legum. Root greyish brown or dark brown, wrinkled lengthwise, internally yellow, and four times sweeter than cane sugar. The roots are dug when sweetest, autumn of the fourth year, preferably of plants that have not borne fruit, a process that exhausts the sweetness of the sap.

Medicinal Part: The dried root.

Solvent: Water, sparingly in alcohol.

Bodily Influence: Demulcent, Expectorant, Laxative, Pectoral.

Uses: Licorice is the well-known root extract for coughs and chest complaints. It is best combined with part, or all, of the following: Black cohosh (Cimicifuga racemosa), Wild cherry (Prunus serotina), Flaxseed (Linum), Ginger root (Zingiber), Lemon and made into an infusion for wheezing, or shortness of breath, pains of the breasts and lungs, dry cough or hoarseness. Can be used alone, however, as the root of this plant is of great esteem and can hardly be said an improper ingredient for mankind. Some of our latest information found in Green Medicine Research Laboratories in Long Island has found active materials in Licorice root with a molecular structure similar to that of hormones from the adrenal cortex (a most important function of the endocrine glandular system), besides being useful in treating chronic skin conditions. From M. B. Kreig's "Green Medicine": "Derivatives from Licorice were given to patients with gastric ulcers, with the result that the ulcers disappeared in 37 per cent of the cases, and were greatly reduced in the remainder according to the researchers." The reason being, Licorice is a beneficial laxative and demulcent, thus removing gastric ulcers causing material from the intestinal tract, and relieving the conditions of the unwanted ulcers.

Used since ancient times, considered a mild demulcent of little value except as a flavouring agent, until more recent research has found the root to be valuable as a source of oestrogenic hormones. Culpeper used Licorice for dropsy and to allay thirst, besides the already mentioned ailments. Too much Licorice is apt to sicken the stomach or even produce vomiting from its relaxing character.

Dose: 1 lb. of Licorice root boiled in 3 pints of water, reduced by boiling to 1 quart, is an all-purpose decoction; 1 teaspoonful three times a day. 1 teaspoonful of the dried root to 1 cup of boiling water can be taken as a herbal tea, made fresh daily. Of the tincture, $\frac{1}{2}$–1 fl. dram.

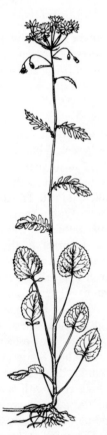

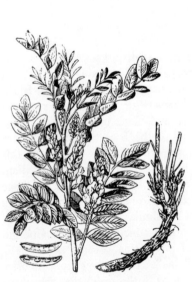

LICORICE Glycyrrhiza glabra, L.
(Medicina, Moscow, 1965)

LIFE ROOT Senecio aureus, L.
(U.S. Agricultural Department,
Appalachia, 1971)

178

Russian Experience: Solodka Gladkaya, smooth (polished) Licorice, grows in many parts of Russia. It is used for commercial, industrial and medical purposes.

Folk Medicine: Domestically very old medicine for Cough, Bronchitis, Stomachic, including Ulcers, Diuretic for inflammation of Kidney and Bladder, Chronic constipation.

Medical: Preparations as extracts, powders and syrups are used for a variety of compounds, not only for its aromatic and sweetening properties; of late, clinically useful for regulating water and salt metabolism (Medicina, Moscow, 1965).

Externally: An ointment for eczema, psoriasis, redness of skin, is made by adding 2 per cent of Licorice juice to an antibiotic formula (Saratov University 1962).

Industrial: Licorice is collected with tractors, transported by train-load, and exported by ship-load for the food and pharmaceutical industry. The uses are many: sweetening and flavouring in the candy and canning industries; soft drinks, beer and liquor; tobacco houses, for taste and appeal in chewing tobacco; fire extinguishers, as it foams when mixed with water.

India Experience: Jethi madh, Madhoka, Mithi lakdi are a few of the common names for Licorice in India. It grows wild in the northern and western sections of India and Pakistan.

Folk Medicine: Generally used in doses of 10–30 grains for Dysuria, Throat conditions, Hoarseness of voice, Bronchitis, Coughs, Asthma, etc.; catarrhal conditions of Bowel, Kidney and Bladder.

Medical: India ardently confirms as Alterative, Expectorant, Emollient, Demulcent, Laxative, Pectoral, Sweet Tonic, Stomachic. In pharmacy the syrup is used for all compounds when aromatics and sweeteners are needed.

LIFE ROOT   Senecio aureus, L.
(N.O.: Compositae)

Common Names: SQUAW WEED, RAGWORT, FALSE VALERIAN, GOLDEN SENECIO, FEMALE REGULATOR, COCASH WEED.

Features: Life root, and various composite herbs of the genus Senecio, are common in most parts of the world. In North America they are found mostly in the eastern states. As this species, medicinally, possess the same properties, it is not necessary to specify them. These perennial, coarse, yellow-flowered plants are allied to the thistles. Can be found in low marshy grounds, and on the banks of creeks. The stems are erect and smooth, 1–2 ft. high; radical leaves are simple and rounded, upper leaves are few, dentate and sessile. Flowers in May and June. Popular with the American Indians, Homoeopaths and Herbalists.

179

Medicinal Parts: The root and herb.

Solvent: Diluted alcohol.

Bodily Influence: Stimulant, Diuretic, Emmenagogue, Pectoral, Astringent, Tonic.

Uses: We of the modern age are bewildered by so many female abnormalities, from grand-daughter to grandmother. The time-honoured "female regulator" (Senecio aureus), of specific use and without complications, is still reliable. Senecio stimulates the pelvic organism, relieving engorgement of women by removing pressure stemming from the perimeum, bladder and rectum. A completely safe aid in gynaecological disorders such as dysmenorrhoea (painful menstruation), menorrhagia (excessive menstruation), suppressed menstruation, atonic leucorrhoea (excessive mucous secretion) and other disturbances of the pelvic organism, including various functional irregularities of menopause. It strengthens flabby uterine ligaments of the fairer sex, and has a place for diseases of men when prostatic enlargement is of the soft, boggy and atonic type. It is also valuable in gravel, stones and diarrhoea.

In pulmonary complaints it is advisable to combine 1 teaspoonful of the fluid extract with other pectorals in sweetened water. The name "Life root" is indicated for many different uses as a household remedy.

Dose: Tincture of Senecio alone, 10–20 drops in water three or four times a day.

Homoeopathic Clinical: Tincture of fresh plant in flower—Amenorrhoea, Ascites, Coryza, Cough, Dropsy, Dysmenorrhoea, Dysuria, Epistaxis, Fainting, Gleet, Gonorrhoea, Haemorrhages, Home-sickness, Hysteria, Kidney (inflammation of), Lumbago, Mania, Menorrhagia, Menstruation (delayed; early, and profuse; obstructed, vicarious), Nails (brittle), Nervousness, Neurasthenia, Phthisis, Prostatitis, Puerperal mania, Renal colic, Sciatica, Spermatic cord (pain in), Wounds.

Russian Experience: Senecio platyphylus (broad leaf), Life root, grows in Russia's Caucasus mountain range; known in their language as Krestovnik. There is no Folk Medicine practice indicated in Russian literature.

Clinically: Extracts of the root and herb are used in powder form and ampoules (Atlas, Moscow, 1962). Clinically given for stomach and intestinal spasm, spasmatic constipation, ulcers, colitis, colic, liver malfunction, bronchial asthma, high blood pressure, angina pectoris, disturbance and circulation of the blood stream due to spasmodic character. Also used in eye practice.

Industrial: To assist the demand for Life root, in Russia Agro-Technics have successful plantations in many parts of central Russia, Bello–Russia and Ukraine.

For 1 acre they seed 5–6 lb. in square nest system; row system, 7–8 lb. The first year's collection of the dried herb is only 100–200 lb. per acre. The third year jumps to 800–1,000 lb. of the dried roots and herb for the same acre.

LINDEN   Tilia cordata, Mill, L.
(N.O.: Tiliaceae)

Common Names: LIME TREE, COMMON LIME, LINDEN FLOWER, AMERICAN BASSWOOD.

Features: Linden, a common name for trees of the genus tilia, in the family tiliaceae, which in Great Britain are commonly called "Limes", and in America "Basswood" (the native species at least), which is Tilia americana, a magnificent forest tree that reaches 130 ft. in height. The genus comprises some thirty species of handsome large- or medium-sized trees, native to the north temperate zone, whose taxonomy is much confused because of free hybridization among many members. All Lindens grow best in rich moist soil, and shed their leaves early in dry locations.

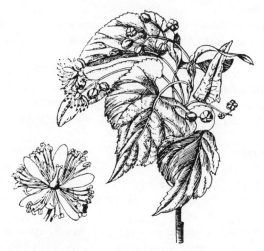

LINDEN   Tilia cordata Mill, L.
(Bello-Russ. Academy of Science, Minsk, 1965)

The species are characterized by prominent winter buds and the lack of a terminal bud; the leaves, which are mostly roundish ovate with oblique and more or less cordate bases, are always toothed and often have tufts of down in the axils of the veins of the lower surface. Flowers are dull white or yellowish, about $\frac{1}{2}$ in. wide, with five sepals and petals and numerous stamens cohering in groups in many species. The flowers

181

appear in June and August and are very fragrant and produce copious amounts of nectar, which is very attractive to bees. The Linden honey is of high quality and rather strong flavour. One of two varieties produce substances poisonous to bees. The fruit is the size and shape of a pea, commonly called Monkey Nuts. The fine wood grain is soft and light, making it ideal for carving, and it was used by the Iroquois Indians. Of no use in construction.

Medicinal Parts: Flowers and leaves.

Solvent: Boiling water.

Bodily Influence: Nervine, Stimulant, Tonic.

Uses: A well known and much used herb for domestic use in nervous conditions and disorders following colds. Promotes perspiration in fevers and relieves cough and hoarseness, helps remove mucus from the lungs and trachea, and provides relief from bronchial catarrh. Advisable to combine with Coltsfoot (Tussilago farfara) for this purpose. The infusion will also flush the kidney, bladder and stomach of unwanted mucus when present, and avoid the development of serious abdominal conditions which are sometimes the cause of lung and windpipe complaints. It is also excellent for female complaints, and has had a great reputation for aid in epilepsy.

Dose: Infusion of leaves or flowers—1 teaspoonful to 1 cup of boiling water, steep $\frac{1}{2}$ hr., cool and drink as frequently as required. Tincture, 15–20 drops as indicated by condition.

Externally: Poultices on boils and other painful swellings.

Homoeopathic Clinical: Tincture of fresh blossom—Dentition, Enuresis, Epistaxis, Leucorrhoea, Lichen, Neuralgia, Peritonitis, Rheumatism, Toothache, Urticaria, Uterus (bearing down in; prolapses of; inflammation of).

Russian Experience: Russian Lippa (Linden) is a most popular tree, there being eleven species throughout Russia, sometimes growing so closely that Lippa foliage is all that can be seen. It is estimated that there are about 2,500,000 acres of pure Linden trees, besides many square miles of assorted trees.

Folk Medicine: As Diuretic (cool or warm), Diaphoretic (hot with honey, or raspberry syrup), Conditions of colds, Inflamed lungs, Headache, Nerve tension or Debility, Sterility, Amenorrhoea. 1 teaspoonful of Linden charcoal and goat's milk is given for Tuberculosis. The leaves and flowers are steeped as a strong tea for throat and cough soreness and used as a gargle.

Externally: Linden tar is used for Eczema, the leaves as poultice for boils and carbuncles.

Industrial: Wine industry uses aromatic Linden flowers; and honey, which is considered the best. The soft elastic tree is excellent material for all kinds of wooden kitchenware, furniture and building material.

182

LION'S ROOT   Nabalus serpentaria, Pursh.
(N.O.: Compositae [subord. Chicoraceae])

Common Names: PRENANTHES SERPENS, WHITE LETTUCE, RATTLESNAKE-ROOT, CANCER WEED.

Features: This member of the Chicory family is an indigenous perennial herb, has a smooth stem and grows 2–4 ft. high. The stem is stout and purplish, with radical leaves, lanceolate, and all irregularly dentate. This plant grows plentifully in moist weeds and in rich soils, from New England to Iowa, and from Canada to Carolina.

Medicinal Part: The whole plant.

Solvent: Boiling water.

Bodily Influence: Astringent, Antiseptic.

Uses: The milky juice of the plant is taken internally, and the root, cut in small pieces or grated, is useful and acts most favourably in cases of dysentery or diarrhoea.

Dose: 1 teaspoonful of the granulated root steeped in 1 cup boiling water. Drink cold 1 cupful during the day, a large mouthful at a time. Of the tincture, 10–20 min.

Externally: In case of snake bites, steep the leaves in boiling water and apply as a poultice.

Homoeopathic Clinical: Tincture of whole fresh plant—Constipation, Ophthalmia.

LIPPIA   Lippia dulcis, Trev.
(N.O.: Verbenaceae)

Common Names: YERBA DUCE, MEXICAN LIPPIA.

Features: Found growing in North America and also in warm regions of Asia and Africa. Cultivated in gardens of England.

Medicinal Part: Leaves.

Solvent: Boiling water.

Bodily Influence: Demulcent, Expectorant, Stimulant.

Uses: This is a stimulating and relaxing agent. The taste is very pleasant but be careful not to use it too freely as it may provoke nausea. The demulcent and expectorant effect to the throat and air passage is soothing to coughs, colds, whooping cough and the freeing of stuffiness in the bronchial tubes and affection thereof, in general. Acting upon the mucous membrane as an alterative. More serviceable combined with syrup of wild cherry or other lung tonics.

Dose: Tincture, 10 drops in water; 1 dram of the tincture will be found sufficient to add to 4 oz. of cough syrup.

Homoeopathic Clinical: Tincture of whole fresh plant—Cough.

LOBELIA   Lobelia inflata, L.
(N.O.: Lobeliaceae)

Common Names: INDIAN TOBACCO, EMETIC WEED, POKE WEED, ASTHMA WEED, GAGROOT, WILD TOBACCO.

Features: A genus of more than 200 species of showy annual or perennial herbs, or sub-shrubs of tropical and temperate regions, belonging to the Bellflower family (Campanulaceae). This plant grows wild in most sections of the United States and is often known as Indian tobacco, because of its taste. However, it is no way related to tobacco and does not contain nicotine or other poisonous properties.

In all species the tubular, five-lobed corolla is irregular with a split on the upper side, an upper lip with two erect lobes, and a lower one with three spreading lobes. Lobelia flowers from July to November; the flowers are small and numerous, pale blue in this species and a variety of red, yellow, white or blue in others. The leaves are alternate, ovate, lanceolate, veiny and hairy; it has a fibrous root and an erect angular, very hairy stem 6 in. to 3 ft. in height. The fruit is a two-celled ovoid capsule containing numerous small brown seeds. More than twenty species attain considerable heights (up to 15 ft. in the high mountains of Africa and Asia). Some dwarf Lobelia plants (L. erina) are cultivated as bedding plants or in hanging baskets.

The proper time for gathering is from the last of July to the middle of October. The plant should be dried in the shade and then preserved in packages or covered vessels, especially if reduced to powder. The people of New England used it long before the time of Samuel Thompson, its assumed discoverer. Contains various alkaloids, lobeline and others. The milky juice is very poisonous to livestock. The whole plant is active, and the stalks are used indiscriminately with the leaves by those who are better acquainted with its properties. The root is supposed to be more energetic, medicinally, than any other part of the plant.

Medicinal Parts: Leaves and stems.

Solvent: Water.

Bodily Influence: Emetic, Stimulant, Antispasmodic, Expectorant, Diaphoretic, Relaxant, Nauseant, Sedative (secondary Cathartic and Astringent).

Uses: The Indians used the root and plant of Red Lobelia for syphilis and for expelling or destroying intestinal worms. The Shoshones made a tea of Lobelia for use as an emetic and physic.

Lobelia is dual in its activities, it is a relaxant and it is a stimulant. In small doses it stimulates, in large doses it relaxes. Lobelia is one of the most valuable herbs used in botanic practice. Much has been written as to whether this herb is poisonous or not but experience, which is far better than theory, has proven that far from being a poison

184

it is an antidote to poison, whether of animal or vegetable variety. Lobelia is an antidote and chiefly used as an emetic and may be prescribed whenever one is indicated. It seems strange that though Lobelia is an excellent emetic, when given in small doses for irritable stomach it will stop spasmodic vomition. It tends to remove obstructions from every part of the system and is felt even to the ends of the toes. It not only cleanses the stomach but exercises a beneficial influence over every part of the body. It is very diffusable, however, and requires to be used with Capsicum, or some other permanent stimulant, to keep alive the blaze which it has kindled.

The action is different on different people and given alone Lobelia cannot cure, but is very beneficial if given in connection with other measures. For irritable conditions of the nervous system it is invaluable and can be relied upon in ordinary convulsions and should be combined with some nervine, such as Lady's slipper (Cypripedium pubescens). As an expectorant it may be used to great advantage in small doses for colds along with decided pulmonary agent Coltsfoot (Tussilago farfara). For spasmodic croup it is invaluable and it has also gained a great reputation for asthma along with nervines such as Blue cohosh (Caulophyllum thalictroides) and Skull cap (Scutellaria lateriflora). It has been successfully used in lock-jaw. Large doses will relax the whole system completely, so that even the smallest muscles cannot be used. This condition is termed the "alarm" and Dr. J. H. Greer, M.D., tells us: "It is uncomfortable although not dangerous, unless poisons should be administered, which are in this condition quickly absorbed." This is not advisable administration for the lay public, however.

Lobelia, in fevers, is suited for phrenitis, meningitis, pneumonia, pleurisy, hepatitis, peritonitis, nephritis, periostitis. This is not a continually used agent but the thought is to clean out, clean up and keep clean the many areas of congested conditions of the vertebral arteries, to pave the way for the use of other remedial nourishment. In bronchial and pulmonary complaints its action is speedily and wonderfully beneficial. Can also be used to subdue spasms, epilepsy, tetanus, cramps, hysteria, chorea and convulsions. Give first of all an infusion of Catnip (Nepa) to the bowels, which of itself will do much to relieve the brain and can be administered even when the patient is delirious. Give Lobelia in small quantities as the case may require, but clean out the waste material and relieve the locked up condition of the body which is causing the trouble. It is a temporary relief in any case when administered internally and if not used with great skill and caution in that way may do as much harm as good.

Dose: 1 oz. of the herb to 1 pint of boiling water makes an ordinary infusion, to be administered in tablespoonful doses every hour or half-hour. A weak infusion given in teaspoonful doses every 10 min. (termed "broken doses") will thoroughly relax the muscular system and prove a great aid in reducing fractures and dislocations, especially if a cloth soaked in the warm infusion is applied over the seat of the difficulty. For convulsions, injections of the herb as infusion is best. Never administer Lobelia where the system is relaxed or when there is congestion. **Externally:** A salve or tincture of Lobelia and other soothing barks and roots can be employed for inflammations and swellings, not recommended for indolent ulcers or dark sores.

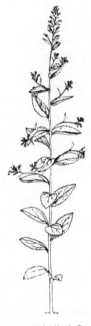 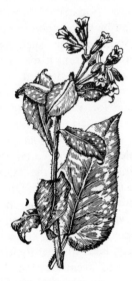

<table>
<tr><td>L<small>OBELIA</small>   Lobelia inflata, L.
(U.S. African Department,
Appalachia, 1971)</td><td>L<small>UNGWORT</small>
Pulmonaria officinalis, L.
(Vishaya Schkolla, Moscow, 1963)</td></tr>
</table>

Homoeopathic Clinical: Tincture of fresh plant; trituration of leaves only—Alcoholism, Alopecia, Amenorrhoea, Angina pectoris, Asthma, Cardialgia, Cough, Croup, Deafness, Debility, Diarrhoea, Dysmenorrhoea, Dyspepsia, Emphysema, Faintness, Gall-stones, Gastralgia, Haemorrhoidal discharge, Hay asthma, Heart (affections of), Hysteria, Meningeal headaches, Miller's asthma, Morning sickness (of drunkards; of pregnancy), Morphia habit, Palpitation, Pleurisy, Psoriasis, Rigid as Seborrhoea, Shoulders (pain in), Tea (effects of), Urethra (stricture of), Vagina (serious discharge from), Vomiting (of pregnancy), Wens, Whooping cough.

Russian Experience: The Russians pronounce Lobelia the same as do

186

the Americans. Lobelia is popular as both a commercial and industrial cultivation in Central Russia—Krasnodar, Voronezh, Moscow and Bello-Russia. The use as Folk Medicine is not indicated in our available literature.

Clinically: The whole plant is used for many critical conditions. The all-important adrenal glands are aroused by stimulating adrenalin into the blood stream; it is not accumulative and can be used repeatedly. Respiratory trouble is soon relieved of symptoms of asthma and spasmodic conditions. Is useful in cases where first aid is needed when shocked by electricity, sun and heat stroke, to force vomiting when poisoned by narcotics, food or medicine, in carbon monoxide poisoning and in infections (Atlas, Moscow, 1962).

Industrial: Agro-Technics have worked out some of the puzzling details of Lobelia in commercial planting. Lobelia is native to the Great Lakes region of North America and due to this fact several nurserymen in Windsor, Canada, failed to grow it successfully. Some interesting facts from Russia may inspire the second attempt. First of all the seeds are so small they must be mixed with fine sand, 1–50, and then planted for fifty to sixty days in the greenhouse (around April). For one flat, 1,500–2,000 seeds are needed. Much care should be taken when watering, as the fine mixture and small seeds can be washed away; they can also be burned out if threatened by too much heat or too much sun, etc. In Russia, June is the time for transplanting the small plants; keep in mind that the feeding area for each plant must be 8×24 in. Seedlings must be 3–4 in. high with five to six well-developed leaves. Lobelia requires care, as does any garden plant and the soil must be cultivated and softened, weeded and fertilized, if necessary, organic preferred. When the green seeds start to form in a mass, this is the time for harvesting. Proper drying is essential and should be done as soon as cut, temperature should be 50–60° F. From 1 acre 1,000–2,000 lb. of dry Lobelia is marketed.

LUNGWORT Pulmonaria officinalis, L.
(N.O.: Pulmonaceae)

Common Names: SPOTTED LUNGWORT, MAPLE LUNGWORT, JERUSALEM COWSLIP, SPOTTED COMFREY.

Features: Lungwort, any of several plants used as folk remedies for lung disease. One is a widely distributed Lichen (Lobaria pulmonaria), that grows usually on tree trunks. Others are hairy perennials that belong to the genus pulmonaria of the borge family (Boraginaceae) and have pink, blue, purple or white flowers, sometimes grown as ornamentals in northern latitudes. This particular perennial species (P. officinalis) is a

187

smooth plant with a stem about 1 ft. high. The flowers are blue, five-angled corolla, funnel-shaped, with stigma, flowering in May. They are without any particular odour.

Medicinal Part: The leaves.

Solvent: Water.

Bodily Influence: Demulcent, Mucilaginous, Pectoral.

Uses: Its virtues seem to be entirely expended upon the lungs and it is certainly an efficaciously reliable agent for all morbid conditions of these organs, especially when there is bleeding from the lung structure and functions. Also valuable as a treatment for coughs, asthma, colds, bronchial and catarrhal affections. Seems to seal the weakened tissue and take away inflammation.

Dose: The infusion of 2 oz. in 1 pint of boiling water is taken in frequent doses of a wineglassful.

Russian Experience: There are two species of Lungwort growing in Russia, Pulmonary obscura or Lungwort obscura and Pulmonaria angustifolia (narrow-leave Lungwort). Both species are used for the same purpose. In this case, as with many other of our Folk Medicines around the world, the people have independently found the useful pro-perties of the plant and named them according to the most influential action on certain parts of the body, such as the attractive Lungwort. Latin name: Pulmonary (Pulm—Lung). Russian name: Legochnitza, (Legkie—Lung). English name: Lungwort (from the lung).

Folk Medicine: The medical properties of Lungwort have long been accepted as Emollient, Mild Astringent, Tonic and a natural source of minerals for stomach and intestinal sickness and lung and pulmonary conditions. There has been recent (1963–5) reports in medical literature of Lungwort being used with other compounds.

Externally: Vulnerary for dressing and washing wounds, swellings and amenorrhoea, as it is antiseptic.

Clinically: Moscow Medical Institute (1963–5) has conducted experimental work and the findings give support to Folk Medicine wisdom and belief. To those of us who like to know what herbal medicine contains, and why it repairs the body's ills, perhaps the following contents of the plant will help us realize that they contain many of the live elements we also are made of, or are necessary for healthy blood. Lungwort contains Vitamins C and B; minerals: iron, copper, silver, manganese, kerotin, titan, nickel, to mention a few of the necessities. Further study by the medical world is expected to produce spectacular findings.

MAGNOLIA   Magnolia virginiana, L. (M. glauca, L.;
M. acuminate, and M. tripetata)
(N.O.: Magnoliaceae)

Common Names: WHITE BAY, BEAVER TREE, SWAMP SASSAFRAS, MAGNOLIA, INDIAN BARK.

Features: A genus of ornamental, widely cultivated evergreen or deciduous trees and shrubs of the family Magnoliaceae. Highly admired by man for its beautiful and fragrant flowers, with little attention given to its medical properties. The thirty-five to forty species are mostly native to the United States, India, China and Japan. They grow in North America in morasses from Massachusetts to the Gulf of Mexico.

They are characterized by large alternate, entire leaves; large, solitary, terminal flowers, often highly fragrant and white, purple pine, or yellowish in colour, and cone-shaped, often red, decorative fruit. This species varies in height from 6–30 ft., being taller in the south than in the north, and flowers from May to August. The bark of both the trunk and the root is employed. The odour is aromatic and the taste bitterish, warm and pungent.

Medicinal Part: The root and trunk bark.

Solvent: Water.

Bodily Influence: Tonic, Aromatic, Astringent, Antiperiodic, Stimulant.

Uses: At one time official in the United States Pharmacopoeia for treating rheumatism. The action is superior to quinine and leaves no evil side-effect, as does quinine, and so can be continued with more safety. Also useful in chills and fever, as a restorative tonic, dyspepsia and for convalescence after fevers. Properly prepared it may be used as a substitute for tobacco (when taken with hygienic measures) and it will break the habit of tobacco chewing.

Dose: In powder, $\frac{1}{2}$–1 dram doses five or six times a day. The infusion is taken in wineglassful doses five or six times a day. The tincture, made by adding 2 oz. of the cones to a pint of brandy, will be found beneficial in dyspepsia and chronic rheumatism.

Homoeopathic Clinical: Tincture of the flower—Asthma, Fainting.

Russian Experience: The Magnolia trees that are seen in Russia are Magnolia fuscata (brown leaves) from China, and Fuscata grandiflora (big leaves) from North America. They are grown both for decorative and medical use.

Folk Medicine: The bark, fruit and seeds are made into Nastoika (with vodka) for Fevers, Heart tonic and Rheumatism (Saratov University, 1963).

Externally: The oil from the flowers and young leaves aids falling hair, and is used as a scalp tonic.

Clinically: Only the extract, 20–30 drops three times daily, for heart trouble and high blood pressure. Larger amounts as local antiseptic for external wounds and pain (Atlas, Moscow, 1962).

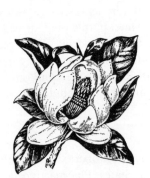

Magnolia   Magnolia glauca, L.,
Magnolia virginiana, L.
(Medicina, Moscow, 1963)

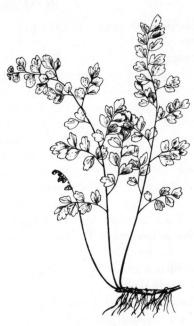

Maidenhair
Adiantum Capillus, L.
(U.S. Agricultural Department,
Appalachia, 1971)

MAIDENHAIR   Adiantum Capillus-Veneris, L.
(N.O.: Filices)

Common Names: Maiden fern, Common polypody.

Features: There are some eighty varieties of this plant, some of which grow abundantly in Canada and the United States. Maidenhair is perennial and is found in deep woods and moist, rich soil. This is a very delicate and graceful flowering fern growing from 12–15 in. high, with a slender, polished stalk. The leaves are aromatic and bitterish.

Medicinal Part: The herb.

Solvent: Boiling water.

190

Bodily Influence: Pectoral, Demulcent, Tonic, Refrigerant, Expectorant.
Uses: Maidenhair has had a long and active life as a helpful agent for pectoral conditions of coughs resulting from colds, nasal congestion, or catarrh and hoarseness, bronchial disorders including shortness of breath, asthma, influenza, pleurisy, etc.
Dose: The infusion of 1–2 oz. to 1 pint of boiling water may be taken frequently in wineglassful doses. Culpeper tells us that it is also used in hair tonic preparations. Should be combined with supporting herbs for more effective results.

MALLOW (COMMON)   Malva sylvestris, L.
(N.O.: Malvaceae)

Common Name: HIGH MALLOW.
Features: Mallow, popular name of plants of the genus Malva, family Malvaceae, including annuals, biennials and perennials. There are about thirty species native to Europe, North Africa and Asia, several of which have been naturalized in North America. Malva sylvestris grows abundantly in fields, roadsides, and waste places.

This species is erect or branching, 1–3½ in. high, with rounded heart-shaped leaves; small flowers are pink-veined against purple appearing clustered or single flowering from May to October. The whole plant abounds in mucilage, more especially the root; odour slight; taste sweetish. The fresh dried leaves are put into decoctions; the root may be dried but it is best fresh, if chosen when there are leaves growing from it.
Medicinal Part: The herb.
Solvent: Water.
Bodily Influence: Demulcent, Emollient.
Uses: As with other mucilagionous herbs the properties of M. sylvestris are an excellent demulcent in coughs, irritation of the air passages, flux, affections of the kidney and bladder, etc. Pliny wrote: "That anyone taking a spoonful of mallows will be free of disease." Parkinson wrote: "Leaves and roots boiled in wine or water or in both with parsley doth help to open the body, for hot agues. Leaves bruised and laid on the eyes with a little honey take away the inflammation from them." The Chinese eat the leaves raw in salad, or boiled as spinach.
Dose: 1 teaspoonful of the herb to 1 cup of boiling water. Drink one or two cupfuls a day. Of the tincture ½–1 fl. dram.
Externally: In inflammatory conditions of the external parts, the bruised herb forms an excellent application, making as it does a natural emollient cataplasm. Our Indians used leaves, soft stems and flowers, steeped and made into a poultice for running sores, boils and swelling.

191

Russian Experience: Malva is known and pronounced in Russia as we do in America. There are several wild species throughout the land. Industry has stimulated cultivation.

Folk Medicine: The medical properties of Malva are appreciated in cases of cathartic excess of the stomach and bowels. Also respiratory ailments of the common cold, sore throat, lung congestion, etc. used as a tea, poultice or Nastoika (with vodka). Malva contains a large amount of mucilage and sugar, plus Vitamin C, minerals, kerotin and colouring matter.

Industrial: For 1 acre 8–10 lb. of seeds are needed, on an average. The following is estimated after a three-year period: roots 1,000–2,000 lb., leaves 1,000 lb.; seeds 200 lb. Ordinary grain seeding is done during the spring, or transplants from the greenhouse, in which case they yield more from the first year harvest.

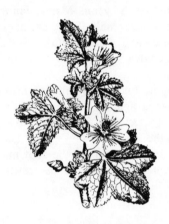

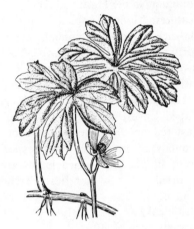

COMMON MALLOW
Malva sylvestris, L.
(Dr. A. J. Thut, Guelph, Canada)

MANDRAKE, AMERICAN
Podophyllum, L.
(Z. A. Popov, Lekarstevennye
Rastenia, Kiev, 1967)

MANDRAKE, AMERICAN Podophyllum peltatum, L.
(N.O.: Berberidaceae)

Common Names: MAY APPLE, HOG APPLE, AMERICAN MANDRAKE, INDIAN APPLE, RACCOONBERRY, WILD LEMON.

Features: In the United States the name is applied to the May apple, Podophyllum pelatum, a herbaceous member of the Barberry family (Berberidaceae), that also has a perennial and sometimes divided root-stock. The American Mandrake is an entirely different plant from White bryony or English Mandrake, dealt with elsewhere. American Mandrake

192

is native to eastern North America and can be found growing throughout the States in moist open woods and pastures.

The jointed dark brown root is about half the size of the finger, is very fibrous and internally yellow. The stem is simple, round, smooth, erect, about 1 ft. high, divided at the top into two petioles, from 3–6 in. long, each supporting two large, peltate, deeply lobed leaves and a solitary nodding white flower 1–2 in. across; flowering in the spring and in flavour resembles the strawberry. The 2-in. fleshy berry is yellow and edible when ripe only and is sometimes used for preserves; rarely develops until July. In the green state the rhizome, foliage, seeds and green fruit are poisonous. The proper time for collecting the root is the latter part of October or early part of November, soon after the fruit has ripened. Its active principle is Podophyllin, which acts upon the liver in the same manner as mercury but is far superior to mercury, and with intelligent physicians it has dethroned that noxious mineral as a cholagogue.

Medicinal Part: Rhizome and the resin extracted from it.

Solvents: Alcohol, boiling water (partially).

Bodily Influence: Cathartic, Hepatic, Hydragogue, Cholagogue, Alterative, Tonic, Emetic, Purgative.

Uses: Its usefulness covers a wide range, brought to our attention by the Indians. It seldom fails in cases of urine incontinence or diseases associated with it. The influence is exercised on every part of the system, stimulating glands to a healthy action, releasing obstructions such as bilious and typhoid febrile disease. In chronic liver diseases it has no equal in the whole range of herbal practice. For all chronic scrofulous, dyspeptic complaints it is highly valuable, acting upon the bowels without disposing them to subsequent costiveness. In cases of determination of blood to the brain, this article, given in cathartic doses, is prompt and will soon restore the equilibrium of the circulation. In old cases of mecurial poisoning it acts promptly; as a tonic and alterative should always be combined with other herbs. The Old Testament recommended Mandrabora (Mandrake) as a cure for sterility. Its most beneficial action is obtained by the use of small doses frequently, because if given in large amounts it can cause violent evacuation and debility. For children, smaller doses should be prescribed, according to age. This herb is powerful in action and should be combined with a supporting herb such as Black root (Leptandra), Senna leaves (Cassia Senna), etc., for better results.

Dose: 1 teaspoonful of the root, cut small, to 1 pint of boiling water. Take 1 teaspoonful at a time as required. Of the tincture, 2–5 min.

Homoeopathic Clinical: Tincture of root gathered after fruit has ripened; of whole fresh plant; of ripe fruit. Solution of resinous extract, Podophyllin—Acidity, Amenorrhoea, Anus (prolapse of), Asthma (bronchial), Bilious attack, Bronchitis, Cataract, Cholera infantum, Cornea (ulcer of), Dentition, Diarrhoea (cramp), Duodenum (catarrh of), Dysentery, Dyspepsia (from calomel), Fevers, Flatulence, Gagging, Gallstones, Gastric catarrh, Goitre, Haemorrhoids, Headache (sick; bilious), Heart (pains in), Hydrocephaloid, Intermittents, Jaundice, Leucoma, Liver (affections of), Ophthalmia, Ovaries (pain in; numbness in; tumour of), Palpitation, Pneumonia, Proctitis, Prostatitis, Pustules, Sciatica, Stomatitis, Strabismus, Taste (lost; perverted; illusions of), Tenesmus, Tongue (burning in), Urticaria, Uterus (prolapse of), Whooping cough, Worms.

Russian Experience: Russian literature refers to the Latin name Podophyllum (Podofil). Mandrake does not grow wild in Russia, but they import American Podophyllum and find the importance of this medical plant worthy of cultivation. American Mandrake, Podophyllum peltatum, and India's Podophyllum emodi are under special Agro-Technic supervision.

Clinically: For chronic constipation, liver and gall-bladder conditions, to promote bile, malignancy of the skin (cancer) (Atlas, Moscow, 1963). For the lymphatic system, spleen, blood conditions, skin malignancies and growths (Naukova dumka, Kiev, 1965).

Industrial: American Mandrake receives the most attention, being cultivated in two ways. One is by planting root sections, which can produce twenty-five to thirty plants, and the other by seeding. Quantity or harvest amount is not revealed in literature to date. Mandrake does not flower before the third year. Requires the correct soil, climate, cultivation, weeding and much attention to water, as it cannot stand dryness.

MAPLE   Acer-rubrum, L.
(N.O.: Aceraceae)

Common Names: SUGAR MAPLE, SWAMP MAPLE, RED MAPLE.

Features: Together with a few shrubs of the family Aceraceae, the species covers about 100 Maples that constitute one of the most widely useful genera of trees, being extensively employed for ornamental purposes. In America, the best known, most widely planted and otherwise most important species is probably the rock, or sugar, Maple (A. saccharum). It is especially found in the rich woods from Maine to Michigan and southwards in the mountains to Georgia, everywhere being noted for the rich colours of its leaves in autumn. There are many varieties of this tree, according to the place of its growth and the taste of the planter. The large Maple, if tapped, yields 3–6 lb. of sap annually, and the genuine Maple syrup cannot be bettered for flavour and nutrition. The flowers are rich in nectar and are sought by bees.

194

Medicinal Parts: The inner bark and leaves.

Solvent: Boiling water.

Bodily Influence: Astringent, Deobstruent, Tonic.

Uses: The American Indians use it as an application to sooth sore eyes, owing to its astringent nature. It is believed the sweetness of the Maple sap was first discovered by an Indian girl. The sap had dripped into a hollow, or pocket, of a tree trunk together with fresh rain water. She drank this liquid and, as with the majority of our useful herb medications, we have the fathers of our country to thank for the prehistoric beginning. The decoction of the leaves or bark strengthens the liver and spleen and relieves the pain which proceeds from them. In fact, Maple bark or leaves are a good medicine for the whole body as they are tonic and soothing to the nerves.

Dose: 1 large teaspoonful to 1 cup of boiling water; 1–3 cups a day may be taken on an empty stomach. A wineglassful every hour or two if there is pain in the liver or spleen is very helpful for some.

Russian Experience: Maple, known as Klen, is represented in many varieties throughout Russia. The American Maple is favoured for decoration in public parks and family gardens because of its grace, elegance and beauty (Bello-Russ. Academy of Science, 1965). Builders and carpenters value Maple wood for its beauty and service.

Folk Medicine: Employ the astringent properties as a tea for general tonic, and specifically for new mothers as a muscle toner. Maple syrup is used as a food and general tonic food supplement.

Externally: Boiled leaves and tea are used as a poultice for boils.

MILKWEED   Asclepias syriaca, L.
(N.O.: Asclepiadaceae)

Common Names: EMETIC ROOT, SNAKE MILK, MILK IPECAC.

Features: Most of the 150 species of the Asclepia family are erect perennial herbs, from 2–4 ft. high. The root is yellowish, large and branching. The leaves are scattered, sessile, oblong, smooth in some plants, very hairy in others and from 1–2 in. in length. The attractive flowers are white and purplish-white, with fruit of three-celled capsule. The genus is named in honour of the Greek God Asclepius (God of medicine).

Milkweed grows abundantly in Canada and the United States in dry fields and woods and flowers from June to September. When the leaves are pulled off, or the stem cut, a milky white liquid rushes to the exposed surface. Asclepius is poisonous to cattle and sheep, but rarely to horses. The Indians used the inside fibres for rope and fishing nets; the milk was collected and rolled until firm enough to make chewing gum. The boiled roots taste like asparagus. The green plant was collected when very small and boiled in two waters to use as greens. We do not advise this for the general public as the amount and correct species is of importance in quantity.

Medicinal Part: The root.

Solvent: Water.

Bodily Influence: Diaphoretic, Expectorant. (Many of the common names are duplicated, this Milkweed (Asclepius) is not the same as Bitter root, (Apocynum androsaemifolium, Dogbane family) often called Milkweed.)

Uses: Medicinally the Indians used Asclepias for inflammatory rheumatism. Today it is still employed for rheumatism, dyspepsia and scrofulous conditions of the blood. A helpful remedy for female complaints, bowel and kidney trouble, asthma and stomach complaints. Used for dropsy

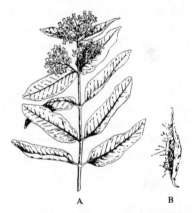

A   B

MILKWEED FAMILY   Asclepiadaceae, L.
A—Common milkweed   B—Seed pod
(Ontario Department of Agriculture, Toronto, Canada, 1966)

as it increases the flow of urine. Effective remedy for gall-stones. J. Kloss ("Back to Eden") says: "Take equal parts of milkweed and marsh-mallow (Althea), steep a teaspoonful in a cup of boiling water, take 3 cups daily, and one upon retiring. It will expel gallstones in a few days, where combined with this. Fomentations applied to the liver and the liver thoroughly massaged at the same time is very effective."

Dose: Bruise 4 oz. of the root and boil in 3 quarts of water, reducing down to 1 quart or less, and take ½ teacupful three times a day. Of the saturated tincture, from 1–2 teaspoonfuls three times a day.

Externally: The fresh milky fluid that weeps from the cut stem will in most cases cause warts to disappear if applied often to the elevated part only.

196

Homeoepathic Clinical: Tincture of the root—Abortion, Bronchitis, Catarrhal fever, Dropsy, Dysmenorrhoea, Hay fever, Headache, Indigestion, Influenza, Pleurisy, Rheumatism, Uraemia, Uterine pains.

MINT   Mentha piperita, L.
(N.O.: Labiatae)

Common Names: BRANDY MINT, CURLED MINT.

Features: The genus mentha consists of probably not more than fifteen true species, but with numerous transitional forms several hundred species have been described. Practically all are native to Eurasia or Australia. The two best-known forms are M. spicata, the spearmint, with narrow, interrupted spikes of pink to pale violet flowers and sessile leaves, and M. piperita, the peppermint, with thicker spikes of purplish flowers and petiole, dark green leaves. This perennial herb is 1–3 ft. high, smooth square stem, erect and branching, generally smooth on both sides, but sometimes hairy on the veins of the lower surface. Both of these species have escaped from North America. They flower from July to September; blossoms are small and purplish. Can be found in rich soils in northern Indiana and southern Michigan states of U.S.A. and Canada. Peppermint oil is distilled from the dried, upper portions of the plant and consists largely of menthol, which is used medicinally, and for flavouring confections, chewing gum and toothpaste. Should be collected in dry weather, August and September, just as the flowers appear. If for oil, just after the flowers have expanded.

Medicinal Parts: Leaves and stems.

Solvent: Water.

Bodily Influence: Aromatic, Stimulant, Stomachic, Carminative.

Uses: A most agreeable and harmless herb for cramps and hiccoughs of infants, children and adults. Our mother of eight children always had mint growing somewhere in the garden as a reliable preparation for unpredictable tummy trouble. A wise and beneficial herbal tea to replace coffee, as it will strengthen the heart muscles instead of having the digestive hindrance and weakening effect of the so widely accepted coffee habit. Peppermint is cleansing and strengthening to the entire system. Get in the habit of having a strong cup of peppermint tea and 10 min. of relaxation when in the need of an inhibiting aspirin. Peppermint is a general stimulant and will act more powerfully on the system than any liquor stimulant, without the degenerative possibilities. Useful to check nausea and vomiting, to expel wind, relieve hysterics and prevent the gripping effect of cathartics. The fresh leaves may be bruised and applied to the stomach for the above mentioned, and the tea taken

197

internally. Also an agent for suppressed menstruation and a remedy for sea sickness.

Dose: 1 teaspoonful of mint, fresh or dried, to 1 cupful of boiling water, steep 3–10 min. Children less, use as needed. Of the tincture, ½–1 fl. dram.

Externally: The bruised leaves bound on the forehead will relieve most headaches.

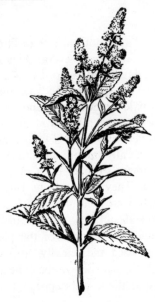

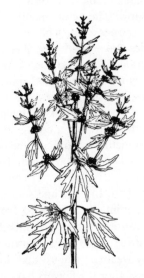

MINT   Mentha piperita, L.
(P. A: Volkova, Dikorastushie,
Moscow, 1962)

MOTHERWORT   Leonurus cardiaca, L.
(Ontario Department of Agriculture,
Toronto, Canada, 1966)

Homoeopathic Clinical: Tincture of whole plant; dilutions of essence— Cough (dry), Headache, Hoarseness, Influenza, Pruritus, Throat (sore), Voice (weakness of).

Russian Experience: Miatta, Mentol, common names for Russian Peppermint. Mint does not grow wild in their country but together with U.S.A., Japan, Italy and France, Russia is among the largest producers of Peppermint for industrial and medical purposes.

Clinically and Home Medicine: The leaves, oil and menthol are used as Anodyne for headaches, Stomach trouble—gas, bloating, wind, heart-burn—Toothache, Antiseptic, inflammations of Lungs, Bronchitis, Sinus, Throat (sore), Colds. Relaxant and Antispasmodic to stop vomiting, nausea, indigestion (Nastoika with vodka). It is useful for sea-sickness, dizziness, diaphoretic, and to promote bile. Used in many compounds as Aromatic, Carminative, Tonic, Relaxant, in the form of teas, tablets, oil, extract (Saratov University, 1965).

198

Industrial: Agro-Technics have details and mechanized procedure of Mint plantations in many parts of European Russia and Bello-Russia. Cultivation was started in the eighteenth century in the Medical Botanics Gardens, for medical purposes only. Today, after much experience, we learn Mint is cultivated through propagation, as seeds require especially favourable conditions and still only a small percentage will thrive. For 1 acre they can collect, on an average, 1,000–2,000 lb. of dry herb, which is cut first in July–August, the flowering season. In some districts it can be cut once again before the frost comes.

MOTHERWORT   Leonurus cardiaca, L.
(N.O.: Labiatae)

Common Names: LION'S TAIL, LION'S EAR, THROWWORT.

Features: There are about ten Eurasian species of this plant, three of them having been introduced into North America from Europe. The genus is of the mint family (Labiatae). Motherwort is an exotic perennial plant found growing in pastures and fields, flowering, with pink or white flowers in dense auxiliary whorls, from May to September. The upper lip of the corolla is shaggy; the calyx has stiff teeth. The rigid stem grows up to 5 ft., bearing some resemblance to Horehound, but has much longer and darker leaves.

Medicinal Parts: The tops and leaves.

Solvents: Water, alcohol.

Bodily Influence: Antispasmodic, Emmenagogue, Nervine, Laxative.

Uses: Motherwort has been employed from time immemorial as a domestic remedy in infusion preparations. It is especially strengthening to the heart when of a palpitation nature. A valuable bitter tonic for almost all conditions of the stomach. Being a true nervine it is excellent for suppressed menstruation and other female trouble, hysteria, urinary cramps, albumen in the urine and scanty muddy urine of typhoid. The unexplained, long-established hidden talent of Leonurus has yet to be scientifically conceived. Experience from lasting results has also given matchless benefits in rheumatism, sciatica, neuritis, sleeplessness, convulsion, delirium and chest colds. Motherwort seems to seek out congested material and eliminate the unwanted material that is causing discomfort. S. Clymer, of "Natures Healing Agents", suggests Leonurus in small doses for prenatal prevention of kidney complications during this period, especially albumen in the urine. Also an agent for unsuspecting worms. Combines well with all herbs and is used for liver affections in combinations.

Dose: Of the decoction, from 1–2 wineglassfuls every 2–3 hr. Of the extract, 3–5 grains.

199

Externally: Hot fomentations made from strong tea will relieve cramps and pain in painful menstruation, etc.

Homoeopathic Clinical: Tincture or infusion of fresh plant—Dysentery, Haemorrhage.

Russian Experience: Pustirnik Serdechny, "Heart Herb", is one of the names for Motherwort, of which there are many species. It seems to be the forgotten herb of Europe. In the fifteenth century it was prominent in herbal books, but in the nineteenth and twentieth centuries it seems to have been forgotten. Its popularity still holds good in Folk Medicine of Rumania as an aid to heart conditions, goitre and epilepsy and also in Britain for hysteria, neuralgia, weakness of heart, shortness of breath.

Folk Medicine of Russia consider the fresh leaves and flowers better than dried. The fresh juice is extracted and prepared for winter use— 2 parts of juice to 3 parts of alcohol (Vishaya Schkola, 1963). For female complaints of amenorrhoea, dysmenorrhoea, sleeplessness, nervousness, TB of the lungs (Bello-Russ. Academy of Science, 1965). For heart neurosis, high blood pressure, goitre, epilepsy, used as a tea (Moscow University, 1963). Instead of Valerian (Valeriana officinalis) the fresh juice of leaves and flowers, 30–40 drops, for calming (Saratov University, 1963).

Clinically: Extract and tablets are combined with many other herbs for neurosis of the heart, high blood pressure (cardiosclerosis, sensitive nerves), slight form of goitre. Experimentally, toxicity is not shown but it is used for improving the central nervous system, heart tone and to regulate blood pressure (Atlas, Moscow, 1963).

Industrial: Commercial cultivation: 7–8 lb. of seed needed for row system; 3–4 lb. for square net procedure. Plantation harvest runs four years, with about 1,000 lb. of dry leaves and flowers to an acre from the first year's crop. For the following three years, 2,000–3,000 lb. per acre are attained, if maintained with loving care.

MUGWORT   Artemisia vulgaris, L.
(N.O.: Compositae)

Common Names: MUGWORT, FELON HERB.

Features: Mugwort grows wild in North America in hedges and waste places. A slender to moderately stout herb, 1–5 ft. tall; the leaves are alternate, five to seven lobes, silvery-white beneath, nearly smooth above. Flowers are small ovid, yellow to purplish, in numerous clusters from July to August. Odour aromatic, leaves slightly bitter.

Medicinal Part: Leaves.

Solvent: Boiling water.

Bodily Influence: Emmenagogue, Diuretic, Diaphoretic.

Uses: Our Indians used the leaves medicinally in decoctions for colds, colic, bronchitis, rheumatism and fever. Safe for suppressed menstruation of mother and daughter, also effective in female complaints of various nature when combined with Marigold (Calendula), Cramp bark (Viburnum opulus), Black haw (Viburnum prunifolium), and Mint (Mentha). Of importance in kidney and bladder inflammations and their many reflected ailments, gout, sciatica, water retention, etc. Culpeper used the herb for counteraction of opium.

Dose: 1 teaspoonful to 1 cupful of boiling water, steeped for 20 min. To be taken in wineglassful amounts.

Externally: After using a poultice of Slippery elm (Ulmus fulva), Cleavers and Bear's foot (Helleborus foetidus), bathe the inflammatory swelling with a strong tea of Mugwort. Some cases of tumours have been known to disappear, as well as abcesses, carbuncles and bruises, if repeated faithfully. Culpeper states: "The fresh juice mixed with hog's grease and whipped into an ointment takes away wens and hard kernals that grow about the neck and throat, and eases the pain, more effective if field daisies be up with it." The Indians also used it externally for wounds and the juice was used for poison oak.

Homoeopathic Clinical: Tincture of fresh root—Catalepsy, Chorea,

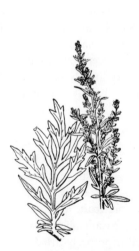

MUGWORT
Artemisia vulgaris, L.
(Bello-Russ. Academy of Science,
Minsk, 1967)

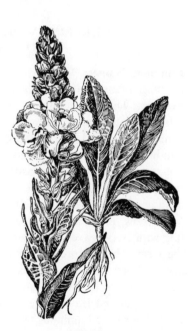

MULLEIN
Verbascum blattaria, V. thapsus
(A. F. Hammerman and others,
Rastenia Tzelitely, Moscow, 1963)

Convulsions, Dysemenia, Epilepsy, Hydrocephalus, Hysteria, Somnambulism, Worms.

Russian Experience: Polin obiknovennaya or Chernobilnik, is common to Russian people as Mugwort, which grows in all parts of Russia and was an accepted home medicine before being thought of as material for books.

Folk Medicine use the leaves, roots and whole plant in female sickness of many varieties—amenorrhoea, dysmenorrhoea, cramps, labour pains, generally as calming, nervine, for convulsions, epilepsy, neurasthnis and other nervous disorders (Atlas, Moscow, 1962); for colds, stones (kidney, bladder, gall-bladder) (Medicina, Moscow, 1965); roots and herb as decoction for tubercular lungs, epilepsy (Moscow University, 1963); decoction of the whole plant for gastric conditions, nervousness, fright, epilepsy, convulsions, female weakness; decoction of the plant in painful and feverish labour after delivery; in female sickness as diuretic and abortive (Bello-Russ. Academy of Science, 1965).

Externally: Decoction of Nastoika (with vodka) for inflammations of mucous membranes, wounds and ulcers (Saratov University, 1962). Decoction of whole plant to bathe children with rickets.

MULLEIN Verbascum blattaria, V. thapsus.
(N.O.: Scrophulariaceae)

Common Names: WHITE MULLEIN, VERBASCUM FLOWERS, WOOLLEN BLANKET HERB, FLANNEL FLOWER, COW'S LUNGWORT, VELVET LEAF.

Features: The genus comprises some 300 species native to Europe, North Africa, western and central Asia. Some species have escaped and are common in the United States, growing in recent clearings, sparsely inhabited fields and along roadsides. They vary greatly in size and form, but most have a columnar aspect, are hairy or woolly, and have yellow, red, purplish or brownish-red flowers arranged in dense terminal spikes or in narrow panicles. The best-known species in America is the common V. thapsus, marked by a stout, erect, unbranched, woolly stem 2–3 ft. tall, with basal leaves, narrowing at the base into wings which pass down the stem. This feature is characteristic of V. thapsus, enabling it to be distinguished from the various other Mulleins. The dense spikes of small yellow flowers bloom in July and August; the fruit, a capsule or pod. The flowers and leaves have a faint, rather pleasant odour, and a somewhat bitterish, albuminous taste. Keeps well if properly dried and stored for winter use.

Medicinal Parts: The leaves and flower (Culpeper used the root also).
Solvent: Boiling water.

202

Bodily Influence: Demulcent, Diuretic, Anodyne, Antispasmodic, Astringent, Pectoral.

Uses: The dried leaves were smoked to relieve lung congestion by the Indians, this being one of their many uses. Herbalists of the space age know of its remedies for coughs, colds and pectoral complaints, including haemorrhages from the lungs, shortness of breath and pulmonary complaints. Mullein has been considered a treatment for haemorrhoids for several hundred years and is still used for this purpose, both internally and as a fomentation. A decoction made with equal parts of Horsemint (Monarda punctata) and Mullein (V. thapsus) and taken three times a day is excellent for kidney diseases.

Dose: 1 teaspoonful of the leaves or flowers to 1 cupful of boiling water. Of the tincture, 15–40 drops in warm water every 2–4 hr., according to condition.

Externally: A very early German remedy for deafness resulting from dried earwax, wax too soft or insufficient wax: "Mullein oil, sun distilled from green Mullein flowers, 3 to 5 drops twice a day until the condition is corrected."

A fomentation of the leaves in hot vinegar and water forms an excellent local application for inflamed piles, ulcers, tumours, mumps, acute inflammation of the tonsils, malignant sore throat, dropsy of the joints, sciatica, spinal tenderness, etc. A mixture of simmered leaves can also be inhaled through a teapot spout for many of the mentioned conditions.

Homoeopathic Clinical: Tincture of fresh plant at the commencement of flowering—Anus (itching of), Colic, Constipation, Cough, Deafness, Enuresis, Haemorrhoids, Neuralgia, Brosopalgia, Urine (incontinence of).

Russian Experience: Mullein, or Koroviak Visoky, is common in all parts of Russia. This herb is seldom mentioned in ancient books, but was a common medicine in the Middle Ages.

Folk Medicine: Leaves and flowers are used as Astringent, Demulcent Expectorant and Tonic in the form of teas, extracts, as Nastoika (with vodka) either straight or in combinations. The uses are many as most natural treatments improve or assist the body as a complete unit instead of the specialized isolated practice of civilized thinking. Mullein is thought of first for pulmonary conditions, colds, shortness of breath, asthma; thus improving heart conditions, nervous disorders, kidney and bladder. Female and venereal diseases associated with, or without, bleeding. Epilepsy and headache in children (Atlas, Moscow, 1962).

Externally: The leaves and flowers simmered and used as a wash for old wounds, broken skin and to kill skin epidermis worms (Vishays Shkolla, Moscow, 1963). Fresh leaves bruised and applied to boils and carbuncles.

Veterinary: For tapeworms of cows the fresh leaves are given internally.

NETTLE   Urtica dioca, L.
(N.O.: Urticaceae)

Common Names: GREAT STINGING NETTLE, GREAT NETTLE.

Features: Nine of thirty species of Urtica, a herbaceous plant or shrub of the Urticaceae family, are found in temperate regions of the United States and Canada, in waste places, beside hedges and gardens. The most common is Urtica dioica, the stinging nettle, which grows to a height of almost 3 ft. The root of this pereninal is creeping and branching. The dull green stem is usually covered with stinging hairs which pierce the skin and emit an acrid fluid when touched, causing pain. When the Nettle is grasped in such a way as to press the hairs to the stem, however, no stinging occurs. The leaves of stinging nettle are coarse, opposite and conspicuously acuminate. The small green flowers can be seen from June to September. Always use your tender leaves. The Scots and Irish use the young leaves for greens, the French prepare seven different dishes from the tops.

Medicinal Parts: The roots and leaves.

Solvent: Boiling water.

Bodily Influence: Diuretic, Astringent, Tonic, Pectoral.

Uses: The Indians used Nettle as a counter-irritant when in pain, by striking affected parts with the branches. A root decoction was made to bathe rheumatic pains and joint stiffness. Pounded leaves rubbed on limbs, and hot poultices of the bruised leaves were also used to dress rheumatic discomfort. Nettle is an excellent styptic, checking the flow of blood from the surface almost immediately upon application of the powdered root or leaves softened and bruised. (If the fresh leaves are left on too long they will encourage water blisters.) For spitting of blood and all haemorrhages of the lungs, stomach and urinary organ, this is one of the most powerful agents in the vegetable materia medica.

Dr. George P. Wood, M.D., and Dr. E. H. Ruddock, M.D., "Vitalogy" (1925) relay the following: "For haemorrhages the express juice of the fresh leaves is regarded as more effective than the decoction, given in teaspoonful doses every hour or as often as the nature of the case requires." In decoction, Nettle is valuable in diarrhoea, dysentery, piles, neuralgia, gravel, inflammation of the kidney. Tea made from the young or dried root is of great help in dropsy of the first stages. A herbal Nettle tea will expel phlegm from the lungs and stomach and will clean the urinary canal. The seeds are used in coughs and shortness of breath.

204

Dose: Of the decoction, from 2–4 fl. oz. Of the powdered root or leaves, 20–40 grains.

Externally: J. Kloss, in "Back to Eden", says: "Use nettle simmered for 30 minutes and massage into the scalp after rinsing the hair to bring back the natural colour." For those suffering from rheumatism, without any relief, rub or stick the troubled part with fresh nettles for a few minutes daily. The relief of joint pain will often surrender to a few moments of unpleasant stinging.

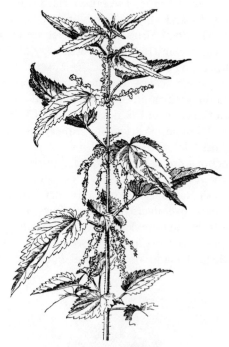

NETTLE   Urtica dioica, L.
(Rastenia Tzelitely, Moscow 1963)

Homoeopathic Clinical: Tincture of the fresh plant in flower—Agalactia, Bee stings, Burns, Calculus (prevention of), Deltoid (rheumatism of), Dysentery, Erysipelas (vesicular), Erythema, Gout, Gravel, Haemorrhage, Intermittents, Lactation, Leucorrhoea, Menorrhagia, Phlegmasia dolens, Renel colic, Rheumatism, Spleen (affections of), Throat (sore), Uremia, Urticaria, Nodosa, Vertigo, Whooping cough, Worms.

Russian Experience: Krapiva (Nettle) grows everywhere in Russia. After 300 years modern science has established and gives credit to one of the secrets of Nettle as an antiseptic.

Folk Medicine: Since the seventeenth century Russian Herbalists have given credit to Nettle as antiseptic, astringent, blood purifier, which are only a few of its properties. From some of the first books on herbs and their uses Nettle ranks high, and still has unalterable thoughts for treatment. Decoction of the whole plant for headache; decoction with honey or sugar to improve the function of the heart, liver, kidney, anaemia, blood purifying, gastritis, tubercular lungs; taken cold after delivery for afterbirth, whooping cough; decoction of the root for whooping cough and any internal bleeding: flower decoction for diabetes.

Externally: "Decomposing flesh will be cleansed, wounds and ulcers healed after treatments of Nettle. The boiled Herb is used to strengthen, stimulate new growths and stop falling hair if used as a hair wash." (Vishaya Schkolla, M., 1963). Bruised fresh leaves are used for rheumatic pain, dropsy, and chest pain (Bello-Russ. Academy of Science, 1965).

Clinically: As extracts and compounds.

Food: The young spring leaves are among the best used as garden greens, and is a main ingredient in Caucasus national recipes.

India and Pakistan Experience: Local name Bichu, Chicru.

Bodily Influence: Diuretic, Astringent, Emmenagogue, Haemostatic, Anthelmintic, Lithotriptic, Antiperiodic.

Uses: Nettle decoctions are used for kidney diseases and haemorrhage, especially from the uterus, and kidneys, consumption and jaundice. Young tops as a fresh Nettle tea are used for intermittent fever, gravel in the kidneys and excessive menstrual flow. Juice is very effective in checking bleeding from the nose, lungs, uterus and other internal organs.

Externally: The pulverized dry herb is used to sniff for nose bleeding (J. F. Dastur, "Medical Plants of India and Pakistan", India, 1962).

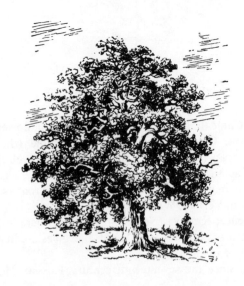

OAK TREE Quercus robur, L.
(N.O.: Fagaceae)

Common Name: TANNERS BARK.

Features: Approximately eighty species of the beech family (Fagaceae) are native to the United States, of which fifty-eight are trees. These forest trees vary in size, according to the climate soil. The pubescence of the leaves and twigs consists of fascicled hairs which are intricately branched. The April flowers appear with, or after the leaves, which later develop into the cup of the fruit known as the acorn. In some areas, Indians would gather 500 lb. per family, which was a year's supply. These were stored and later used for bread, pudding, soup, etc., prepared fresh from the ground acorn. White Oak bark is chiefly used in medicine. It has a brownish colour, fainty odorous, very astringent, with a slight bitterness.

Medicinal Parts: The bark, acorn.

Solvents: Alcohol, water.

Bodily Influence: Astringent, Tonic, Haemostatic, Antiseptic.

Uses: It may be of use to know that a decoction of acorns and bark added to milk and taken resists the forces of poisonous medicines, or when the bladder becomes ulcerated by taking them, and shows voidance of bloody urine. The bark is an agent in chronic diarrhoea, chronic mucous discharges, passive haemorrhages, and wherever an internal astringent is required. White Oak bark as an infusion is best known as a goitre remedy, and is still being used for excess of stomach mucus, which causes the common complaint of sinus congestion, post-nasal drip, etc. It relieves the stomach by paving the way for better internal absorption and secretion, thus improving metabolism. The distilled water of the buds before they become leaves can be used either externally or internally for inflammation, burning fevers and infections; also used for leucorrhoea, womb troubles, haemorrhoids and prolapsed rectum (sitz bath). The Oak bark tea acts like a resin in a strengthening way on the outer vessels; often dangerous fistules on the rectum are dissolved and healed by this method, occasionally using the diluted tea as a colonic.

Dose: A decoction is made from 1 oz. of bark in 1 quart of water, boiled down to 1 pint, and taken in wineglass doses.

Externally: Excellent as a gargle for sore or relaxed throat. For neck enlargements, fomentations are beneficial if applied often. Indian tribes are known to have allowed acorn meal to go mouldy in a dark, damp place and then scrape the mould off for application to boils, sores and other inflammations.

Homoeopathic Clinical: Tincture of acorns (peeled and crushed or shredded); spirit distilled from tincture (Spiritus glandium quercus); water extract of acorn with addition of alcohol (Aqua glandium quercus)— Alcoholism, Breath (offensive), Constipation, Diarrhoea, Dropsy (splenic), Fistula, Dizziness, Gout, Intermittent fever, Leukaemia splenica, Spleen (affections of).

Russian Experience: Oak, or in Russian "Dub", grows wild and besides being used medicinally is also widely used in industry, especially in the food and tanning trades.

Folk Medicine: Oak bark should be collected in the early spring while the sap is active. The bark must be from young branches, twigs and thin young trunks. Decoctions are used for diarrhoea, menstrual disturbance; tea and decoction with honey for tubercular lungs, gastritis, bleeding from the bladder and bloody urine, and as a gargle for swollen or irritated tongue; coffee of acorns for scrofula, children's skin rash, hysteria.

Externally: Antiseptic for malignant wounds containing decayed cells. A tea solution prepared for painful bleeding and itching haemorrhoids. Can also be used to stop falling hair and dandruff. Leaves and bark for inflammation of burns.

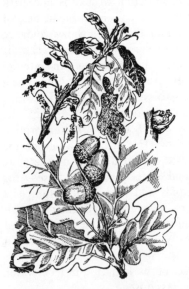

OAK TREE Quercus robur, L.
1—Spring flowering twig 2—Branch
with fruits 3—Flower
(Vishaya Schkolla, Moscow, 1963)

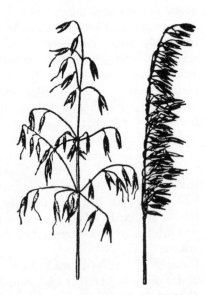

OATS Avena sativa, L.
Left—Spreading Right—One-sided
(Botanica, Moscow, 1949)

208

OATS   Avena sativa, L.
(N.O.: Gramineae)

Common Name: GROATS.

Features: Widely distributed in most parts of the world, in field cultivation. The Oats of commercial and general use are the seeds of Avena sativa with the husk removed. The crushed or coarsely flaked grain is known as oatmeal. The tincture and powder is used in herbal combinations of tonics and capsules.

Medicinal Part: Seeds.

Solvent: Water.

Bodily Influence: Nervine, Tonic, Stimulant, Antispasmodic.

Uses: Cheerfulness is health; its opposite, melancholy, is disease. The cliché, "He's feeling his oats", usually refers to a spirited horse who has been fed on Oats. It is a recognized natural food, appealing in taste and nourishment, and has long been used as a family remedy in an infusion, usually accepted by patients of weak digestion when other foods fail. The properties of Avena sativa in tincture of Oats beards has had recognition by people of all lands as a naturalizer to the sexual gland system. An important restorative in nervous prostration and exhaustion after all febrile diseases, it seems to support the heart muscles and urinary organs. Instead of coffee a drink made from equal parts of Oak beards, roasted acorns and chicory, in equal proportions, is a welcome and beneficial change.

Dose: The tea is made by steeping 1 teaspoonful of the beards in a cup of hot water for 10 min. or more, then straining and adding honey if desired. Taken a mouthful at a time throughout the day.

Externally: Culpeper recommends oatmeal boiled in vinegar as an application for the removal of freckles and spots on the face and body.

Homoeopathic Clinical: Tincture of fresh plant in flower—Alcoholism, Cholera, Debility, Influenza, Neurasthenia, Opium habit, Palpitation, Sexual excess, Sleeplessness, Tuberculosis.

Russian Experience: In Russia, Oves (Oats) are highly regarded for both human and domestic animal consumption, having a great value as both food and medicine, when thought is given to the subject, it does seem this was intended.

Folk Medicine: Employ its virtues in decoctions and tea (grain and Oat straw) as Diuretic, Diaphoretic, Carminative and Febricide (to reduce fever). Recommended as an all-round food for the sick, weak and healthy.

Externally: Hot Oat straw compresses applied to painful areas when in pain from kidney stone attack will soon bring about welcome relief. Oat straw and oak bark decoctions are used for excessive foot perspiration.

209

Oat straw steam baths are used for children with rickets and scrofula, and as a cosmetic aid to a fresh, healthy skin.

ONION   Allium cepa, L.
(N.O.: Liliaceae)

Common Name: ONION.

Features: There are various species of Allium, a genus of the Lily family; specifically. A. cepa, a bulbous, rooted biennial herb. It is probably native to western Asia, as it is mentioned in old Egyptian writings and the Pentateuch. The Onion has spread to all countries occupied by man. They can be planted as soon as the ground can be worked in early spring, or it may be cultivated during the winter where the temperature does not fall to freezing point. The flowers appear early in summer.

Medicinal Part: The bulb.

Solvent: Water.

Bodily Influence: Stimulant, Carminative, Condiment, Diuretic, Expectorant.

Uses: As a domestic medicine the Onion, in various preparations, has come to the rescue in colds and croups. Roast the Onion until soft, extract the liquid, add honey to taste, mix well and give in teaspoonful to tablespoonful amounts as age and condition calls for. If desired the whole roasted Onion can be eaten with honey. The Onion is also effective internally and externally in catarrhal pneumonia, abscesses, convulsions of children, suppurating tumours. If a child has worms, after fasting for a morning give a decoction of Rue (Ruta graveolens), Onion seeds, Onion extract and honey. Prepare the mixture the night before by pouring boiling water over the preparation and then straining. If taken on an empty stomach it will often clear the system of the unwanted creatures. Mix Onion with Rue and honey as a cure for the bite of venomous creatures and mad dogs. Should be applied externally, and taken internally, often. In Holland they macerate the Onion, and the tincture is taken for gravel and dropsical affections.

Externally: The juice of a grated or bruised Onion, or leek, with the addition of a little salt, when laid on fresh burns or scalds draws out the fire and prevents them from blistering. Used with vinegar it diminishes skin blemishes. Herbalists of long ago used the above for pain and ringing in the ears.

Homoeopathic Clinical: Tincture of the onion, or of whole fresh plant gathered from July to August—Anus (fissure of), Ascites, Catarrh, Cold, Coryza, Cough, Diarrhoea, Facial paralysis, Feet (easily galled), Hay fever, Hernia, Influenza, Laryngitis, Panaritium, Pneumonia, Trauma, Whitlow, Whooping cough, Yellow fever.

Russian Experience: Luke and Chesnock, Onion and Garlic, are inseparable from Russian daily life as a food, but also have great importance as a medicine.

Folk Medicine: A custom of the old timers was to wear a piece of Garlic or Onion around the neck, chest high, on a string. The fragrance was not agreeable but that, they insisted, was the very thing which kept sickness from colds, infections, etc. at bay. Prof. B. P. Tokin's interest was aroused enough to do some experiments on this Old Babushka (old wives' tale). Scientifically, some merit was found for this seemingly

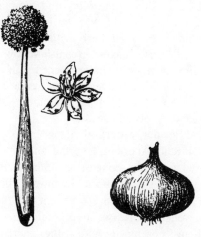

ONION   Allium cepa, L.
(Botanica, Moscow, 1949)

foolish caper. He found that the plants produce a special chemical antiseptic for self-protection and defence which is known in Russia as Fi-ton-ci-tis (English, Phy-to-chi-nin), a substance isolated from the leaves of certain grasses; said to have an effect on carbohydrate metabolism resembling that of insulin. Botanist B. M. Kozo-Poliansky also made tests and found that many plants contain volatile oils with atmospheric protection. He feels that the plant has stronger protection than that of the juice against the enemy who penetrates the first line of defence. For your own simple proof, crush Onion or Garlic and put under a glass. Next to this place culture or fungus and in a few minutes all bacteria or fungus (micro-organism) will perish.

After experiments (1942–5) the fumes are clinically used to treat wounds and ulcers (Vishaya Scholla, Moscow, 1963). Folk Medicine use the Onion as Stimulant, Antiseptic, Diuretic, Tonic and Carminative. For atony of the intestine, and as a result of it high blood pressure, and for Avitaminosis and Hypovitaminosis (Atlas, Moscow, 1962).

211

PARSLEY   Petroselinum sativum, Hoffm.
(N.O.: Umbelliferae)

Common Names: PARSLEY BREAKSTONE, GARDEN PARSLEY, ROCK PARSLEY.

Features: Parsley belongs to a small genus of the Mediterranean plant, Umbelliferae, cultivated since antiquity, and now grown in various forms in all of the civilized world. Parsley is a many-branched, bright green, smooth stemmed, biennial herb with ternately pinnate decompound, sometimes with crisp leaves; greenish-yellow flowers. The root is the official part. French chemists have succeeded in obtaining an essential oil named apiol which has proved a good replacement for quinia in intermittent fever and for ergot as a parturient.

Medicinal Parts: Leaves, roots and seeds.

Solvents: Leaves and powder, water; oil, alcohol.

Bodily Influence: Diuretic, Aperient, Expectorant.

Uses: Is chiefly used for renal congestion, inflammation of the kidney and bladder, for gravel, stones, urine retention, the culprit of many malfunctions. The root or leaves are excellent for the liver and spleen when jaundice and venereal diseases ar present. Also useful in epilepsy. A worthy ingredient, combined with other herbs such as Buchu (Borosma), black haw (Viburnum prunifolium), Cramp bark (Viburnum opulus), for female troubles. Drink as much as 3 cupfuls a day.

Parsley is high in Vitamin B and potassium, a substance in which cancerous cells cannot multiply. Should be considered among the preventive herbs. The seeds contain apiol, which is considered a safe and efficient emmenagogue and is used in amenorrhoea and dysmenorrhoea. Of assistance in intermittent fever or agues.

Dose: Of the oil, for diuretic purposes, 3–4 drops a day. Of the infusion, 2–4 cupfuls.

Externally: Often the bruised leaves are applied to swollen glands and swollen breasts to dry up milk. Hot fomentations wrung out of the tea will relieve insect bites and stings.

Homoeopathic Clinical: Tincture of whole fresh plant when coming into bloom—Catheter fever, Cystitis, Dysuria, Gleet, Gonorrhoea, Gravel, Intermittent fever, Night blindness, Priapism.

Russian Experience: Petrushka, Parsley, a common vegetable in all gardens, is used as food and home medicine. Preparations of tea and decoctions from the root, leaves and seeds are administered for dropsy, kidney and bladder, female corrective, indigestion, liver, spleen ailments, prostatitis.

Externally: The fresh juice is used as a non-toxic insect repellent in the summer time.

PARTRIDGE BERRY   Mitchella repens, L.
(N.O.: Rubiaceae)

Common Names: WINTER CLOVER, SQUAW BERRY, ONE BERRY, CHECKER BERRY, DEER BERRY, etc.

Features: A member of the Madder family (Rubiaceae). Partridge berry is indigenous to North America and found in dry and swampy woods from south-western Newfoundland to Minnesota, south to Florida and Texas, and in Guatemala.

The shining leaves are roundish or heart-shaped, $\frac{1}{2}$–$\frac{3}{4}$ in. long, which sometimes look like clover; they are opposite on the stem and may be marked with white lines, and they remain green throughout the winter. The fragrant white or pink paired flowers, $\frac{1}{2}$ in. long, are joined at the base and usually have four hairy petals; seen in bloom from June to July. The scarlet berry, which remains on the plant all winter, is $\frac{1}{4}$ in. in diameter, containing usually eight bony seeds. The berry is edible but is nearly tasteless. It may be grown in the wild garden or as a tarrarium plant.

Medicinal Part: The whole herb.

Solvents: Dilute alcohol, boiling water.

Bodily Influence: Astringent, Diuretic, Tonic, Parturient.

Uses: One of several common herbs that the Indian squaw used weeks before confinement, in order to render parturient safe and easy. It is best to combine with other herbs, and advisable to consult a herbal physician of experience for safe, proper and effective preparation. In all urinary diseases it is highly beneficial; the berries are used for dysentery.

Dose: 1 teaspoonful of the herb to 1 cupful of boiling water. Drink 1–2 cupfuls a day. Of the tincture, $\frac{1}{4}$–$\frac{1}{2}$ fl. dram.

Externally: The berries are also highly spoken of as an ointment for sore nipples. The application is made by boiling a strong decoction of the leaves down to a thick liquid and then adding cream to it.

Homoeopathic Clinical: Tincture of whole plant—Bladder (irritation of), Dysmenorrhoea, Dysuria, Kidney (pain in), Metritis.

PASSION FLOWER   Passiflora incarnata, L.
(N.O.: Passifloraceae)

Features: Passiflora is a genus of some 400 species, most of which are native to the New World tropics. The plants are mostly herbaceous or woody climbing, tendrilled vines. The striking flowers, often several inches across, have sepals on the rim of the cup, five petals and showy corona. The flower is almost white except for the purple centre and the blue crown banded in the middle. There are usually five stamens developed on a column above the perianth, and above these is the pistil, with three knob-like stigmas and an ovary bearing numerous ovules on three particular placentae. Spanish explorers and missionaries fancied it had a resemblance to the crown of thorns or to the halo of Christ, hence the name Passion flower.

Medicinal Parts: Plant and flower.

Solvent: Diluted alcohol.

Bodily Influence: Anodyne, Nerve sedative, Diuretic, Antispasmodic.

Uses: When in need of help for nervousness, without pain, such as unrest, agitation and exhaustion, Passiflora is helpful. It is useful in controlling convulsions, particularly in the young, as indicated by muscular twitching and also for asthenic insomnia in childhood and the elderly; irritative and neuralgic pains with debility, nervous headache,

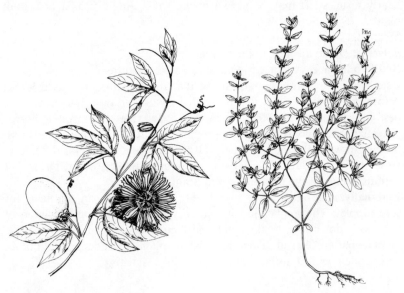

PASSION FLOWER
Passiflora incarnata, L.
(U.S. Agricultural Department,
Appalachia, 1971)

PENNYROYAL (American)
Hedeoma pulegiodes, L.
(U.S. Agricultural Department,
Appalachia, 1971)

214

hysteria, spasms such as epilepsy, etc. When these are present Passion flower tones the sympathetic nerve centre, improving circulation and nutrition to the centres. It is given by physico-medicalists in cases usually placed under bromide medication. The result will be a more restful sleep and a feeling of freshness on awaking.

Dose: Best prescribed in tincture or tablets. Tincture of Passion flower alone, 15–60 drops in water according to age and condition, repeated as necessary.

Homoeopathic Clinical: Tincture of fresh or dried leaves gathered in May; fluid hydroalcoholic extract; powdered inspissated juice—Burns, Cholera infantum, Convulsions, Delirium tremens, Dentition, Epilepsy, Erysipelas, Exophthalmos, Levitation, Sciatica, Sleeplessness, Tetanus neonatum.

PENNYROYAL (American)   Hedeoma pulegioides, L.
(N.O.: Labiatae)

Common Names: SQUAW MINT, THICKWEED, HEDEOMA, STINKING BALM, AMERICAN PENNYROYAL.

Features: Our Pennyroyal (Hedeoma) should not be confused with the European Pennyroyal (Mentha pulegioides). Squaw mint is an indigenous annual plant with a fibrous, yellowish root, and an erect, branching stem, from 6–12 in. high. The leaves are $\frac{1}{2}$ in. or more long, opposite, obscurely serrate, hairy beneath and on short petioles. The flowers are small and light blue, appearing from June to September. They thrive particularly in limestone country, in barren woods and dry fields. Is common to nearly all parts of the United States. The mint-like fragrance is felt in the air for some distance. The taste is aromatic, pungent. It is said to be very obnoxious to fleas.

Medicinal Part: The herb.

Solvents: Alcohol, boiling water (partially).

Bodily Influence: Diaphoretic, Diuretic, Corrective, Nervine.

Uses: The warm infusion, used freely, will promote perspiration. It has long been used by women to promote menstruation. Hot footbaths are taken several days before due date and two cups of Pennyroyal tea, especially before going to bed, for scanty or suppressed flow. Also for nervousness and hysteria, cramps, intestinal pains of colic and griping, colds, and as a sweating and cooling drink in fevers. The infusion may be freely taken several times a day. The tincture of the oil of Pennyroyal is often employed in whooping cough and spasms, to be taken in doses of 2–10 drops.

Dose: 1 teaspoonful of the herb to 1 cupful of boiling water. Of the tincture, $\frac{1}{2}$–1 fl. dram.

Externally: Equal parts of the oil and Linseed oil make a valuable application for burns. Pennyroyal is also used as a hot fomentation in rheumatic affections, applied externally.

Homoeopathic Clinical: Tincture of the whole fresh plant—Amenorrhoea, Dysmenorrhoea, Leucorrhoea.

PINK ROOT Spigelia marilandica, L.
(N.O.: Loganiaceae)

Common Names: INDIAN PINK, CAROLINA PINK, MARYLAND PINK, WORM GRASS.

Features: Pink root is indigenous to America. A perennial that inhabits the southern states and is seldom found north of the Potomas. The Cherokee Indians used to collect the herb, for the market, in the northern part of Georgia, but since their removal the supply comes from the far south-west.

The yellow root is very fibrous and sends up several erect, smooth,

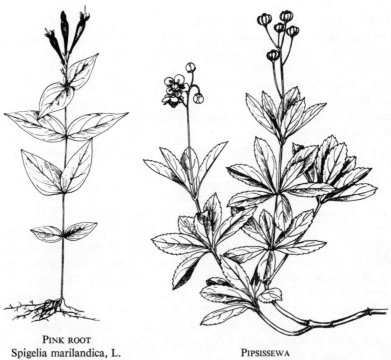

PINK ROOT
Spigelia marilandica, L.
(U.S. Agricultural
Department, Appalachia,
1971)

PIPSISSEWA
Chimaphila umbellata (L.) Nutt.
(U.S. Agricultural Department,
Appalachia, 1971)

216

purplish colour stems, from 6–20 in. high. The leaves are opposite, lanceolate and smooth. The flowers are few in number, growing on one side of the stem only. The outside of the flower growth is above the leaf line of the plant.

Medicinal Part: The root.

Solvents: Dilute alcohol, boiling water (partially).

Bodily Influence: Anthelmintic, in large doses Narcotic.

Uses: Pink root was used by our Indians as an anthelmintic before the discovery of America. We still use the ancient preparation for the same purpose. It is non-poisonous to the body but should be used according to age, and with other herbs. The following is a formula of wide acceptance from J. E. Meyers, Herbalist:

> 1 part Pink root (Spigelia marilandica)
> 1 part Senna leaves (Cassia)
> 1 part Anise seeds (Pimpinella anisum)
> 1 part Male fern (Aspidium filix mas.)
> 1 part Turtlebloom (Chelone glabra)

1 teaspoonful of above mixture to 1 cupful of boiling water. Drink 1 cupful as often as indicated; children 1 tablespoonful. If the creatures persist, administer the decoction at full moon, as they are more active and therefore vulnerable to treatment at this time. Excessive doses or too strong cathartics are to be avoided as they may cause dizziness and dry throat.

Dose: If the powder is used instead of the infusion, 10–20 grains can be mixed with the formula.

Homoeopathic Clinical: Tincture of root—Mania, Strabismus.

PIPSISSEWA   Chimaphila umbellata, (L.) Nutt.
(N.O.: Ericaceae)

Common Names: GROUND HOLLY, PRINCE'S PINE, WINTER GREEN—not to be confused with Winter green (Gaultheria procumbens).

Features: This small evergreen is indigenous to the northern temperate regions of both hemispheres. The perennial herb grows in dry shady woods, flowering in May through to August, with light purple flowers of pleasant fragrance. The root is creeping with several erect stems, woody at their base and 4–8 in. high. The leaves are dark green above, pale below, 2–3 in. long, on short petioles. When fresh and friction rubbed they are fragrant; not noticeable when dried. Contains resin, gum, lignin and saline substances.

Medicinal Part: The whole plant.

Solvents: Diluted alcohol, boiling water.

Bodily Influence: Diuretic, Tonic, Alterative, Astringent.

Uses: As a remedy for dropsy, kidney and bladder troubles this well-known wild herb has enjoyed long and admirable reputation. In folk and domestic usage the combination of agents was made into an infusion, but is best given in the tincture.

Tincture of Pipsissewa (Chimaphila umbellata), 2–15 drops
Tincture of Poke root (Phytolacca decandra), 2–10 drops
Tincture of Prickly ash (Xanthoxylum americanum), 5–20 drops
Tincture of Stickwort (Agrimonia eupatoria), 10–30 drops

15 drops three or four times a day with plenty of water.

A small amount of Dandelion root (Leontodon taraxacum), Yellow dock (Rumex crispus), Golden seal (Hydrastis canadensis) added to the above compound will aid conditions of scrofulous and other blood troubles where the urinary organs are particulary weak. Pipsissewa is often preferred because of its acceptability to the stomach for conditions when the urine is scanty and contains offensive pus or pus and blood mixed, when the urine is scalding or burning, in chronic urethral and prostatic irritations, chronic relaxation of the bladder and chronic prostations with catarrh of the bladder, also effective for skin disease and in gonorrhoeal rheumatism.

Dose: 1 teaspoonful of the plant to 1 cupful of boiling water, three times a day. Of the tincture, 2–15 drops in water as frequently as required.

Homoeopathic Clinical: Tincture of root and leaves, or of fresh plant in flower—Acne, Breast (atrophy of; cancer of; tumour of), Cataract, Cystitis, Diabetes, Dropsy, Fevers, Glands (enlarged), Gleet, Gonorrhoea, Intermittents, Jaundice, Kidneys (disorders of), Lactation (disorder of), Liver disorders, Nephritis, Proctitis, Prostatitis, Pterygium, Ringworm, Scrofula, Stricture, Syphilis, Toothache, Ulcers (malignant), Urinary disorders, Whitlow.

Russian Experience: The wintry pine forests of Russia are perfect for this evergreen shrub, which Folk Medicine call Zimolubka (Loving winter).

Folk Medicine: Use decoction or Nastoika (with vodka) for tenderness and pain of the muscles due to heavy lifting. Also for penetrating pain of areas involved after childbirth and bloody urine.

PLANTAIN   Plantago major, L.
(N.O.: Plantaginaceae)

Common Names: PLANTAGO MAJOR, RIPPLE GRASS, WAGBREAD, WHITE MAN'S FOOT.

Features: Most of the 200 or more widely distributed species of Plantain are weedy herbs, or subshrubs of the family plantaginaceae. Plantago Major is the best-known backyard Plantain, abundant in most of North America. It is native to Europe, but was spread so rapidly by human explorers in America that the Indians called it "White man's foot".

The leaves all radiate from the base but in some species are broader than in others (but both are good). They are dark green in colour and strongly ribbed lengthwise. The flower stem is stiff and smooth and attains heights of 6–18 in. The head is short and studded with tiny four-parted dull white flowers with long slender stamens.

Medicinal Part: The whole plant.

Solvent: Water.

Bodily Influence: Alterative, Astringent, Diuretic, Antiseptic.

Uses: Plantain was used by the Indians both internally and externally; we have adopted their uses of it for cooling, soothing and healing. Plantain is acceptable to most people. It is excellent for healing fresh or chronic wounds or sores, used both internally or externally. Omitting the scientific names, the body still responds to the clandestine ingredients of organic treatment.

Plantain is a superior remedy for neuralgia; take 2–5 drops of the tincture every 20 min.—usually a few drops will give relief. The green seeds and stem boiled in milk will generally check diarrhoea and bowel complaints of children. Culpeper used the seeds as treatment for dropsy, epilepsy and yellow jaundice. The clarified juice, and/or seeds, made into tea or jelly-like water taken by itself or mixed with other herbs relieves intestinal pain of ulcers, spitting of blood, excessive menstrual flow and inflammation of the intestines. For kidney and bladder trouble, including bed-wetting, and pain in the lumbar region, Plantain is of use; also to clear the ear of mucus. If venereal diseases are in the first stages a strong decoction of Plantain, leaves and root, one or two times a day in wineglassful amounts will often leave the afflicted a new admirer on the long list of Plantain users. It is also useful in scrofula, haemorrhoids, leucorrhoea. Make a strong tea and let steep 30 min.; for haemorrhoids inject a tablespoonful or more several times a day and after bowel evacuation. As feminine wash, 2 tablespoonfuls of Plantain to 1 pint of water, simmer covered, cool, strain, add enough water to fill container.

Dose: 1 teaspoonful of Plantain to 1 cupful of boiling water. Of the tincture, $\frac{1}{2}$–1 fl. dram.

Externally: The juice of the leaves will counteract the bite of rattle-snakes, poisonous insects, etc. Take 1 tablespoonful every hour, at the same time applying the bruised leaves to the wounds. Also to check external bleeding, erysipelas, ulcers, eczema, burns and scalds. Can be used as a strong tea to bathe the area often. Apply poultice to rheumatic-like pain, or add large amount to bath water for relief. The leaves dipped in cider vinegar and dried overnight then placed on the feet before

219

putting stockings on will aid leg pains. An ointment can be made by slowly boiling for 2 hr. 2 oz. or granulated Plantain in 1 pint of soy bean, coconut, peanut or other soluble oil.

Homoeopathic Clinical: Tincture of whole fresh plant; tincture of root— ciliary neuralgia, Diabetes, Diarrhoea, Dysentery, Earache, Ear (inflammation of), Emissions, Enuresis, Erysipelas Erythema, Haemorrhoids, Impotence, Neuralgias (of herpes), Polyuria, Snake bites, Spleen (pains in), Tobacco habit, Toothache Urination (delayed), Worms, Wounds.

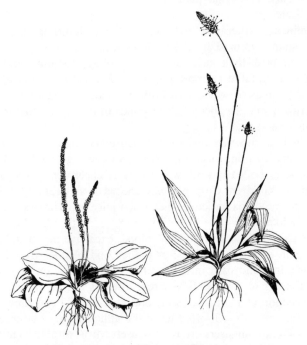

PLANTAIN   Plantago major, L.
(Ontario Department of Agriculture, Toronto, Canada, 1966)

Russian Experience: Wild Plantain is known to the Russians and their native name is "Podoroshnik", meaning near the road or along the road. Plantain grows easily in any climate and soil. Among almost thirty species Plantago lanceolate is cultivated commercially in France, Spain and the United States of America. This and Plantago major are given the most credit. Our herb has an old and honourable history as an Arabian and Persian medicine for dysentery and all other stomach and intestinal trouble. Ancient Roman and Greek medicine valued and gave credit to the healing power of the Plantago.

Folk Medicine: Usually prepared as a tea from the fresh or dried herb,

220

or as conserved juice of freshly picked leaves and flowers with the faithful vodka (Nastoika) after they have extracted the day's supply of the fresh plant. Seeds are used for inflammation of the stomach, intestines, ulcers and to reduce stomach pain. Their use coincides with the Fathers of Antiquity for all stomach conditions, gastritis, loose bowels, stomach ulcers, internal wounds, abscesses and internal bleeding. To induce appetite a drink of Plantain is given, also for kidney, bladder and heart conditions, coughs, tuberculosis of the lungs, red inflamed skin, headache and snake bites. Plantain is rich in minerals and Vitamins C, K, and factor "T" which helps to stop bleeding (Medicine, Moscow, 1963).

Clinical Testimonials: After observation of many cases of stomach sickness, it was found that chronic ulcers responded to treatment with the fresh juice of Plantain, or Nastoika (C. A. Minsoyan, A. J. Perihanian, E. C. Rudakova, M. J. Sumtzeva (Mrs.)). Also used for dysentery, dyspepsia (A. A. Goremik, Mrs.); to correct acid condition of the stomach and regulate secretion of the stomach (N. J. Krivtzova, Mrs.); the Russian Ministry of Health recommends Plantain for chronic colitis and acute stomach conditions of gastritis, enteritis, enterocolitis (Moscow University, Moscow, 1963).

Externally: Extensive clinical research and experiments have proved that fresh Plantain juice is suitable for dressing wounds, ulcers, furnicles, boils (M. P. Rasman) and as a powder for abscesses, ulcers, wounds of bleeding and chronic skin conditions (Bello-Russ. Academy of Science, 1965).

PLEURISY ROOT   Asclepias tuberosa, L.
N.O.: Asclepiadaceae)

Common Names: BUTTERFLY WEED, SWALLOW WORT, WIND ROOT, TUBER ROOT, PLEURISY ROOT.

Features: A handsome perennial herb of the Asclepiadaceae family, common in dry, gravelly and sandy soils throughout the United States and Canada. The large, irregular, yellowish-brown, tuberous roots have a nauseous, bitter taste when fresh, but are better when dried. The hairy stems, which rise to a height of 2–3 ft., bear alternate, lanceolate, hairy leaves, dark green above and pale beneath. The flowers are numerous, erect and of a beautifully bright orange-yellow colour, flowering in June and August, and are followed by erect, long, narrow, pubescent pods. Ascepin is the active principle.

Medicinal Part: The root.

Solvent: Boiling water.

Bodily Influence: Pleurisy root is used for the condition which the name suggests. The influence is active to the accumulated, excessive, life-weakening mucus build-up of pleurisy, pulmonary and gastro intestinal tract.

Uses: Pleurisy root is much used in decoction and/or infusion for the purpose of promoting perspiration and expectoration in diseases of the respiratory organs, inflammation of the lungs, catarrhal affections, consumption. It mitigates the pain and relieves the difficulty of breathing without being a stimulant. The root is also used for acute rheumatism and dysentery, colds, la-grippe, all bronchial congestions, bilious and burning fevers. "It is especially a child's remedy, being feeble in its action in small doses, though quite certain. When freely given, it is one of the most certain diaphoretics we have, even in small doses of one drop it will markedly increase the true secretions from the skin" (Dr. Lloyd Feller).

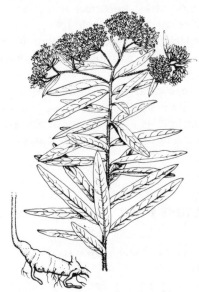

PLEURISY ROOT   Asclepias tuberosa, L.
(U.S. Agricultural Department, Appalachia, 1971)

Dose: Children may be given 1–5 drops in hot water, depending on age and condition, every 1–2 hr. If restless, add some Skull cap (Scutellaria) but reduce this after perspiration is established. Be sure to keep the patient warm. Infusion of 1 teaspoonful of cut or powdered herb to 1 cupful of boiling water, steeped for $\frac{1}{2}$ hr. Give every 3–4 hr. for adults, in proportion for children. Of the tincture, 4–40 drops every 3 hr. or less, depending on age and condition.

Homoeopathic Clinical: Tincture of fresh root—Alopecia, Asthma,

222

Bilious fever, Bronchitis, Catarrh, Chancre, Colic, Cough, Diarrhoea, Dysentery, Headache, Heart (affections of), Influenza, Ophthalmia, Pericarditis, Pleurisy, Pleurodynia, Rheumatism, Scrofula, Syphilis.

POKE ROOT   Phytolacca decandra, L.
(N.O.: Phytolaccaceae)

Common Names: PIGEON BERRY, GARGET, SCOKE, COAKUM, INKBERRY, POCAN.

Features: Poke, a strong-smelling pereninal herb of the family phytolaccaceae. Poke is native to the United States, from Maine to Florida and westward to Minnesota and Texas. Found in dry fields, hillsides and roadsides. The root matures to a very large size; it is easily cut or broken and the fleshly fibrous tissue is covered with a thin brownish bark. The stems are annual, about 1 in. in diameter, round, smooth, green when young and grow 3–12 ft. in height. The small greenish-white flowers appear in July and August, surrounded by dense foliage, followed by dark purple berries which ripen in late summer and autumn and are nearly globular, each containing ten carpels. The berries are only collected when fully matured. The young shoots and seedlings are often eaten; the former like asparagus, the latter like spinach. Make sure the root is scrupulously removed before using as a table vegetable. Phytolaccin is its active principle. Poke has had a long history of usefulness in medicine; it is toxic in too large amounts and persons using it should understand both its value and its limitations.

Medicinal Parts: Root and berries.

Solvents: Dilute alcohol, boiling water.

Bodily Influence: Emetic, Cathartic, Alterative, Deobstruent.

Uses: Preparation and dosage vary considerably with the condition of the root. Thurston, Hammer and other physio-medical practitioners recommended that only the green root should be used, owing to its rapid deterioration. Poke helps greatly in detoxicating the system from poisonous congestions. It stimulates metabolism and is useful for medication of the undernourished. Poke has creditable influence when the lymphatic glands, spleen and particularly the thyroid glands, are enlarged (excellent in goitre, internally and externally), hardening of the liver and reduced biliary flow. The root excites the whole glandular system and is very useful in the removal of mercurio-syphilitic affection, scrofula and chronic skin diseases.

Very few, if any of the alteratives have superior power to Poke if properly gathered and prepared for medicinal uses. Both the berries and root have high recognition for the treatment of rheumatism and arthritis, especially when used with Black cohosh (Cimicifuga) and

223

Prickly ash (Xanthoxylum flaxizeum-rue family). Poke is indicated, and should be combined in formulas, for throat conditions when membrane is dark in colour, tonsils swollen, shooting pains through the ear with difficulty in swallowing.

Dose: Tincture of Phytolacca alone, 2–5 drops, as frequently as indicated by symptoms. As a decoction, 1 tablespoonful of the root, leaves or berries cut small to 1 pint of boiling water, steeped 10 min. Take a mouthful at a time several times a day. The juice of the ripe berries preserved in syrup form may be used in teaspoonful doses every 3 hr.

Externally: Dr. Wood and Dr. Ruddock in "Vitology" (1921): "The juice of the berries dried in the sun until it forms the proper consistency for a plaster, applied twice a day has cured cancer." It is a dependable agent in the treatment of mammillary swelling from which so many women suffer following childbirth, making nursing impossible. In such cases, a mixture of Phytolacca, 3 parts to 1 part of glycerine, will abate the swelling in its beginning, or when suppuration has taken place it will help and bring about granulation. In bone enlargements and bone growths from injuries, when in a chronic state apply a solution of Poke root tea, made fresh daily. This will also relieve itching skin.

Homoeopathic Clinical: Tincture of fresh root dug in winter: tincture of the ripe berries; tincture of fresh leaves; solution of the resinous extract, Phytolaccin—Abortion (threatened), Albuminuria, Angina pectoris, Anus (fissure of), Asthma, Barber's itch, Boils, Bone (disease of; tumours of), Breasts (affections of), Cancer, Cholera, Cicatrix, Ciliary neuralgia, Constipation, Corpulence, Cough, Dentition (difficulty), Diarrhoea, Diphtheria, Diplopia, Dysentery, Dysmenia, Ears (affections of), Erythema nodosum, Eustachian tubes (affections of), Glands (enlarged), Gleet, Glossitis, Gonorrhoea, Gout, Granular conjunctivitis, Haemorrhoids, Headache, Hearing (altered), Heart (affection of; hypertrophy of; fatty), Impotence, Influenza, Intestinal catarrh, Itch, Lactation (abnormal), Laryngismus, Leucorrhoea, Lichen, Liver (affections of), Lumbago, Lupus, Mercury (effects of), Mouth (ulcer), Mumps, Neuralgia, Nipples (sore), Nursing (painful), Orchitis, Ozaena, Panophthalmitis, Paralysis (diphtheritic), Parotitis, Prostatitis, Prostate (affection of), Rectum (cancer of), Respiration (abnormal), Rheumatism (Syphilitic, Gonorrhoeal), Ringworm, Rodent ulcer, Salivation, Sciatica, Sewer gas poisoning, Spinal irritation, Spleen (pain in), Stiff neck, Syphilis, Syphilitic eruptions, Tetanus, Throat (sore; diphtheritic, herpetic; glandular), Toothache, Tumours, Ulcers, Uterus (affection of), Warts, Wens.

Russian Experience: Phytolacca decandra is not native to Russia. Poke was brought from North America to the Black Sea regions of Caucasus and Crimea. The natives have adopted Fitalaka Americana (or from Folk Medicine, Lakonos Americana) as the identifying name.

Folk Medicine soon found use for the American import as diuretic, laxative, vermifuge, emetic. They use it as tea, decoction and Nastoika (with vodka) for ulcer conditions, kidney and bladder trouble.

Clinically: Experiments prove that taken internally in small doses it is very relaxing and calming; large doses create disturbing effects of shortness of breath and convulsions.

Externally: Nastoika used as rheumatic liniment.

POPLAR   Populus tremuloides, Michx.
(N.O.: Salicaceae)

Common Names: WHITE POPLAR, AMERICAN ASPEN, QUAKING ASPEN.

Features: About thirty-five species of Poplars compose the family Salicaceae, all of which are trees. The Poplar grows throughout the United States and Canada, from sub-tropical to sub-arctic regions and from sea level to timberline. They are medium- to large-sized trees with simple, deciduous leaves of dull, whitish, dark green with white veins, attached alternately to the twigs. In several species, the leaf stalk, or petiole, is laterally compressed and the leaves tremble or quake in the slightest breeze. The flowers of a tree are of a single sex and male and female flowers occur on separate trees in drooping catkins which develop from floral buds before the leaves appear in the spring. The fruits are one-celled capsules which contain numerous small seeds with long tufts of silky hairs that facilitate their distribution by wind. The bud of this species and Populus canadensis are commonly called Balm of Gilead.

Medicinal Parts: Leaves, bark, buds.

Solvent: Boiling water (soak buds in alcohol, then boiling water will expel their properties).

Bodily Influence: Tonic, Diuretic, Stimulant, Febrifuge.

Uses: A preferred agent to Peruvian bark, and Quinine, with the same results but less after-effect. A well-established bitter tonic to restore digestive disturbances caused by disease or old age. The relaxing effect to the system relieves headache due to liver or stomach conditions of flatulence and acidity. In all cases of faintness, hysteria, neuralgia, diabetes, hay fever, cholera, infants' diarrhoea, Poplar is indicated. It has much value for obstruction of the urine when not due to prostatitis. In uterine, vaginal and renal weakness, 2–15 drops of Poplar (Populus tremuloides) combined with 10–20 drops of Uva ursi (Arctostaphylos), taken three times a day, is a useful mixture.

Dose: 1 teaspoonful of the leaves, buds or bark to 1 cupful of boiling water, 1–2 cupfuls a day. Of the tincture, $\frac{1}{2}$–1 fl. dram.

Externally: If the skin is bathed once a week with a solution of Poplar it has excellent cosmetic benefits, acting as a tonic and conditioner.

For serious skin conditions such as cancer, ulcers, gangrenous wounds, eczema, burns and strong perspiration, bathe the skin with a fresh solution daily for results.

Homoeopathic Clinical: Tincture of inner bark; solution of Populin—Ardorurinea, Bladder (catarrh of), Gleet (chronic), Prostatic affections.

PRICKLY ASH BARK   Xanthoxylum fraxineum, Mill.
(N.O.: Rutaceae)

Common Names: YELLOW WOOD, TOOTHACHE TREE, SUTERBERRY, PRICKLY ASH BERRIES.

Features: This beautiful little tree grows 8–15 ft. high and is native to North America from Canada to Virginia and west to the Mississippi. This perennial shrub is of the Rue family (Rutaceae) and grows in woods, thickets and on river banks. The branches are armed with sharp scattered prickles; when the bark is cut it shows green in the outer part

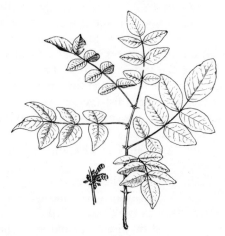

PRICKLY ASH BARK   Xanthoxylum americanum, Mill.
(U.S. Agricultural Department, Appalachia, 1971)

and yellow in the inner. The flowers appear before the leaves, in April and May, and are small and greenish. The fruit is an oval capsule, varying from green to red and blue-black in colour, and grows in clusters on the top of the branches. The taste is very pungent, causing salivation, and there is little odour when the tree is cut. Xanthoxyline is its active principle.

Medicinal Parts: The bark and berries.

Solvents: Boiling water, dilute alcohol.

226

Bodily Influence: Stimulant, Diaphoretic, Alterative, Nervine, Sialagogue.
Uses: Excellent, innocent, tonic used for convalescence from fevers and other diseases. It promotes general perspiration, invigorates the stomach and strengthens the digestive organs when slow, which permits unwanted sluggish fermentation, at the same time equalizing the circulation. For more effectiveness the infusion, or tincture preferably, of 5–10 drops Prickly ash (Xanthoxylum) 3 drops Golden Seal (Hydrastis) and 1 drop Capsicum should be given shortly before meals in warm water. In chronic cases the tincture is more desirable than the infusion and may be used where there is lack of hepatic and pancreatic activity, chronic muscular rheumatism, lumbago, scrofula, temporary paralysis, chronic female trouble and syphilis. J. Kloss in "Back to Eden": "The berries are stimulant, antispasmodic, carminative acting mostly on the mucous tissue removing obstructions in every part of the body."

Prickly ash will increase the flow of saliva and moisten the dry tongue often found in liver malfunctions, and is helpful in paralysis of the tongue and mouth. The fresh bark chewed will give relief in the most inveterate cases of toothache; also the inside bark steeped in whisky and the tincture applied. In all the above mentioned, if the stomach is irritable and sensitive, Prickly ash may not be kindly received and then the tincture should be given in warm water.

Dose: 1 teaspoonful of the bark, cut small or granulated, to 1 cupful of boiling water; drink a mouthful at a time throughout the day, more according to case. Of the tincture, 5–20 drops.

Externally: The powdered bark is applied directly on indolent ulcers and old wounds. Coffin recommends 1 oz. of the pulzerized powder to 4 oz. of olive oil, heated, and used as a massage night and morning, for rheumatic pain.

Homoeopathic Clinical: Tincture of fresh bark—After-pains, Asthma, Coccygodynis, Dysmenorrhoea, Earache, Fibroma, Headache, Hemiplegia, Hysteria, Jaw joint (pain in), Lactation, Menstruation (painful), Nerves (injured), Nervousness, Neuralgia, Ophthalmia, Sciatica, Toothache, Ulcers.

PRIVET   Ligustrum vulgare, (Common); Ligustrum amurense (Amur)
(N.O.: Oleaceae)

Common Names: PRIVY, PRIM.
Features: A common name of shrubs and small trees of the genus Ligustrum, in the olive family (Oleaceae) comprising approximately fifty species. The common privet (L. vulgare), with its numerous cultivated varieties, is hardy in the north, is planted as a hedge plant and is locally naturalized in eastern North America, from New England to Virginia and

227

Ohio. Found growing in wild woods and thickets. This smooth shrub is 5–6 in. high, the leaves are dark green, 1–2 in. in length, about half as wide, entire, smooth, lanceolate, and on short petioles. The small, white and numerous flowers show themselves in June and July; the spherical black berries are ripe in August and September. The bark is said to be as effective as the leaves and contains sugar, mannite, starch, bitter resin, bitter extractive, albumen, salts and a peculiar substance called ligustrin.

Medicinal Part: The leaves.

Solvents: Boiling water, dilute alcohol.

Uses: A decoction of the leaves is valuable in chronic bowel complaints, ulcerations of the stomach and bowels, or as a gargle for ulcers of mouth and throat and where there is bleeding of either bowel or mouth. Useful in diarrhoea and summer complaints of children; as a decoction for offensive ulcerated ears with offensive discharges and excessive flow of urine. A solution as a vaginal douche is toning to the tissue and will expel offensive discharge. Of the decoction, 1 teaspoonful to 1 cupful of boiling water, ½ cupful three times a day. Of the powder, 15–20 grains.

PYROLA Pyrola rotundifolia, L.
(N.O.: Pyrolaceae)

Common Names: FALSE WINTERGREEN, SHIN LEAF, CANKER LETTUCE. PEAR LEAF PYROLA.

Features: There are several kinds of Pyrola growing in North America: Green pyrola (Pyrola vivens), Pink pyrola (Pyrola asarifolia), Shin leaf (Pyrola elliptica) and Round leaved pyrola (Pyrola rotundifolia), which is the one most used in herbal practice. Pyrola is common in damp and shady woods in various parts of the United States.

The herb is a low perennial evergreen. The leaves are radical, ovate, nearly 2 in. in diameter, smooth, shining and thick, resembling Pipsissewa (Chimaphila umbellata) and used similarly. The petioles are much longer than the leaf. The large, white, fragrant and drooping flowers are many and in blossom from June to July. The fruit is a five-celled many-seeded capsule.

Medicinal Part: Whole plant.

Solvent: Boiling water.

Bodily Influence: Astringent, Diuretic, Tonic, Antispasmodic.

Uses: Administer internally for gravel, ulcerations of the bladder, bloody urine and other urinary diseases; useful in the relief of a scrofulous taint from the system; also for epilepsy and other nervous affections. The decoction will be found beneficial as a gargle for sore throat and

228

mouth, and as an external wash for sore or ophthalmic eyes. It is also used in injections for whites and various diseases of the womb.

Dose: 1 teaspoonful of the herb to 1 cupful of boiling water, steeped 10 min. or more and taken three times a day at meal times. Of the extract, 2–4 grains.

Externally: The decoction is much used in all skin diseases and as a poultice for ulcers, swellings, boils, felons and inflammations.

Russian Experience: In Russia Groushanka (Roundleaf) can be found growing among bushes of the Coniferous forests. They use the herb in Folk Medicine, homoepathically and clinically in the the form of teas, decoctions, Nastoika, extracts for throat conditions, stomach and back pain as a result of too much and too heavy lifting, and scurvy.

Externally: As application for recent and long-standing skin lesions.

RAGGED CUP   Silphium perfoliatum, L.
(N.O.: Compositae)

Common Names: INDIAN CUP PLANT, INDIAN GUM.

Features: This plant is common to the western states of North America and a member of the Aster family. The pitted root is large, long and crooked, with smooth herbaceous stem, 4–7 ft. high. The leaves of this perennial plant are opposite, ovate, 8–14 in. long by 4–7 in. wide. The flowers are yellowish, which are perfected in August, and the fruit a broadly ovate winged achenium. Ragged cup is common to the western states and is found growing in rich soil. The root yields a bitterish gum, somewhat similar to frankinscense, which is frequently used to sweeten the breath.

Medicinal Parts: The root.

Solvents: Alcohol, water.

Bodily Influence: Tonic, Diaphoretic, Alterative.

Uses: A strong infusion of the root, made by long steeping, or an extract is said to be among the best remedies for the removal of ague cake, or enlarged spleen. As nearly as can be ascertained the spleen, liver and stomach are dependent on each other and the derangement of either or all is closely associated. Also useful in intermittent and remittent fevers, internal bruises, debility, ulcers, liver affections and as a general alterative, restorative. The gum is said to be a stimulant and antispasmodic.

Dose: 1 teaspoonful of the root, cut small or granulated, to 1 cupful of boiling water. Drink 1 cupful during the day, a large mouthful at a time. Of the tincture, 5–20 drops.

RASPBERRY   Rubus idaeus, L.
(N.O.: Rosaceae)

Common Names: AMERICAN RASPBERRY, WILD RED RASPBERRY.

Features: A native to North America and Europe, the Raspberry, due to popularity, has been cultivated since the sixteenth century. Species of Raspberries are seen in most temperate parts of the world. The plants are perennial, but they have a characteristic biennial growth habit. The canes are generally erect, freely branched and prickly 3–4 ft. high, and covered with small, straight, slender prickles. The leaves are pale green above, grey-white beneath, doubly serrated with a rounded base, about 3 in. long and 2 in. broad. The small, white, pendulous flowers bloom in May or June in simple clusters with the ripening of the Raspberry in June and July. The fruit is not a true berry, but aggregates composed of a number of drupelets.

Medicinal Parts: Leaves and berries.

Solvents: Water, alcohol.

Bodily Influence: Astringent, Stimulant, Tonic.

Uses: Raspberry has long been established as a remedy for dysentery and diarrhoea, especially in infants. It is mild, pleasant, soothing. It will remove cankers from mucous membranes, at the same time toning the tissue involved, be it of the throat (as a gargle) or alimentary tract. It is much used in relief of urethral irritation and is soothing to the kidneys, urinary tract and ducts.
Compound of:

> Tincture of Bayberry (Myrica cerifera), 5–10 drops
> Tincture of Raspberry (Rubus idaeus), 10–40 drops

in water three or four times a day, is a useful solution for the uterus and to stop haemorrhages. Raspberry leaf tea can be taken freely before and during confinement; it will strengthen and prevent miscarriage and render parturition less laborious. The infusion will also relieve painful menstruation and aid the flow; if too abundant it will decrease without abruptly stopping it. Infuse with Prickly ash (Xanthoxylum fraxineum) and Blue cohosh (Caulophyllum thalictroides) and take $\frac{1}{2}$ cup three times a day. Raspberry leaves as a feminine douche for leucorrhoea is made by 1 tablespoonful of the leaves simmered in 1 pint of water for 10 min., covered, cooled and added to container of room-temperature water.

Dose: Tincture of Raspberry alone, 30–60 drops in water as required. Infusion, 1 teaspoonful to 1 cupful of boiling water; steep at least 3 min.

Externally: The infusion is a valuable wash in sores, ulcers and raw surfaces, as an astringent.

Russian Experience: Malina (Raspberry) is a most popular aromatic berry. This wild plant alone covers vast areas of the country. It is used and also cultivated for wine, food, medicine (domestic and clinical). Folk Medicine employs the most common and simple things of their surroundings. If an analysis was made these simple herbs would not be described as the same, as their content and structure draws from many vital sources which nature alone can provide.

Folk Medicine: Tea, decoction, Nastoika (with vodka) are employed for colds, coughs and as a diaphoretic, when required. Berries are

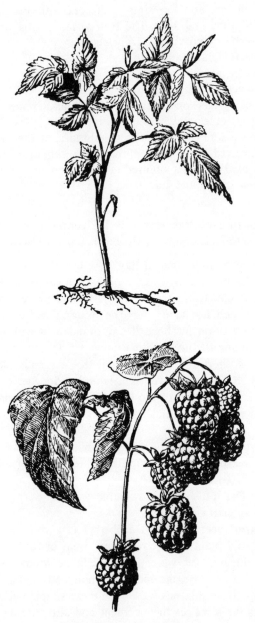

RASPBERRY   Rubus idaeus, L.
(Botanica, Moscow, 1949)

enjoyed by most and have a therapeutic value for La Grippe. Also stem twigs as tea for the above and difficulty in breathing.

Clinically: Used in syrups to improve the taste of other compounds and as a tonic itself.

RED CLOVER   Trifolium pratense, L.
(N.O.: Leguminosae)

Common Names: PURPLE CLOVER, TREFOIL, CLEAVER GRASS, COW GRASS.

Features: True Clover, plants of the genus Trifolium, family Leguminosae, number about 250 species. It is believed that the true clovers originated in south-eastern Europe and south-western Asia Minor, although more than eighty species are listed as indigenous to North America. The clovers are herbaceous annuals or perennials, depending on insect pests or to unfavourable climatic conditions.

Red clover is an upright perennial 18–36 in. in height that behaves as a biennial under most eastern conditions. The colours of the flowers of the many species include white, pink, purple, red, yellow and combinations of shades thereof. The flowers are borne on conspicuous heads, with 55–200 florets for such species as Red clover. The leaves, composed of three leaflets, grow on alternate sides of the stem. The leaflets themselves are broad, oval, pointed and frequently show a white spot. The hairy stem supports the generous numbers of separate blossoms at the end of the flower stalk.

Common in pastures, lawns, roadsides and meadows throughout the United States and Canada. Harvesting varies, depending on the species. Agriculturally they are classified as winter annuals.

Medicinal Parts: The blossoms and leaves.

Solvents: Boiling water, alcohol.

Bodily Influence: Alterative, Sedative, Deobstruent.

Uses: A quote from Herbalists of the past: "The likelihood is that whatever virtue the Red Clover can boast for counteracting a scrofulous disposition and as antidote to cancer, resides in its highly elaborated lime, silica and other earthy salts." It is not recognized, however, by orthodox medical profession as being of use. It possesses very soothing and pleasant-tasting properties and promotes healthy granulation.

Admirable for malignant ulcers, scrofula, indolent sores, burns, whooping cough and various spasm, bronchial and renal conditions. The warm tea is very soothing to the nerves. J. Kloss, in "Back to Eden", gives a splendid formula for the above. Combine with equal parts of:

Blue Violet (Amara dulcis)
Burdock (Arctium lappa)
Yellow Dock (Rumex crispus)
Dandelion (Leontodon taraxacum)
Rock Rose (Helionthemum canadense)
Golden Seal (Hydrastis canadensis)

As you can see, Red clover can be used alone, or supported by many other effective herbs.

As a gargle for sore and inflamed throat, make a strong tea and gargle four to five times a day, swallowing a fresh mouthful after each cleansing. Also of use for rectal and vaginal irritation, making sure to hold in the solution for several minutes before releasing.

Dose: Internally as an infusion, 1 teaspoonful of clover to 1 cupful of boiling water, steeped 30 min. or more. Take 4–6 cupfuls a day, children less. Of the tincture, 5–30 drops in water, according to age and purpose.

Externally: Red clover blossoms have been long and successfully used in the form of a salve for the removal of external cancer and indolent ulcers. A tea is also helpful to bathe the affected part, making it fresh daily.

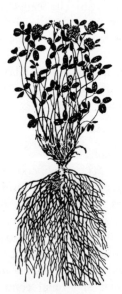

RED CLOVER   Trifolium pratense, L.
(N.O. Leguminosae)
(Botanica, V. A. Teterev, Moscow,
1949)

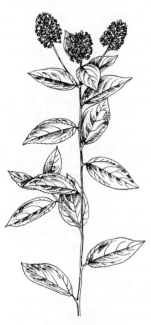

RED ROOT
Ceanothus americanus, L.
(U.S. Agricultural Department,
Appalachia, 1971)

234

Homoeopathic Clinical: Tincture of flower heads—Cancer, Constipation, Cough, Mumps, Pancreas (affections of), Throat (sore; mucus in), Uvula (pain in).

Russian Experience: For Russian clover change the "O" to "E". Clever, and your Russian friends will recognize and perhaps add to your knowledge of its use. There, species grow wild, but several are cultivated.

Folk Medicine: Clever flowers are used as tea, decoctions, Nastoika (with vodka) for children of all ages when anaemic, as the properties are nutritious, aiding general weakness and shortness of breath. A female assistant to stop bleeding of amenorrhoea. Decoction of herbs for coughs.

Externally: Clover is known to Russians as being a strong natural antiseptic, and is adaptable as poultices for burns and abscesses. Fresh leaf juice is used for external eye wash. Decoction of leaves and salt as a poultice for headache.

RED ROOT   Ceanothus americanus, L.
(N.O.: Rhamnaceae)

Common Names: NEW JERSEY TEA, WILD SNOW BALL, RED ROOT, MOUNTAIN SWEET.

Features: A genus of shrubs and small trees of Rhamnaceae. There are about thirty-five species native to North America. C. americanus, known as New Jersey tea and Red root, is common from Canada to the Gulf states of America.

The plant's root is large with a red or brownish bark, and body of dark red colour. The stems are 2–4 ft. high, slender, rather smooth above and cordate at the base. The flowers appear in June and August in small showy clusters, which are often panicled. The leaves are serrated or entire and simple. The three-celled drupaceous fruit when dry separates into three stone-like seeds. Found growing in dry woodlands, bowers, etc.

Many of the species and their hybrids, of various colours, are popular ornamental shrubs. The wild Red root was put to use by the Indians during the American civil war as a leaf tea. The official root contains a large amount of prussic acid, which has been given the name "Ceanothine" and used as its active principle.

Medicinal Part: The root.

Solvent: Boiling water.

Bodily Influence: Astringent, Expectorant, Sedative, Antispasmodic.

Uses: Ceanothus is one of the few remedies which has a direct affinity for the malfunction of the spleen, and is of special help in all ailments where there is despondency and melancholy. Some consider its action of less influence than Fringe tree (Chionanthus virginica) but both are effective and can be combined if in doubt as to which one to use. It is an indirect herbal agent for diabetes. Especially useful in nervousness when mentally disturbed, bilious sick headache, acute indigestion and nausea due to inactivity of the liver.

> Tincture of Golden seal (Hydrastis canadensis), 7–10 drops
> Tincture of Fringe tree (Chionanthus virginica), 3–7 drops
> Tincture of Red root (Ceanothus americanus), 10–20 drops

Dose: 15–30 drops in water before meals and at bedtime. Red root is also used with results in dysentery, asthma, chronic bronchitis, whooping cough, consumption and venereal diseases, also as a gargle for swollen tonsils and canker sores. A strong tea will often prevent the condition from reappearing if the area is swabbed and a solution as a gargle used every 2 hr.

Dose: 1 teaspoonful of granulated root to 1 pint of boiling water, steep 20–30 min. Drink 1 cupful of tea before each meal and before going to bed. Of the tincture of Ceanothus alone, 10–20 drops in water before meals and at bedtime.

Externally: The astringent action of Red root as a strong tea for haemorrhoids will decrease the tissue if used often.

Homoeopathic Clinical: Tincture of fresh leaves—Diarrhoea, heart (disordered), Intermittent fever, Jaundice, Leucorrhoea, Leucocythemia, Menses (suppressed), Side (pain in), Spleen (affection of).

SAGE—Salvia officinalis, L.
(N.O.: Labiatae)

Common Names: GARDEN SAGE, WILD SAGE.

Features: Sage is a name covering both the common garden herb (S. officinalis) and other plants of diverse families, somewhat resembling it in colour or odour. Sage is native to southern Europe, but has been naturalized in North America for the last three centuries as a garden and wild herbal shrub. This perennial has erect, branched semi-shrubby hoary down. The majority of the leaves are grey-green, opposite, entire and reticulate veined; with the base leaves of a woolly white. The flowers, blue with white and purple streaks, blossom in whorls of varying lengths, springing from a common stem, in June and July, and this is the proper time to carefully gather the leaves and tops to dry for future use. Found in stony places throughout the U.S.A.

The strong aromatic camphorous odour is a characteristic of Sage, and it has a warm, slightly bitter taste. Highly prized as winter foliage for livestock. Sage is well known for seasoning, dressing, soups, roasts, etc. A volatile oil may be obtained by distilling the plant.

Medicinal Part: The leaves.

Solvents: Dilute alcohol, boiling water (partially).

Bodily Influence: Tonic, Astringent, Expectorant, Diaphoretic.

Uses: An old English proverb: "He that would live for aye must eat sage in May." The infusion is much valued in cases of gastric debility, checking flatulency with speed and certainty. The warm infusion will activate its diaphoretic tendency. In fevers it should be given in cold infusions as a substitute for fruit juice. Use 2 teaspoonfuls in 1 pint of boiling water, steep 1 hr., cool, strain and when cold take every hour or two until sweating subsides.

The express juice taken for a considerable time is excellent in rheumatic pains and was formerly used as an agent against venereal disease, but since the introduction of mercury its use has been set aside.

When conditions advance to consumption, fast, use 3 tablespoonfuls of the juice with a little honey; this will usually stop the spitting of blood. For foul ulcers or old lesions, use as indicated by case.

The infusion as a gargle for sore, ulcerated, strained, relaxed vulva, etc., of the throat is worth remembering, used alone or with cider vinegar, honey, Sumach (Rhus glabrum).

From Dr. Brown (1895): "It is called by some a most capital remedy for spermatorrhoea, and for excessive venereal desire, and I am one of those who know from experience in my practice that it is grand for what is termed sexual debility when its use is indicated."

Dose: Tincture, 16–40 drops three or four times a day. Decoction, 1 teaspoonful of leaves to 1 cupful of boiling water, hot or cold depending on condition of its use.

Externally: The decoction is used to cleanse old ulcers and wounds, and massaged into the scalp if troubled with dandruff, falling hair or loss of hair if the papilla (root) is dormant and not destroyed.

Homoeopathic Clinical: Tincture of fresh leaves and blossom tip— Cough (tickling), Phthisis, Night sweats.

Russian Experience: The Middle Ages gave much credit to the power of Shalfey (Sage) as a food and medicine. Many couplets like the following have been written about it:

> "Contra vim mortis
> Crescit salvia in hortis."

> ("Against power of death
> Sage grows in the garden.")

> "Cur moriatur homo
> cui salvia crescit in hortis."

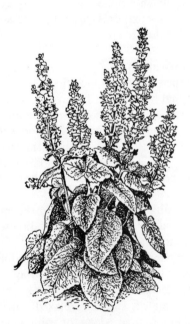

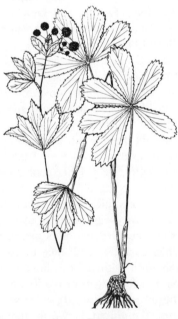

SAGE
Salvia officinalis, L.
(P. A. Volkova, Dikorastushye,
Moscow, 1960)

SANICLE
Snakeroot, Sanicula marilandica, L.
(Wild Plants, Canadian Agricultural
Department, Ottawa, 1964)

238

("Why man would die
When sage grows in the garden.")

Over 500 species grow wild, some being cultivated in south Russia and west Siberia as food and medicine aromatics.

Folk Medicine and Clinical: Aromatic, Astringent, Antiseptic, Carminative, Disinfectant (against inflammations).

Commercial: Systematically Agro-Technics sow 7–8 lb of seed per acre and in five years' time they can harvest two or three times a season, gathering up to 600 lb. per acre the first year and 1,200 lb. the following season. With exceptional climate conditions and care it is possible to gain 3,000 lb. per acre.

SANICLE   Sanicula marilandica, L.
(N.O.: Umbelliferae)

Common Names: BLACK SNAKEROOT, POOL ROOT, AMERICAN SANICLE, WOOD SANICLE.

Features: Sanicle, of the Parsley family, is an indigenous perennial common to the United States and Canada. The fibrous root is aromatic in taste and odour, with a smooth reddish furrowed stem, 1–3 ft. high. The leaves are digitate, mostly radical and on petioles, 6–12 in. long, nearly 3 in. across, glossy green above, less colour underneath. The flowers bloom in June and July, and they are mostly barren white, sometimes yellowish, fertile ones sessile.

Medicinal Parts: The root and leaves.

Solvent: Water.

Bodily Influence: Vulnerary, Astringent, Alterative, Expectorant, Discutient, Depurative.

Uses: Used by the Indians in intermittent fevers and for treating a variety of skin conditions. The action upon the system very much resembles Valerian, possessing (besides the previously mentioned) nervine and anodyne properties.

J. Kloss in "Back to Eden": "This is one of the herbs that could well be called a 'Cure All', because it possesses powerful cleansing and healing virtues, both internally and externally." It heals, stops bleeding, diminishes tumours, whether of a recent or long-standing nature. The properties when administered seem to seek the ailment most in distress, be it of the throat, lungs, intestines or renal tract, reproductive organs. You name it. Sanicle will find it. Its qualifications are many as a cleansing and healing herb, both of man or animal.

For throat discomforts, gargle a strong tea with honey as often as necessary. The fresh juice can be given in tablespoonful doses in

239

treatment of dysentery, and strong decoction of the leaves made by boiling 1 oz. of the leaves in 1½ pints of water, reduced to 1 pint, can be taken constantly in wineglass doses till haemorrhage ceases.

Dose: 1 teaspoonful of the root or leaves, cut small or crushed, to 1 cupful of boiling water. Take 1 cupful ½ hr. before meals. If haemorrhaging, it is best to refrain from food until bleeding stops. Of the tincture, 15–30 drops. Of the powder, 1 dram.

Externally: For cutaneous or subcutaneous skin conditions, chapped hands or bleeding skin ulcerations use a fresh preparation daily for chronic conditions until they improve. Internally and externally, can be combined with other supporting herbs.

Homoeopathic Clinical: Amenorrhoea, Asthma, Bee stings, Boils (blind), Borborygmus, Coccyx (soreness of), Condylomata, Conjunctivitis, Constipation (of children), Cornea (ulceration of), Coryza, Cough, Dandruff, Debility, Diabetes, Diarrhoea, Digestion (slow), Dropsy (during pregnancy), Eczema, Emaciation, Enuresis, Excoriations, Foot sweat, Gastritis, Gum (suppressed), Itching, Leucorrhoea, Liver (soreness of), Lumbago, Melancholy, Milk (thin), Mouth (sore), Neuralgia, Neurasthenia, Night terrors, Nose (crusts in), Ophthalmia (tarsi), Os utteri (dilated), Ossification (too early), Ozaena, Perspiration (excessive), Potbellied children, Pregnancy (sickness of; dropsy of), Rectum (cramp in), Rheumatism, Rickets, Scurvy, Sea sickness, Shoulders (rheumatism of), Throat (sore), Tongue (ringworm of; burning), Toothache, Uterus (prolapse of; soreness of; tumour of), Vomiting (of milk; of water), Wrist (boils on).

SARSAPARILLA   Aralia nudicaulis, L.
(N.O.: Araliaceae)

Common Names: RED SARSAPARILLA, SMALL SPIKENARD, SPIGNET, QUAY, QUILL.

Features: There are several species of Sarsaparilla, which are indigenous to Central America, southern Mexico, northern South America, and such West Indian islands as Jamaica. The name Sarsaparilla is derived from the Spanish zara (shrub) and parrilla (little vine), known in the south as bamboo brier. Aralia racemosa, American Sarsaparilla, is a member of the Ginseng family.

The Sarsaparilla of commercial use consists of very long roots having a thick bark of a greyish or brownish colour, with many slender rootlets, deeply furrowed longitudinally. When cut, sections show a brown, hard bark with a porous centre portion. The roots that have a deep orange tint are the best and the stronger the acrid and nauseous qualities the better are the properties of the root. Height 1–2 ft., bearing several bunches of yellowish-green flowers, followed by clusters of small berries resembling, to some extent, the common Elderberry.

Chemically we know the root contains salseparin, a colouring matter, starch, chloride of potassium and essential oil, basserin, albumen, pectic and acetic, and the several salts of lime, potash, magnesium and oxide of iron. The taste is mucilaginous with scarcely any odour.

Medicinal Part: The root.

Solvents: Water, dilute alcohol.

Bodily Influence: Alterative, Diuretic, Demulcent, Stimulant, Antiscorbutic.

Uses: Alfred Metraus, Swedish anthropologist, found Amazon Indians using Sarsaparilla to cure general debilities and he said that it was invigorating to the entire system. Indian hunting expeditions subsided for long periods on Sarsaparilla root.

In the mid-1800s Sarsaparilla was something of a national phenomenon in the United States as a spring tonic to eliminate poisons from the blood and purify the system from all left-over infections of winter. It is dependably useful in rheumatism, gout, skin eruptions, ringworm, scrofula, internal inflammation, colds, catarrh, fever and to relieve gas from stomach and bowels.

When in need of an excellent antidote for deadly poisons, cleanse

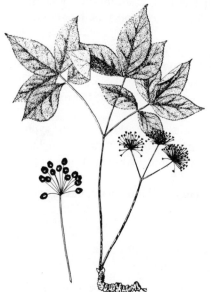

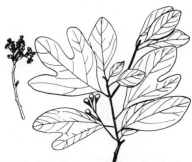

WILD SARSAPARILLA
Aralia nudicaulis, L.
(Wild Plants, Canadian Agricultural
Department, Ottawa, 1964)

SASSAFRAS   Sassafras albidum
(Nutt.) Nees.
(U.S. Agricultural Department,
Appalachia, 1971)

241

stomach with an emetic, causing vomiting, and drink copiously of the tea. As an alterative tea it is best prepared with Burdock (Lappa). One of the best herbs to use for infants infected with venereal diseases. They can be cleansed without the use of mercurials. Also wash the pustules of sores with a tea made of the root and administer inwardly by mixing the powdered root with food.

Dose: 1 oz. of the root boiled in 1 pint of water, taken in wineglassful amounts three times a day. For colds, etc., it should be used as a syrup, 1 teaspoonful to 1 tablespoonful four times a day, depending on age and condition. Of the tincture, 20–40 drops four times a day.

Externally: As a strong tea for skin infections.

Homoeopathic Clinical: Triturations and tincture of the dried rhizome—Asthma, Bladder (affections of), Bones (affections of), Breast (scirrhus of), Bright's disease, Calculi, Climaxis, Constipation, Dyspepsia, Dysuria, Enuresis, Eruptions, Eyes (affections of), Faintness, Glands (enlarged), Gonorrhoea, Gout, Gravel, Hands (chapped), Headache, Hernia, Herpes (of prepuce), Hiccough, Intermittents, Marasmus, Masturbation (effects of), Melancholia, Mercury (abuse of), Mycosis, Nipples (retracted), Renal colic, Rhagades, Rheumatism (gonorrhoeal), Seborrhoea, Spermatic cords (swelling of), Spermatorrhoea, Strangury, Syphilis, Ulcers, Warts.

Russian Experience: In the Russian Far East a shrub known as Aralia manchurian is used as a general tonic of Nastoika (with vodka) for physical and mental exhaustion.

India and Pakistan: Known as Country Sarsaparilla, or Indian Sarsaparilla, it grows in many parts of India and Pakistan. The roots are considered a substitute for American Sarsaparilla.

Bodily Influence: Demulcent, Alterative, Blood Purifier, Diuretic, Tonic, Diaphoretic.

Uses: As an appetizer and for dyspepsia, fever, skin diseases, syphilis, leucorrhoea, diseases of the genito-urinary tract, chronic cough, etc.

Dose: Powdered roots, 10–60 grains with milk. Also used as syrup and decoctions from the root.

Externally: Ointment for swelling, rheumatic pains, boils, carbuncles.

SASSAFRAS   Laurus sassafras (Nutt.) Nees.
(N.O.: Lauraceae)

Common Names: SAXIFRAX, SALOOP, AGUE TREE, CINNAMON WOOD.

Features: The generic name of three species of trees, two native to eastern Asia, one to eastern North America, in the laurel family Lauraceae. In the United States and Canada, Sassafras extends from Maine, southern Ontario and Michigan to Texas and Florida. May approach 100 ft. in height and 6 ft. in diameter, but it is usually smaller, sometimes shrubby.

The bark is dark red-brown, deeply furrowed, soft and brittle with short, corky, layered fracture, with many oil cells. The young twigs are green. The heart wood of Sassafras is dark or orange-brown and resistant to decay. The leaves, bright green above, downy beneath, are 4–6 in. long, oval, especially on older branches often mitten shaped, or three-lobed on younger shoots or twigs. In autumn they turn various shades of yellow, orange, pink and deep red. The small greenish flowers appear in April or early May before the leaves. The fruit pistil, which ripens into a blue drupe, is eagerly devoured by the birds. The bark has an aromatic, agreeable taste, and similar fragrance.

In the book "Trees and Shrubs of Massachus, 1894", Sassafras has the credit of having aided in the discovery of America. The wind-swept fragrance of the trees encouraged Columbus to persuade his mutinous crew that land was near.

Sold in some areas under the name of Salap or Saloop.

Medicinal Parts: The bark of the root.

Solvents: Boiling water, alcohol.

Bodily Influence: Stimulant, Diaphoretic, Aromatic, Tonic, Diuretic, Alterative.

Uses: Early explorers and settlers in the New World were told by the Indians that it would cure diverse ills, and it was eargerly sought and shipped to Europe. In domestic practice it enjoys a wide field of application and use, especially as a so-called spring renovator to thin and purify the blood. J. H. Greer, M.D., tells us: "Sassafras should not be used by thin-blooded persons." It would accentuate the positive.

It is used as corrective in rheumatism, varicose ulcers; given in painful menstruation it soon relieves the sufferer, and is effective in afterpains of childbirth and in all skin eruptive diseases. It is antagonistic to narcotic effect of alcohol. The essential oil will often relieve most painful toothache. Sassafras is used with other compounds to improve the flavour and render their properties more cordial to the stomach.

Dose: Infusion of 1 oz. of crushed or chipped bark to 1 pint of boiling water. Of the tincture, 15–30 min.

Externally: A poultice of the root is a good application for ill-conditioned ulcers. The oil may be used as an ingredient in liniment, and provides an excellent application for bruises and swellings.

SAW PALMETTO Serenoa serrulata, Hook, F.
(N.O.: Palmae)

Common Names: FAN PALM, DWARF PALMETTO, SABAL.

Features: Found in profusion near the Atlantic Ocean in Georgia and

Florida, on a strip of coast hundreds of miles in length and from one to five miles wide.

The small, stout evergreen shrub is supported by a large underground trunk. The edge of the leaves has the appearance of a saw, hence its name. Saw palmetto fruit. The berries are very abundant, closely resembling the black olive in size and shape, being dark purple or nearly black in colour. They ripen from October to December.

People of the areas learn to love the fruit, as it is very sweet and juicy and richer in nutrition than the raw sugar cane. The aromatic odour is pronounced and easily distinguished. Contains volatile oil, alkaloid, resin, dextrin and glucose.

Medicinal Part: The berries.

Solvents: Dilute alcohol, boiling water.

Bodily Influence: Sedative, Diuretic, Expectorant, Tonic, Anti-catarrhal. Nutritive.

Uses: Attention was brought to this herb because of the remarkably good animals that fed upon its fruit. Used under observation as a natural treatment for mankind, the berries were found to improve the digestion, increase flesh strength and weight. It is highly recommended in all wasting diseases as it has a marked effect upon all the glandular tissue. Especially used in atrophy of the testes, prostrate and all diseases of the reproductive glands.

Serenoa is of great service for colds in the head, irritated mucous membrane of the throat, nose and air passages, and chronic bronchitis of lung asthma. Of use in renal conditions and diabetes.

Among the most beneficial agents of the Materia Medica.

Dose: 1 teaspoonful of the dried berries to 1 cupful of boiling water. Of the tincture, up to 1 fl. dram.

SENEGA   Polygala senega, L.
(N.O.: Polygalaceae)

Common Names: SNAKEROOT, MILKWORT, RATTLESNAKE-ROOT, MOUNTAIN FLAX.

Features: Polygala is a genus of more than 500 annual and perennial herbs and shrubs of the family Polygalaceae. Most species are subtropical but nearly 200 are North American. P. senega, known as Mountain flax or Senega snakeroot, grows from New Brunswick to Alberta and southward to Georgia and Arkansas. This indigenous plant has a perennial, firm, hairy, branching root, with a thick bark, and sends up several annual stems, which are erect, smooth, 8–14 in. high, occasionally tinged with red. The leaves are alternate, nearly sessile lanceolate with a sharpish point, smooth. The new, small white

244

flowers consists of five sepals, three petals and the capsules are small, two-celled and two-valved.

Found in rocky woods and on hillsides, flowering in July. The English name is Milkwort. The botanical name means "much milk", which has been applied to some species for the increase of milk flow. Its chemical constituents are polygalic, virginic, pectic, tannic acids, an oil, gum, albumen, salts of alumina, silica, magnesium and iron. For medicinal purposes, gather in the autumn just before the frost; the taste is bitter, though somewhat sweet.

Medicinal Part: The root.

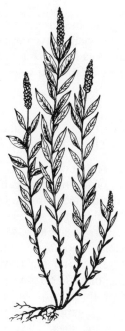

SENEGA   Polygala senega, L.
(U.S. Agricultural Department, Appalachia, 1971)

Solvents: Water, dilute alcohol.

Bodily Influence: Diaphoretic, Diuretic, Expectorant, large doses Emetic and Cathartic.

Uses: In the early part of the eighteenth century Scottish physician Tennant heard from the Senega Indians of the use of Senega in cases of snake bites, and investigated its merits. He discovered that an infusion of the dried roots would actively promote salivation, desirable in chronic catarrh, croup, asthma and lung disorders of pleurisy and pneumonia, but that it is too irritating for recent coughs of active inflammatory

245

diseases. It increases the secretions and circulation and is indicated where there is prostration from blood poisoning, smallpox, asthma, diseases of the lungs, bronchitis, chronic catarrh, croup, dropsy and rheumatism.

Dose: 1 teaspoonful of the root, cut small or granulated, to 1 cupful of boiling water. Of the tincture, 15–20 drops. Of the powder, 5–20 grains.

Homoeopathic Clinical: Tincture of powdered dried root—Ascites, Asthma, Bladder (irritable; catarrh of), Bronchitis, Constipation, Cornea (opacity of), Cough, Enuresis, Facial paralysis, Hay fever, Influenza, Iritis, Oesophagus (stricture of; catarrh of), Phthisis mucosa, Pleurisy, Pneumonia, Snake bites, Sneezing (fits of; at end of cough), Throat (sore), Whooping cough.

Russian Experience: Senega is known and pronounced the same as in North America. Cultivated in south Russia for experimental observation and study of the medicinal roots and rhizomes for expectorant influence in chronic bronchitis and long-established respiratory illness.

SENNA   Cassia marilandica, L.
(N.O.: Leguminosae)

Common Names: WILD SENNA, LOCUST PLANT.

Features: Cassia is a genus of leguminous plants inhabiting the tropical parts of the world consisting of trees, shrubs, or herbs. American Senna is to be found from New England to Carolina, growing in rich soils.

The leaves have long petioles, ovate at base; each petiole has eight or ten leaflets, which are oblong, smooth, 1–2 in. long and quite narrow. The flowers are a bright yellow and the leaves are gathered while in bloom from June to September. The fruit is a legume, 2–4 in. long, and contains a quantity of thick pulp which is mildly laxative and cathartic and is used in the composition of the confection of Cassia and of Senna. It belongs to the sugar class of laxatives, its properties being due, for the most part, to the water-attracting properties of the sugar while in the intestinal canal.

Medicinal Part: The leaves.

Solvents: Water, alcohol.

Bodily Influence: Laxative, Vermifuge, Cathartic.

Uses: Senna sometimes causes griping effects. To modify this, combine Senna leaves with one of the aromatic herbs Ginger, Anise, Caraway, Fennel or Coriander. Can also be used in combination with Pink root (Spigelia marilandica). Should not be used in cases of inflammation of the stomach.

Dose: Of the tincture, 1–2 tablespoonfuls. Of the powder, 10–20 grains. Of the infusion, ½–1 cupful steeped 30 min.

Homoeopathic Clinical: Colic (flatulent) of infants, Exhaustion, Nitrogenous waste, Sleeplessness, Sneezing, with heat.

Russian Experience: In Russia Senna leaves are known as Alexandre leaves, or Cassia. The species Cassia acutifolia grows in Russia, having the same properties as the American variety.

Use: For treating conditions of constipations they prefer the buds with oils; this can be used repeatedly without side-effect. The leaves alone are rather harsh, so a compound of Cassia with similar herbs is recommended.

India and Pakistan: Many varieties of Senna grow in India and Pakistan, one being Cassia angustifolia (Indian Senna).

Uses: Their traditional use is not only as a laxative, but also for biliousness, gout and rheumatism, in the form of decoctions, infusions, powder and confections. Warning: it should not be administered for inflamatory conditions of the alimentary canal, fever, piles, menorrhagia, prolapse of the rectum and uterus or pregnancy.

Externally: For skin diseases and pimples use a paste of the dried leaves made with vinegar.

SHEPHERD'S PURSE   Capsella bursa pastoris, Medik.
(N.O.: Cruciferae)

Common Names: MOTHER'S HEART, PICKOOCKER, SHEPHERD'S SPROUT, CASE WORT.

Features: This common herb of the mustard family (Cruciferae), found originally in Europe, is now naturalized in most parts of the world. This is a small herb which grows abundantly in fields, looking like ordinary pepper grass, only the seed pods resemble small pear-shaped purses or pouches of flattened pods at the end of its branching stem with a prominent vein on each face, and contain many orange-brown seeds. The few stem leaves are arrowhead shaped, stalkless and smooth edged or toothed. The usually branched stem may grow 2 ft. tall. The slender stalked flowers have four small white petals and six stamens and are borne in clusters that elongate as the seeds mature. The taste of the herb is like cabbage; odour is unpleasant.

Medicinal Part: The whole herb.

Solvent: Water.

Bodily Influence: Astringent, Diuretic, Antiscorbutic.

Uses: To collect the seed pods for a nutritious meal is unheard of today, nevertheless the body-building elements which our fathers of America knew by test and experience still remain. They roasted the seeds and combined with other meal for pinole bread. The leaves were used raw, or for pot herbs like spinach. The medicinal properties of

247

the herb are chiefly manifested by their action upon the kidney and bladder; there they act as a stimulant and moderate tonic for catarrh of the urinary tract indicated by much mucus in the urine. Has been successfully used in cases of haemorrhage after childbirth, excessive menstruation and for internal bleeding of lungs, colon, haemorrhoids, etc. Combined with Agrimony (A. eupatoria) it is of use for bed-wetting (enuresis). Excellent for diarrhoea and intermittent fever.

Culpeper writes: "The juice being dropped into ears, heals the pains, noise, and mutterings thereof. A good ointment may be made of it for all wounds, especially wounds in the head." Parkinson states: "Some do hold that the green herb bruised and bound to the wrists of the hands and soles of the feet will help yellow jaundice."

Dose: Infusion, 1 teaspoonful of the herb to 1 cupful of boiling water, steeped for $\frac{1}{2}$ hr. Take 1 or 2 cupfuls a day as required. Of the tincture, 20–40 drops two or three times a day.

Externally: Used as a fresh juice, or bruised leaves for external bleeding and bruises.

Russian Experience: Pastushya Sumka has the same meaning as Shepherd's purse. From one plant 64,000 seeds are shed periodically in one season and can thrive on any soil. So you can see why the continuation of the plant's generation is prolific; actually it grows all over

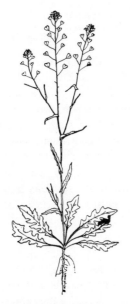

SHEPHERD'S PURSE
Capsella bursa pastoris, Medik.
(Ontario Department of Agriculture,
Toronto, Canada, 1966)

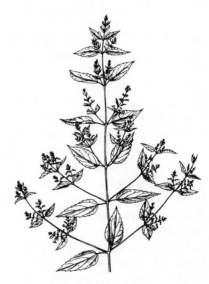

SKULL CAP
Scutellaria lateriflora, L.
(U.S. Agricultural Department,
Appalachia, 1971)

248

the country. Known as a medicine in ancient Roman and Greek times it retained its popularity all over Europe into the Middle Ages. Later it was shamefully forgotten. However during the last world war, when Russia could not import Canadian Golden seal interest was renewed in Shepherd's purse. Since this time the herb has again played a prominent role in Folk Medicine and clinical use. Some districts use the leaves for soup and salad and the seeds instead of mustard (Bello-Russ. Academy of Science, Minsk, 1965).

Folk Medicine: Stomach trouble of diarrhoea, dysentery and gastritis, gall-bladder, kidney and bladder, liver colics, disturbed metabolism, venereal disease, lung TB, bleeding lungs, malaria. For stomach ulcers and bleeding ulcers and also for typhus it is used with vodka (Nastoika).

Clinically: In gynaecology it is used for female bleeding, bloody urine and bleeding from the stomach.

SKULL CAP   Scutellaria lateriflora, L.
(N.O.: Labiatae)

Common Names: BLUE SKULL CAP, BLUE PIMPERNEL, HOOD-WORT, MAD-DOG WEED, SIDE FLOWER, SKULL CAP HELMET FLOWER, AMERICAN SKULL CAP.

Features: Indigenous to North America, this little herb is very abundant throughout the land, growing in damp places, meadows, ditches and by the sides of ponds, from Connecticut, south to Florida and Texas.

This small perennial, with fibrous yellow roots, has an erect and very branching square stem, 1–3 ft. in height. The tooth-edged leaves grow opposite each other on short stalks. It derives its common name from the helmet-shaped upper lid of its small seed pods; the pale blue flowers bloom in pairs just above the leaves in July and August.

The whole plant is medicinal and should be gathered while in flower, dried in the shade and kept in well-closed tin vessels, as it deteriorates rapidly from age and heat. Chemically it contains essential oil, yellowish-green fixed oil, a volatile matter, albumen, an astringent principle, lignin, chloride of soda, salts of iron, silica, etc.

Medicinal Part: The whole herb.

Solvents: Dilute alcohol, boiling water.

Bodily Influence: Tonic, Nervine, Antispasmodic, slightly Astringent.

Uses: Skull cap, by its action through the cerebro spinal centres, is a most valuable remedy for controlling nervous irritation. In many cases of hydrophobia it has been known to eventually render the patient free from disturbances, also in cases of insomnia, excitability, restlessness, wakefulness, St. Vitus dance, hysteria, epilepsy convulsions, shaking palsy, rickets, bites of poisonous insects and snakes, and all nervous affections. It supports the nerves, quietening and strengthening the system. It is also effective in reducing temperature and inducing perspiration in feverish children.

Skull cap was known to the original people of the New World and our country people as Hood-wort or Mad-dog weed.

For persons troubled by undue sexual desires, Skull cap taken freely and persistently will prove a most efficient regulator without damage of any character. When given with Pennyroyal (Hedeoma pulegioides) as a tea, it is also successfully used as a female remedy for cramps and severe pain caused by suppressed menstruation due to colds.

The following formulae have been proved effective by prominent herbalists and doctors of both the past and present:

Weakness of the heart:
> Tincture of Skull cap (Scutellaria lateriflora), 3–15 drops
> Tincture of Golden seal (Hydrastis canadensis), 7–10 drops
> Tincture of Cayenne pepper (Capsicum) 2–4 drops

In warm water as often as required.

For irritable and nervous conditions:
> Tincture of Lady's slipper (Cypripedium pubescens), 10–20 drops
> Tincture of Skull cap (Scutellaria lateriflora). 2–15 drops

In warm water every 2–4 hr.

For hydrophobia and bites of poisonous snakes:
> Tincture of Cone flower (Echinacea angustifolia), 15–20 drops
> Tincture of Skull cap (Scutellaria lateriflora), 2–15 drops

In water, in doses as frequently as indicated.

For insomnia or exhaustion, whether from excessive application to business or due to alcoholism:
> Tincture of Skull cap (Scutellaria lateriflora), 2–12 drops
> Tincture of Passion flower (Passiflora incarnata), 15–40 drops

In water every 3 hr., or more frequently depending on age and condition.

Tincture alone, 3–12 drops in water as indicated.

Infusion: 1 teaspoonful of the cut or powdered herb steeped in 1 cupful of boiling water for $\frac{1}{2}$ hr.; take every 3–4 hr. for adults; in proportion for children.

Homoeopathic Clinical: Tincture of fresh plants—Ardor urinea, Brain, (irritation of), Chorea, Delirium tremens, Dentition, Flatulence, Headache (nervous), Hiccough, Hydrophobia, Hysteria, Night terrors, Sleeplessness, Tobacco heart.

Russian Experience: Scutellaria baikalensis Georgi is one species of Skull cap growing in Siberia, Russian Far East, north China, Mongolia and Japan. In Russia Shlemnic Baikalski (Skull cap) is not mentioned in medical Folk Medicine literature, but a lot of interest is shown in it because Chinese, Mongolian and Tibetan practice accept the properties. Chinese medicine administers Skull cap as stimulant, tonic, sedative and nervine in the treatment of cramps, convulsions, epilepsy and heart conditions, to reduce fever, for severe rheumatism and pain, and to expel tape worms. Extensive study and experiments confirm Tibetan and Chinese practice (Tomsk University, Siberia, Russia).

Clinically: To reduce high blood pressure, heart conditions, including pains in the heart, disorders of the slowly progressive central nervous system, headaches, head noise, sleeplessness. All experiments indicate that the preparation is not toxic.

SKUNK CABBAGE   Symplocarpus foetidus, Nutt.
(N.O.: Araceae)

Common Names: SKUNK WEED, POLECAT WEED, SWAMP CABBAGE, COLLARD.

Features: Skunk cabbage, a common plant of the order of Araceae, is native to the United States and is also found in Asia. The perennial root is large, abrupt or tuber with numerous crowded, fleshy fibres, which extend some distance into the ground. The first sign of this unusual-looking plant can be seen while the snow is still on the ground. The spathes push through the mud, having a twisted point overhanging the orifice. They are fleshy, curiously mottled with purples, greens and yellows, and protect a round spadix in which perfect flowers are imbedded.

The dull flowers are seen in March and April and maturing its fruit in August and September, forming a roughened, globular mass, 2–3 in. in diameter, and shedding its bullet-like fruit, $\frac{1}{3}$–$\frac{1}{2}$ in. in diameter, which are filled with a singular solid, fleshy embryo.

The flowers are the first pollen bearers to attract the bees. The seeds and roots have an extremely disagreeable odour. Chemically it is known to contain fixed oil, wax, starch, volatile oil and fat, salts of lime, silica, iron and manganese.

Medicinal Part: The dried root.

Solvents: Water, alcohol.

Bodily Influence: Stimulant, Expectorant, Antispasmodic, Diuretic, slight Narcotic influence.

Uses: A well-known and often-used medicine from the earth, Skunk cabbage is much valued in spasms of asthma, tuberculosis, all bronchial and lung affections, including whooping cough, hay fever, pleurisy and pulmonary consumption. Used also to control the involuntary conditions of hysteria, fits, epilepsy and convulsions.

Dose: In small doses the powder may be mixed with honey: $\frac{1}{2}$–4 oz. of honey, in $\frac{1}{2}$–1 teaspoonful amounts. For infusions, the root, cut in small pieces, 1 teaspoonful steeped in 1 cupful of boiling water for $\frac{1}{2}$ hr. When cold, 1 tablespoonful at a time throughout the day as required. Dose of the tincture, 3–15 drops.

Externally: An ointment for external tumours which stimulates granulations and eases pain.

SLIPPERY ELM   Ulmus fulva, Mich.
(N.O.: Ulmaceae)

Common Names: SLIPPERY ELM, RED ELM, INDIAN ELM, AMERICAN ELM, MOOSE ELM.

Features: The deciduous Elm can be found in Central and North America and Asia. There are about twenty species belonging the the Elm family (Ulmaceae). Slippery, or Red, elm is smaller than the rest of the elm family (60 ft. or less) with a wide open crown. The bark and leaves are characteristically rough, deeply furrowed; under layers ruddy brown, protecting the white aromatic fibres used medicinally; odour distinct; taste mucilaginous. The leaves are extremely rough on top, deep yellowish olive-green, lighter and sometimes rusty beneath; flowering in March or April before the leaves appear; fruit nearly round in outline, winged without hairy fringe, ripening in the spring at intervals of two to four years.

Medicinal Part: The inner bark (fresh or dried).

Solvent: Water.

Bodily Influence: Demulcent, Emollient, Nutritive.

Uses: Slippery elm is an agreeable emulsive drink in any disease. The finely powdered bark prepared as an ordinary gruel has shown definite results as a demulcent in catarrhal affection of the whole digestive and urinary tracts, and in all diseases involving inflammation of the mucous membrane of the stomach, bowels and kidneys, and will sustain ulcerated and cancerous stomach when nothing else will. The bark may be chewed and the fluid swallowed for irritation of the throat. It has remarkable soothing, cleansing and healing qualities on all the parts (internally or externally) it comes in contact with and it is interesting to learn that its nutritious value is equivalent to oatmeal.

J. Kloss, in "Back to Eden", gives us another use for Slippery elm bark: "An excellent treatment in female troubles in the following: Make a thick paste with powdered Slippery elm with pure water, shape into

252

pieces about one inch long and one inch thick. Place in warm water for a few minutes. These are called vaginal suppositories. Insert three, afterwards inserting a sponge with a string attached. Let it remain 2 days, then remove the sponge and give douche which will remove the Slippery elm. This is an excellent treatment for cancer and tumours of the womb, all growths in the female organs, fallen womb, leucorrhoea, or inflammation and congestion of any part of the vagina or womb and as a rectal suppository, renewed after bowel elimination."

As a nourishing gruel for children and adults, take 1 teaspoonful of the powder, mix well with the same quantity of honey or maple syrup, add 1 pint of boiling water, soya bean milk, nut milk or milk, slowly mixing as it is poured on. May be flavoured with cinnamon or nutmeg to suit the taste. As a tea, 1 teaspoonful of the inner bark to 1 cupful of boiling water, steeped for 1 hr. or overnight. Can be simmered, strained and then used. This will be like a thick syrup; use small amounts often.

Externally: For poultice, the ground powder or bark should be used, softened with water containing a little glycerine. As a mixture 2 parts Slippery elm, 2 parts Corn meal, 1 part of each of Blood root, Blue flag, Ragweed, Chickweed and Burdock. Mix well, add warm water to required consistency and use on abscesses, fresh wounds, inflammation, congestion, eruptions, enlarged prostate, swollen glands of the neck, groin, etc. If applied to a hairy surface, coat the face of the poultice with olive oil. Always use clean white cotton and change often if drainage is noticed.

Homoeopathic Clinical: Pounded dried inner bark; decoction of dried bark; tincture of fresh bark—Constipation, Deafness, Haemorrhoids, Herpes, Pain, Syphilis.

SOLOMON'S SEAL (AMERICAN) Polygonatum commutatum,
P. multiforum, (Walt.) Ell.
(N.O.: Liliaceae)

Common Names: DROP BERRY, SEALWORT, SEAL ROOT.

Features: Solomon's seal consists of about thirty species of usually hardy perennial herbs of the Liliaceae family. Native to moist, shady woods in the north temperate zone. They grow in colonies, each simple (in some species branched) arching stem 12–18 in., arising in the spring from a thick, fleshy, many-jointed white rhizome, on which, when the stem dies away in the winter, a round scar is left, the "seal" (though this name may derive from the pattern on a cross-section of the stem). The leaves are simple, linear to ovate, sometimes in whorls but mostly alternate, opposite and in two close ranks. The small white or greenish bell-shaped three partite flowers are seen in May and June; later the globular bluish-black berries. Taste is mucilaginous, sweet, then acrid.

Medicinal Part: Rhizome.

Solvent: Boiling water.

Bodily Influence: Astringent, Demulcent, Tonic.

Uses: From Herbalists of the past: "If any of what age or sex so ever chance to have any bones broken in what part of their bodies so ever their refuse is to stamp the root here of and give it unto the patient, in ale to drink, which sodereth and glues together the bones in very short space and very strongly, yea though the bones be but slenderly and unhandsomely placed and wrapped up."

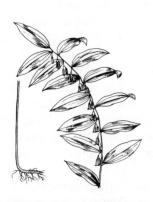

SOLOMON'S SEAL (AMERICAN)
Polygonatum biflorum (Walt.) Ell.
(U.S. Agricultural Department,
Appalachia, 1971)

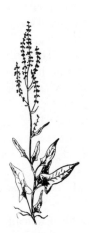

SORREL
Rumex acetosa, L.
(Ontario Department of Agriculture,
Toronto, Canada, 1966)

As a successful decoction used for pectoral affections, menorrhagia, female debilities, whites, inflammation of the stomach and intestines. Will relieve pain and heal haemorrhoids if a tea solution is injected three or four times a day. An agent for obvious conditions such as erysipelas, itch, etc.; also of use in neuralgia and ruptures when taken internally and an external poultice applied to painful area.

Dose: 1 oz. of the root to 1 pint of boiling water, taken in wineglassful amounts.

Externally: The extract from the root is used to diminish freckles and discoloration of the skin. If the fresh root is used, proceed with caution and dilute with water until you find individual acceptance. Used for congested blood caused from bruises, and will close fresh and bleeding wounds.

Russian Experience: Koopena Medical, Solomon's seal, grows through-out the country. Folk Medicine have used its properties for many centuries. Recently modern science of Russia has been interested (Zemlinsky, 1951; Hoppe, 1958).

Folk Medicine and Clinical: Decoction of the dried rhizome for stomach and duodenal ulcer (Popov, 1964) (Bello-Russ. Academy of Science, 1965).

Externally: The fresh juice of the rhizome and decoction of it dried is useful for old and fresh wounds. Fresh juice for freckles (Cholovsky, 1888).

SORREL   Rumex acetosa, L.
(N.O.: Polygonaceae)

Common Names: MEADOW SORROW, SOURGRASS, RED TOP SORREL.

Features: Introduced from Europe and now widely distributed in North America. Sorrel is a name applied to several unrelated plants having in their leaves an acid sap that gives them a sour flavour. It is a low perennial, sprouting from slender running root stocks, and has red pigment in root, inflorescences, and often in leaves, which are halberd to linear shaped. The plants are one-sexed and either pollen or seed bearing. Acidity may result from the presence of one or more of several organic acids, citric, malic and oxalic being the most common.

Medicinal Part: The leaves.

Solvent: Water.

Bodily Influence: Diuretic, Antiscorbutic, Refrigerant, Vermifuge.

Uses: Sorrel is known to the natives of our country as an agent for the stomach, and they use the fresh leaves as pot herbs or in salads. In herbal practice we also agree that Sorrel resists the putrefaction of the blood and is indicated for conditions of inflammation of fever, and to quench the thirst. Also a cordial to the heart.

The life-giving properties of Sorrel to the system is not received with the same acceptance for intestinal worms; they have no resistance to the properties of Sorrel and their presence could cause many misunderstood symptoms.

The root in decoction or powder is effective for all the above purposes, plus jaundice, gravel and stones of the kidney and bladder. The boiled root is used for profuse menstruation and stomach haemorrhage. If there be any sign of scurvy, Sorrel is your food.

Externally: For cutaneous tumours, tetters, ringworm, boils, etc., the express juice with a little cider vinegar applied often will prove effective, if at the same time Sorrel is taken internally.

Homoeopathic Clinical: Tincture of the leaves—Convulsions, Gastritis,

Oesophagus (inflammation of), Paralysis, Throat (sore), Uvula (elongated).

Russian Experience: The Rumex family grows abundantly in Russia. Shavel (Male Rumex acetosella L.) is often found in areas of what seems to be complete Sorrel beds.

Uses: Decoction for internal bleeding, compress for external bleeding (Bello-Russ. Academy of Science, 1965).

SPIKENARD   Aralia racemosa, L.
(N.O.: Araliaceae)

Common Names: INDIAN SPIKENARD, AMERICAN SPIKENARD, PETTY MORREL, LIKE OF MAN, SPIGNET, OLD MAN'S ROOT, WILD LICORICE.

Features: Spikenard is a perennial plant of the Ginseng family Araliaceae. Found from Quebec to south-eastern Manitoba, south to Georgia and Kansas, in rich wooded areas. The root stalk is light brown, thick and fleshy, with prominent stem scars and furnished with numerous long, thick roots, which have a spicy taste and have been used in flavouring root beer. The large, compound, rather-imposing leaves, sometimes nearly 3 ft. long with broad leaflets, grow alternately from a slightly zig-zag stem; and are light green with deeply furrowed indentations the length of the leaf. The flowers are small and greenish-yellow or greenish-white, and are in many-branched, long clusters. The dark purple berries are pleasantly flavoured and can be made into jelly.

Medicinal Parts: Root, rhizome.

Solvent: Water.

Bodily Influence: Alterative, Diaphoretic, Expectorant.

Uses: Our North American Indians used the whole root as food. For many years Spikenard has been used as an addition to cough syrups, with other agents according to the nature of the cough. For irritable conditions, combine with 1 oz. of Wild cherry syrup (Prunus serotina); for old coughs, 1 oz. of Elecampane; for relaxed coughs, 1 oz. Coltsfoot (Tussilago farfara). Any one of the above to be mixed with 1–2 oz. of the tincture of Spikenard (Aralia racemosa) in syrup form. The alterative properties are of use in general uric acid disorders of rheumatic conditions. Often used by our Indians a few months before the time of delivery to shorten pain and delivery; every misery we miss is a new blessing. Spikenard is combined with many other well-known herbs to build or purify the bloodstream, the true cause of pimples, acne, eruptions, etc.

Dose: The infusion of ½ oz. in 1 pint of boiling water is taken in wineglassful doses. Of the tincture, 1–2 fl. drams.

Homoeopathic Clinical: Tincture of fresh wild plant in bloom—Asthma,

Cough, Diarrhoea, Haemorrhoids, Hay fever, Leucorrhoea, Prolapsus ani.

Russian Experience: In the far east of Russia, Manchuria and China, a shrub known as Aralia manchuria grows up to 15 ft. in height and is of the same family as the American Spikenard.

Uses: The properties of the plant are very close to Ginseng. They use the roots as a general tonic and stimulant, especially for physical and mental exhaustion.

Clinically: In Khabarovsk, far eastern Russia, they produce the extract for clinical use.

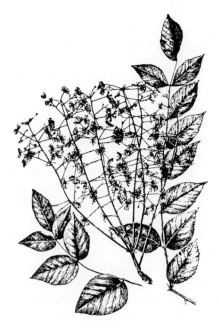

ARALIA MANCHURIA, L.
(Medicina, Moscow)

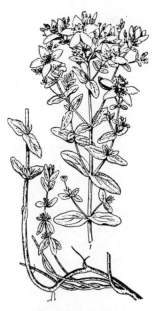

ST. JOHN'S WORT
Hypericum perforatum, L.
(Naukova Dumka, Kiev, 1964)

ST. JOHN'S WORT   Hypericum perforatum, L.
(N.O.: Hypericaceae)

Common Names: JOHNSWORT, ST. JOHN'S GRASS, KLAMATH WEED.

Features: This plant grows abundantly in the United States and Europe. An ornamental herb to our meadows, often considered a pest when too freely mingled in corn and wheat fields. It is said that St. John's wort is well known among bakers, as a small quantity added to the flour improves the quality of bread.

257

The upright, woody, slender stem reaches a height of 1–2 ft. The leaves are stalkless, ½ in. long, growing in pairs on opposite sides of the stem. The dark green leaves are full of transparent holes, which can be plainly seen when the leaf is held up to the light, and sometimes marked with black spots on the underside. From June to August, at the tops of the stalks and branches, stand the yellow flowers of five petals apiece, rather close clustered with many yellow threads in the middle, which when bruised yield a reddish juice like blood, after which come small round heads, wherein is contained a small blackish seed smelling like resin. The fruit is a three-celled capsule.

Medicinal Parts: The tops and flowers.

Solvents: Boiling water, alcohol.

Bodily Influence: Expectorant, Diuretic, Astringent, Sedative.

Uses: An old custom of our Indians was to dry Hypericum and use it as a meal, as they did Acorn. They were also known to eat the fresh leaves for their soothing effect. In many cases of bronchitis, has been known to eliminate all signs of the condition. A family remedy to overcome bed-wetting if taken every night before going to bed. Dose, ½ teaspoonful of leaves and flowers to ½–1 cupful of boiling water, steeped 1 hr.

St. John's wort can be administered to all, whatever age or sex, and was at one time found in almost every country household. For treatment of dysentery, diarrhoea, bleeding of the lungs, worms, jaundice, suppressed urine, and/or pus in the urine, hysteria and nervous irritability. It will help correct irregular menstruation along with proper diet. A specific for deep, low pain of the coccyx (the vertebrae at the base of the spine), head complaints arising from watery matters of obstructions of phlegm in the head, or from the gases rising to the head, stomach spasm, slight obstructions of phlegm on the chest and lungs are healed at once by tea made of St. John's wort. The tea with a small amount of Aloe powder is of special influence on the liver, which can be observed chiefly in the urine; whole flakes of morbid matter are sometimes washed away with it.

J. Kloss, in "Back to Eden", gives us the following: "The seeds steeped in boiling water will expel congealed blood from the stomach caused by bruises, falls, or bursting veins. For this purpose use a heaping teaspoonful of the seeds to a cup of boiling water, and take a large mouthful of the tea often, throughout the day."

Dose: Of the tincture, 8–15 drops in water before meals. As a tea, 1 teaspoonful of the tops and flowers, cut small or granulated, to 1 cupful of boiling water; sweeten to taste with honey.

Externally: The fresh bruised flowers added to olive oil and placed in a glass container to age in the sun for ten days to two weeks, after which time fresh flowers replace the old ones, and simmered in original container on a bed of straw, to keep the glass from breaking, is excellent for swollen breasts and hard tumours, sciatic pain, ulcers, old sores and all wounds. Can be applied as a fomentation of boiled flowers and tops for the above mentioned when caught unprepared.

Homoeopathic Clinical: Tincture of whole fresh plant—After-pains, Asthma, Bites, Brachial neuralgia, Breast (affections of), Brain (concussion of), Bruises, Bunions, Compound fractures, Corns, Coxalgia, Diarrhoea, Gunshot wounds, Haemorrhoids, Headache, Hydrophobia, Hypersensitiveness, Impotence, Labour (effects of), Meningitis, Mind (affections of), Neuralgia, Operations (effects of), Panaritium, Paralysis, Rheumatism, Scars, Sciatica, Spastic paralysis, Spinal concussion, Spinal irritation Stiff neck, Tetanus, Ulceration, Whooping cough, Wounds.

Russian Experience: Zveroboi, "Killing the beast" or "Beast Killer", grows in many parts of Russia. After eating Zveroboi (Hypericum) in the summer time, sheep, cattle, horses and pigs develop white spots and become extremely sensitive to sunshine, eventually developing skin eruptions. The animals will recover if kept in a dark place but a successful precaution is to paint them with non-toxic dark dye. This can also happen with dry Hypericum (Medicine, Moscow, 1963). We are pleased to say our skin type is not sensitive in this way. This is a very old herbal remedy that has been on the forgotten list for too long. Of late, the rediscovery can explain its complicated chemical compound and its wide use in medicine and industry.

Folk Medicine: For generations, Folk Medicine has used Zveroboi in many serious cases of acute and chronic stomach disorders, gastroenteritis, liver, jaundice, kidney and bladder, ulcers, TB anaemia, scrofula, rheumatism, boils, carbuncles, haemorrhoids, coughs, and all inflamed processes. In many female disorders, including excessive bleeding, preventive in bleeding and to dry wounds, ulcers (Bello-Russ. Academy Minsk, 1965). To break bed-wetting, 1 cupful of tea before retiring (Naukova Dumka, Kiev, 1963). A strong decoction of mouthwash to heal gums and offensive mouth odour. Simmer 1 tablespoonful of the flowers in ½ glassful of water for 10 min., cool, strain and gargle a mouthful before meals, three times a day.

Externally: Medical Academy of Russia introduced a special external preparation, "Imanin", for skin conditions and burns, which is now used nationwide (Vishaya Schkola, Moscow, 1963). Extract with Sunflower or Sweet almond oil for skin ulcers and skin conditions: 1 part flowers to 2 parts of oil; keep at least three weeks. The fresh crushed flowers or juice can be used for skin conditions of recent lesions, broken skin, bruises, eruptive skin, etc.

Clinically: Used as Astringent, Disinfectant, Antiseptic, Styptic, Tonic, in the forms of extracts, tinctures, decoctions and tea.

Industrial: Depending on strength, colours of yellow, green, red and pink are made and used for fabric dyes. Collection of wild Hypericum cannot

259

keep up with the growing demand so in Russia they have special plantations. Two or three months before spring seeding they mix the seeds with wet sand and keep in freezing compartments at 0°C. They plan on 3-4 lb. of seed per acre. Once it is planted, the life is good for four or five years. Zveroboi is harvested when the flower is in full bloom; after thirty to forty-five days it can again be harvested, sometimes yielding as larger and richer crop than the first. The first year they collect on the average up to 2,000 lb. of dry herb; in following years 3,000-4,000 lb. It comes to the State collecting stations and is processed as tea, extracts and other preparations.

STAR GRASS   Aletris farinosa, L.
(N.O.: Haemodoraceae)

Common Names: AGUE ROOT, CROW CORN, TRUE UNICORN ROOT, COLIC ROOT.

Features: Star grass is the name given to a variety of plants which have star-shaped flowers. Among them is Aletris farinosa, a perennial herb, indigenous to North America and which grows in low, sandy soils and at the edges of woods.

The tuberous rhizome and bitter fibrous root is covered by smooth, lanceolate leaves lying on the ground in a flat rosette from which arises a tall, stiff stem, terete and sometimes 3 ft. high, with narrow bract-like leaves. It is crowned by a variegated, spike-like raceme of bell-shaped white flowers, just touched with yellow, and having an appearance of crinkliness, like crepe, as they grow old, and is covered with a rough powder externally. Flowers in May to August. The fruit is a triangular capsule.

Medicinal Part: The dried root.

Solvent: Alcohol is its best solvent.

Bodily Influence: Tonic, Diuretic.

Uses: Star grass contains a vegetable agent that has helped to balance the female generative organism in dysmenorrhoea by stimulating and toning the uterus to normal action; also relieves pain. In menorrhagia it controls excessive flow, also engorged conditions of the uterus and prolapsus of the organ. Containing Vitamin E as a preventive to miscarriage it is dependable and free from affects during the entire period of gestation.

The following is prepared by S. Clymer, "Natures Healing Agents": Prenatal care for miscarriage:

Tincture of Star grass (Aletris farinosa), 2-40 drops
Tincture of Black haw (Viburnum opulus), 5-20 drops

Tincture of Blue cohosh (Caulophyllum thalictroides), 5–15 drops
Tincture of Squaw vine (Mitchella repens), 5–15 drops

In hot water as required.

In menorrhagia, dysmenorrhoea and pain due to menstrual disfunctions:

Tincture of Star grass (Aletris farinosa), 10–40 drops
Tincture of Squaw vine (Mitchella repens), 5–15 drops
Tincture of Milkwort (Polygala vulgaris), 1–15 drops

In water three or four times a day.

Though an intensely bitter tonic, the decoction or tincture is of great effect in dyspepsia, general or local debility, flatulence, colic (hence its common name), hysteria, etc.

Homoeopathic Clinical: Tincture of root—Abortion, Anaemia, Colic, Constipation, Convulsions, Debility, Dysmenorrhoea, Dysuria, Endometritis, Fever, Haemorrhoids, Hysteria, Indigestion, Leucorrhoea, Menorrhagia, Myalgia, Pregnancy (vomiting of), Sterility, Uterus (pain in, prolapse of).

STILLINGIA Stillingia sylvatica, L.
(N.O.: Euphorbiaceae)

Common Names: QUEEN'S ROOT, YAW ROOT, QUEEN'S DELIGHT, SILVER LEAF.

Features: Stillingia is a native of the southern part of the United States. This perennial herb has an unequally tapering, rarely branched root; the internal bark is thick, spongy, fibrous with resin cells, easily separated from porous, radiate wood. The somewhat angled stem is 2–4 ft. high, which when broken gives a milky sap, like Milk weed. The leaves are sessile, of a silver colour on the underside and somewhat leathery, and tapering at the base. The flowers are yellow and arranged on a terminal spike. The fruit is a three-grained capsule. The root should be used soon after being gathered as age impairs its properties, due to a very acrid oil, known as the oil of stillingia.

Medicinal Part: The root.

Solvents: Alcohol, water (partially).

Bodily Influence: Alterative, Expectorant, Diuretic, Diaphoretic, Sialagogue, Cholagogue, Antivenereal, in large doses: Emetic, Cathartic.

Uses: The oil by itself should not be used internally. It is a most pronounced glandular stimulant and for this reason is of great use, especially when combined with Sarsaparilla as an alterative preparation. For bronchitis and ordinary sore throat, tetter and as an accepted ingredient by all who know of its possessions in the treatment of syphilis, scrofula, hepatic and cutaneous affections. If there is no response to treatment the reason will probably be because the root used is too old.

As a blood purifier in the form of a fluid extract for the above mentioned:

> Tincture of Stillingia (S. sylvatica), 5–20 drops
> Tincture of Burdock (Arctium lappa), 10–20 drops
> Yellow dock (Rumex crispus), 5–15 drops
> Blue flag (Iris versicolor), 5–15 drops
> Tincture of Pipsissewa (Chimaphila umbellata), 5–10 drops

A tincture of Prickly ash (Xanthoxylum fraxineum), 10–20 drops, can also be added.

Dose: Of the tincture, 15–30 drops in water four times a day. Stillingia root alone, cut small or granulated, 1 teaspoonful to 1 cupful of boiling water; drink cold 1 cupful during the day, a large mouthful at a time.

Homoeopathic Clinical: Tincture of the root after flowering—Bones (disease of; nodes on), Clergyman's sore throat, Elephantiasis, Haemorrhoids, Headaches (syphilitic; mercurial; catarrhal), Hip joint disease, Influenza, Larynx (affections of), Nodes, Periostitis, Psoriasis, Rheumatism, Scrofula, Syphilis.

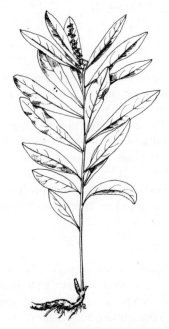

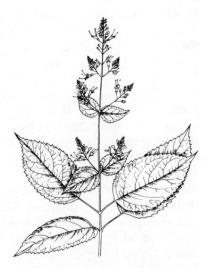

STILLINGIA   Stillingia sylvatica, L.
(U.S. Agricultural Department,
Appalachia, 1971)

STONEROOT   Collinsonia canadensis, L.
(U.S. Agricultural Department,
Appalachia, 1971)

STONEROOT   Collinsonia canadensis, L.
(N.O.: Labiatae)

Common Names: HARDROCK, HORSE-WEED, HEAL-ALL, RICH-WEED, OX-BALM, HORSE-BALM, KNOB-ROOT.

Features: Stoneroot, of the mint family, is native to North America, growing in moist weeds from Canada to Carolina. Collinsonin is the active, concentrated principle of the knobby root which has a four-sided stem 1–4 ft. in height, terminating in several branches at the top which produce large, numerous, greenish-yellow flowers of peculiar balsamic fragrance, and flowering from July until September. The leaves are few, opposite, 6–8 in. long, and 2–4 in. broad. The whole plant is generally used, but the root is the most important.

Medicinal Parts: The whole plant, fresh root (dried).

Solvent: Boiling water.

Bodily Influence: Diaphoretic, Diuretic, Tonic, Astringent.

Uses: As a general diuretic, and is considered a certain remedy in cases of gravel and stones in the bladder. It is not surprising that, due to the power to break up exudation in the valves throughout our system, Stoneroot is receiving much attention as a remedy in functional, vascular diseases of the heart, very often caused by uric acid accumulation and catarrh generally. Its action has a strong influence over all the mucous tissues. Collinsonin is valuable for haemorrhoids and all diseases of the rectum. Often called a clergyman's friend, as a gargle or tincture added to honey and taken four or five times a day it will relieve hoarseness in a few hours. Also helpful in chronic bronchitis, headache, colic, cramps, dropsy, indigestion, etc. Combine with other indicated herbs, or use by itself.

Dose: Largest amount 5 grains; average amount 2 grains three times daily. Of the tincture, 5–20 drops three times daily. As a tea, in 1 cupful of boiling water.

Externally: As a fomentation and poultice the leaves are used for bruises, wounds, sprains, contusions, cuts, ulcers, sores, etc. Made into an ointment for rectal application.

Homoeopathic Clinical: Tincture of fresh root, titration—Constipation, Diarrhoea, Dropsy (cardiac), Dysentery, Dysmenorrhoea, Dyspepsia, Haemorrhages, Haemorrhoids, Heart (affections of), Irritations, Labour, Pregnancy (affections of) Proctitis, Pruritus vulvae, Rheumatism.

STRAWBERRY LEAVES   Fragaria vesca, Fragaria americana, L.
(N.O.: Rosaceae)

Common Name: STRAWBERRIES.

Features: A genus of Fragaris (family Rosaceae), one of several native plants of North America highly prized for their fruit. F. vesca, or Wood strawberry, is a perennial herb and is highly aromatic but with small fruit. Strawberries vary in size, shape, colour, texture, etc. One of the many species of this low or trailing vine is popular to the majority.

Medicinal Parts: Leaves, root, berries.

Solvent: Boiling water.

Bodily Influence: Mild Astringent, Diuretic.

Uses: The effectiveness of the common Strawberry leaf for eczema, the outward appearance of acute or chronic blood contamination, is still on the active list of blood purifying, and blood building agents of created purpose. Use a strong téa or decoction of leaves or roots sweetened with honey and use freely for children and adults for intestinal malfunctions of diarrhoea, dysentery, weakness of the intestines, affections of the urinary organs; will also prevent night sweats, acting as a general tonic to the individual out of step with internal occupancy. A strong tea used as a gargle will strengthen the gums.

Dose: 1 teaspoonful of fresh or dried herb to 1 cupful of boiling water, steeped 15 min. Take 4–5 cupfuls a day; children wineglassful amounts. For a more effective agent, combine with equal parts of Dandelion

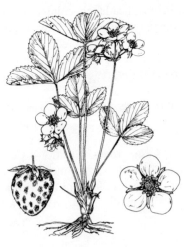

STRAWBERRY LEAVES
Fragaria virginiana, Dushesne fragaris
Veska, Fragaria americana, L.
(U.S. Agricultural Department,
Appalachia, 1971)

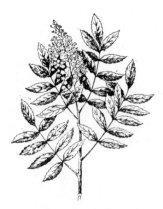

SUMACH   Rhus glabra, L.
(Medicina, Moscow, 1965)

(Taraxacum), Burdock (Lappa) and just enough Rhubarb (Rheum) to assure regular bowel evacuation. Dose of the tincture, 5–15 drops in water three times a day.

Externally: A strong decoction to cleanse and heal eczema and other skin conditions.

Homoeopathic Clinical: Tincture of the ripe fruit; infusion of the root—Anasarca, Biliousness, Chilblains, Convulsions, Erysipelas, Gonorrhoea, Psilosis (or Sprue), Tape worm, Tongue (strawberry; swollen), Urticaria, Weaning.

Russian Experience: Zemlianika, Strawberry, grows in wooded settings throughout Russia and is highly praised as dietetic and medicine. However, some people's systems cannot tolerate Strawberries and they can cause skin rash, itching, redness, etc. If there are indications of this, treatment should be avoided in any form, tea jam, pie, etc. (Saratov University, 1962).

Folk Medicine use the fresh and dried leaves and berries for anaemia, general weakness, bleeding, tape worm, kidney and bladder, children's diarrhoea (Atlas, Moscow, 1963). Also of use for kidney and liver stones, female bleeding, scurvy and vitamin deficiency. To some extent for reducing high blood pressure.

SUMACH   Rhus glabra, L.
(N.O.: Anacardiaceae)

Common Names: SMOOTH SUMACH, INDIAN SALT (powder on the berries), SCARLET SUMACH, MOUNTAIN SUMACH, DWARF SUMACH.

Features: There are several species of Sumach and care should be taken in their identification, as some are poisonous. But this, the blue Glabrum, may be easily distinguished by the colour acidity of the berries and their appearance in cone-shaped bunches. R. glabrum is a shrub 6–15 ft. tall, consisting of many straggling branches covered with a pale grey bark, having occasionally a reddish tint. The leaves are alternate, consisting of from six to fifteen lanceolate, acuminate, shining and green above, whitish beneath, turning red in the autumn. When the green leaves or limbs are cut or broken, a milky juice exudes. The flowers are greenish-red on spikes followed by long bunches of hard, red down-covered berries, extremely sour to the taste, which is due to malate of lime.

They can be found growing in thickets and waste grounds of Canada and the United States, flowering June to July, the fruit maturing in September and October. The berries should be gathered before the rain washes away the acid properties which reside in their external, downy efflorescence.

Medicinal Parts: The bark and fruit.

Solvents: Boiling water, alcohol.

Bodily Influence: Bark—Astringent, Tonic, Antiseptic; Berries—Refrigerant, Diuretic.

Uses: The American Indians crushed the fruit to make a refreshing drink, and also dried the berries for winter use. For application to skin diseases, they made a poultice of the bruised leaves and fruit. Where conditions of mucous membranes are irritated, as in dysentery, scalding of the urinary passage, Sumach is appreciably reliable. The infusion as an injection of the bark (being stronger) and tea taken internally will give prompt relief in leucorrhoea, rectal conditions, chronic diarrhoea and rectal haemorrhage. Of use in malaria and all kinds of fevers, canker in the mouth and as a gargle for sore throat. Sumach is often combined with Slippery elm (Ulmus fulva) and White pine bark for scrofula. The tea is cleansing to the system, and Sumach berries with Blueberry (Vaccinium myrtillus) are most effective in diabetes. A syrup may be made with the berries by covering them with boiling water, steeping for 1 hr., straining, adding honey, boiling into a syrup, and bottling for future use.

Dose: 1 teaspoonful of either the bark, leaves or berries steeped ½ hr. in 1 cupful of boiling water. When cool, 2–4 cupfuls a day. Of the tincture, 10–20 drops.

Externally: For old sores and skin ulcers and wounds apply poultice of bruised leaves and fruit, or a strong tea, and bathe area as needed.

Homoeopathic Clinical: Tincture of fresh bark, roots or berries—Debility, Diarrhoea, Dreams (annoying), Dysentery, Epistaxis, Haemorrhages, Headache, Mouth (ulcers in).

Russian Experience: The species Sumach (Rhus cariaria) grows in south Russia and south Asiatic Russia. From the raw material estimated extract contains 33 per cent tannin (Medicine, Moscow, 1965). Sumach can be very irritating, especially on hot summer days, when a simple touch of the leaves can inflame the skin in various individual ways.

Uses: Russian Homoeopaths and Chinese medicine use Sumach for rheumatism (Moscow University, Moscow, 1963) and for internal bleeding, diarrhoea, enteritic colitis (Atlas, Moscow, 1963).

Externally: Tannin extracts are used for burns, fresh wounds, chronic ulcers, eczema, and as a gargle for inflammation of the throat (Atlas, Moscow, 1963).

SUNDEW Drosera rotundifolia, L.
(N.O.: Droseraceae)

Common Names: ROUND LEAF, SUNDEW, FLYTRAP, DEWPLANT.

Features: A genus, Drosera, of carnivorous plants with ninety species throughout the world. D. rotundifolia is common in North America in damp, sandy soil near bogs from Labrador to Florida, Alaska to California; sometimes so abundant the dew-beds are aglow with glistening red.

The fibrous black rootlets are reddish inside. The leaves are round on long stems extending from the root, the top side of each leaf bearing as many as 200 red tentacles, each tipped with a gland exuding an exceedingly sticky drop of fluid. The flat little rosette of spatulate leaves is formed around a dainty white flower on a stem 1–2 in. tall. The tentacles are expanded until the pressure of a small insect's body is held by the sticky drops, which its weight bends over the prey, enclosing it in a sort of stomach. Digestive juices, analogous to pepsin, are excreted, and the insect is dissolved and absorbed.

Medicinal Part: The whole herb.

Solvent: Boiling water.

Bodily Influence: Stimulant, Expectorant, Demulcent, Antispasmodic.

Uses: In the conditions for which Sundew is used it is almost as if the dew-drops are quenching the dry and tickling condition of the respiratory organs. Considered a prophylactic (prevents the spread of disease) in whooping cough and controls the spasms and characteristic coughs; also indicated in laryngitis, for tobacco cough, some types of asthma, chronic bronchitis and catarrh, when attended with dryness of the mucous membranes and irritable states of the nervous system. Excellent in the early stages of consumption when attended with a harassing cough without expectoration.

S. Clymer gives us a formula that proves very effective:

Tincture of Sundew (Drosera rotundifolia), 2 to 5 drops
Tincture Queen's root (Stillingia sylvatica), 1 to 40 drops
Tincture Passion flower (Passiflora incarnata), 3 to 10 drops

In water as frequently as necessary.

Dose: 1 teaspoonful of the herb, cut small, to 1 pint of boiling water; take a mouthful at a time as required. Of the tincture alone, 3–6 drops in water as indicated. External application may cause water blisters on the skin.

Homoeopathic Clinical: Tincture of the active fresh plant, Amblyopia, Asthma, Bronchitis, Catarrh, Consumption, Cough, Coxalgia, Epilepsy, Haemorrhage, Headache, Laryngitis, Measles, Nausea, Sciatica, Vomiting, Whooping cough.

Russian Experience: Rossianka Round Leaf and Rossianka English (Drosea) grows in many parts of Russia including the far east and Siberia. Commercially collected in Bello-Russia, Siberia and northern Russia in June and July when the plant is in full flower. Long orange needles are used to extract crystalline plumbagin (1928). Plumbagin, which suppresses some pathogenic fungus and bacterial growths, was discovered in other plants in 1828. In northern Russia farmers used the plant in boiling water to disinfect milk containers. The plant also contains peptic ferment of antispasmodic properties, which explains the calming effect for spasmodic and whooping cough.

Folk Medicine: For nervous headache, sickness and disorders due to nerve maladjustment, plague, diphtheria, and as Nastoika (with vodka) for malaria (Bello-Russ. Academy of Science, 1965). Prepared as extracts, decoctions, tea and Nastoika.

Dose: 10–20 drops of extract three times daily. As a tea, 1 teaspoonful steeped in cupful of boiling water, three times a day in tablespoonful amounts.

Externally: Fresh juice for warts (Moscow University, Moscow, 1963).

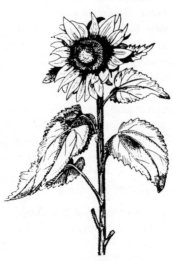

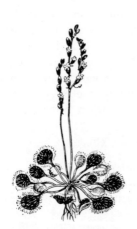

SUNDEW   Drosera rotundifolia, L.
(Vishaya Schkolla, Moscow, 1963)

SUNFLOWER   Helianthus annuus, L.
(Bello-Russ. Academy of Science,
Minsk, 1965)

SUNFLOWER   Helianthus annuus,
(N.O.: Compositae)

Common Name: SUNFLOWER.

Features: This plant belongs to a large composite genus, Helianthus, so called because its golden-rayed flowers are likened to the sun. Perhaps the Sunflower seeds' nutritional richness is due to the flower's amazing ability to follow and face the sun from morning to night. Scientists call this ability heliatropic. The robust annuals (H. annuus) are never known

268

in the wild state, they existed in cultivation in pre-Columbus America. The root system of the sunflower is quite extensive and goes down deep, so extracting many of the trace minerals not always present in top soil.

The leaves are numerous, rough, very large, and somewhat heart-shaped. The disc is very broad and brownish, and its tubular florets develop four-sided, very oily achenes (a small dry carpel containing a single seed, which does not burst when ripe). The yellow petals are daisy-like in pattern. The plant reaches 15 ft in height and is often planted as a concealing border. The Sunflower is the state flower of Kansas in the United States, and a floral symbol of Peru in South America.

Medicinal Part: The seed.

Solvent: Boiling water

Bodily Influence: Diuretic, Expectorant, Nourishing.

Uses: Our Indians used the mineral-grasping root in combination with other roots for snake bites, and a warm decoction was used as a wash for rheumatism and inflammations. They boiled the flower heads to extract the oil and used it as a hair tonic. As a nourishing meal, the roasted shells or seeds were crushed and sifted; the same was also made into a hot beverage; the parched and crushed seed was used for bread meal. Herbalists use the plant in syrup or infusions for coughs, bronchitis, clergyman's sore throat, pulmonary difficulties, early stages of consumption and disease of the kidneys. Infusion of the pith stalk used as a wash will often act effectively in early stages of inflammatory sore eyes, the same being taken internally. Sunflower leaves have also been used for the treatment of malaria. The sun-drenched, deep-rooted Sunflower is known to contain the following (as quoted from the Alumni Research Foundation):

Phosphorus: Essential for building bones, teeth, activating and regulating enzymes, proper fat and carbohydrate digestion, and is a vital building material for all body cells.

Calcium: Our bodies need calcium for building strong bones, hard teeth, good muscle and tissue tone, well-being of nerves and proper clotting of blood.

Iron: Found in good amount and while iron is most essential for the formation of healthy, red blood corpuscles, evidence also points to the necessity of copper being present even though in minute quantities for the proper utilization of iron. There are very few foods in which copper is found in any amount, however Sunflower seeds present a rich source.

Fluorine, Iodine: Iodine has always been associated with sea foods, sea salt and sea moss or vegetation, but it is also found in Sunflower seeds. Natural fluorine, so essential for hard tooth enamel formation, is present in amounts of 2.6 parts per million. Fluorine is also needed in the development of the skeleton since no normal bony substance can be formed without it.

Potassium: Without it, life as we know it would not exist. It is very predominant in brain tissue and appears to be vital in the proper functions of this organ and of the nervous system.

Magnesium: Magnesium takes part in the formation of the albumen of the blood and is also found in greater amounts than calcium in muscular tissues, brain and nervous tissue and lungs.

Sodium: It is interesting to note that Sunflower seeds are unusually low in sodium, containing only 0.4 mg.

Protein: Sunflower seeds contain up to 30 per cent protein, plus all of the amino-acids needed for building and repairing the body cells. This protein is 98 per cent digestible and has a biological or utilization value of 64.5 per cent and does not putrefy as does animal protein.

Thiamine: Sunflower seeds contain a good amount of Vitamin B, this being essential for normal growth and metabolism, maintenance of appetite, nerve functioning, and for good mobility and tone of the stomach and intestines.

Niacin: Niacin is another important vitamin that is also known as the pellagra preventive vitamin. A lack of this vitamin affects the skin, digestive and nervous system of the body. Sunflower seeds are a very good source of this vitamin.

Vitamin D: Every 100 g. of Sunflower seeds contains 92 U.S.P. units, or 23 per cent of an adult minimum daily requirement. This vitamin is necessary for controlling the metabolism of calcium and phosphorus in bone building and teeth formation. While no definite minimum daily requirement has been established, it has been shown that this vitamin appears to be important in the prevention of sterility and for increasing endurance. Further tests have also indicated its value in heart conditions and in some countries it is used to treat heart trouble (due to the unsaturated fatty acids, the opposite of which, saturated fats, form high cholesterol in the bloodstream). Sunflower seeds are used by those who know and respect this vital source of natural nourishment for snacks, soups, meatless loafs and desserts.

Dose: Prepared as medication, 2 oz. of Sunflower seeds to 1 quart of water; boil down to 12 oz. and strain; add 6 oz. of Holland gin and 6 oz. of honey. The dose is 1–2 teaspoonsfuls three or four times a day. The oil contained in the seeds has also been found to possess similar properties, and may be given in doses of 10–15 drops or more, two or three times a day. Make sure the seeds are fresh, as old and rancid oil is detrimental.

Russian Experience: The Russian name is Podsolnechnik, "Under the Sun". Sunflowers are inseparable from Russian daily life as a plant of decoration, food and medicine. It may be difficult for the new generation to believe that the Sunflower originated in North America. Archaeological discovery reveals Sunflower seeds found in clay containers over 3,000 years old, indicating that the original people of this continent knew how to cultivate and use this essential plant. In 1510 the Spaniards were the first to bring the Sunflower species to Spain, where Madrid Botanic Garden started its cultivation for decorative purposes only, as the flowers resembled giant Chamomile and Daisys. Botanist Lobelius, in the sixteenth century, gave us the first botanical description, named Helenithus annuus, which was also grown for decoration only. A Russian Tzar, Peter the Great, first observed the Sunflowers while visiting Holland. His order for seed supplies were filled and Russia soon started cultivation, at first experimentally in St. Petersburg Botanic Garden but soon small farms in the Ukraine and central Russia were producing comparatively larger and healthier species, due to the rich black soil. Peter the Great truly succeeded, as the plants grew to over 15 ft. A pleasurable discovery soon found persons of all ages enjoying the seed-meat as dried or roasted tit-bits when entertaining. The pressed oil was found to be superior and the handsome plant soon had another purpose. The practical usefulness of the Sunflower brought about The Academy of Science Review in 1779 when Russia's capital was St. Petersburg. There botanical and commercial description of Russia's Sunflower was established.

In 1835 a practical gardener in the Ukraine cultivated the first commercial Sunflower plantation. Within fifteen to twenty years the waste areas of central Russia, Ukraine, south Russia and many parts of Siberia were covered. It is hard to imagine a garden without a Sunflower plant (Vishaya Schkolla, Moscow, 1963). For the past 100 years the Russians have known the Sunflower as a source of nourishment as well as a decorative flower.

Folk Medicine of Bello-Russia use the whole head (basket) of the Sunflower when the seeds begin to ripen. They cut this into small pieces, add soap chips, Nastoika (vodka) and place in the sun for nine days. The aged liniment is used externally for rheumatic pain. Decoctions made from the flowers are taken internally as Nastoika, 1 part flowers to 5 parts vodka, 30-40 drops three times a day. Soft, pulpy stem parts are used as tea for fevers (Bogdanovich, 1895).

Clinical: Many oil preparations of ointments, liniments and medical compounds; decoction of the seeds for jaundice, malaria, heart conditions, diarrhoea, kidney and bladder (Bello-Russ. Academy of Science, Minsk, 1965); oil as dietic food is a part of daily life; decoction or tea from flowers and leaves for malaria (Atlas, Moscow, 1963).

The Sunflower serves as an illustration of how a plant can travel around the world and come back as a new-found food thought, somehow

271

transformed but still native of one's own country. Nutrition takes many forms and sources and the towering Sunflower is one of the almost perfectly balanced foods, yet to be experienced by the majority.

SWAMP BEGGAR'S TICK Bidens connata, Muhl.
N.O.: Compositae)

Common Names: COCKHOLD HERB, BEGGAR'S TICK, SPANISH NEEDLES, DEVIL'S PITCHFORK.

Features: This is a common weed, found in wet grounds, rich fields, swamps and ditches from New England to Missouri. The herb has a smooth stem, 1–3 ft. high. The leaves are lanceolate, opposite, serrate, acuminate, and decurrent on the petiole. The terminal florets are yellow, and can be seen in August; the fruit is a wedge-formed achenium.

Medical Part: The herb.

Solvent: Boiling water.

Bodily Influence: Emmenagogue, Expectorant, Antispasmodic, Diaphoretic.

Uses: Dr. Brown (1857): "The root and seeds are emmenagogue and expectorant; the seeds, in powder or tincture have been used in amenorrhoea, dysmenorrhoea, and some other uterine derangements, and an infusion of the root has proved beneficial in severe cough." It has been used with great success for palpitation of the heart and for croup. For the latter affliction a strong infusion of the leaves sweetened with honey and administered in tablespoonful doses every 15 min. until vomiting is produced is regarded as a cure. The leaves, heated to the form of a poultice and laid upon the throat and chest in cases of bronchial and laryngeal attacks from exposure to cold, etc, are very beneficial.

Dose: 1 teaspoonful of the root, cut small or granulated, to 1 cupful of boiling water. Drink cold 1 cupful during the day, a large mouthful at a time. Of the tincture, 5–20 drops. Either Bidens bipinnata, (Spanish needles) or Bidens frondosa (Beggar's tick) can be employed, both having the same medical properties.

Russian Experience: A variety of Bidens grow throughout Russia. Chereda (Bidens triparita) has the most attention medicinally and commercially. The well-dried leaves keep their natural colour, have specific aroma and astringent, slightly bitter taste.

Folk Medicine employed the silent qualities of Chereda long before words were expressed on paper. Decoctions were used for tension of fear, blood purifying, liver trouble, colds, inflammation of the bladder, headache, eczema (internally as tea, decoction, extracts), external bathing for skin irritations, nervous upset children to induce sleep (Bello-

Russ. Academy of Science, Minsk, 1965). Tea used for scrofula, rickets, diathesis, gout and as a diuretic and diaphoretic. For improved metabolism, 1 tablespoonful to 1 cupful of boiling water, steeped 10 min. and strained. Dose, 1 tablespoonful eight times a day (Moscow University, Moscow, 1963).

Clinical: In the form of Nastoika, extracts and decoctions in combinations of compounds for treatment of internal and external ailments. Pharmacopeia of late has given attention to Bidens triparita (Atlas, Moscow, 1963).

Industrial: The wild collection of Bidens falls short of the demand. Cultivation is very successful: they seed 12–14 lb. per acre and harvest up to 2,500 lb. of dry herb. Cutting starts just before the buds flower and when the plant is about 50 cm. high, using only the leaves and tops (Medicine, Moscow, 1965).

Commercial: Beautiful cream shades of brown, orange and yellow are used for dying wool and silk.

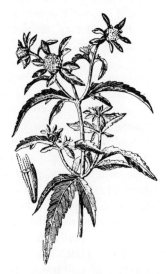

SWAMP BEGGAR'S TICK
Bidens triparita, Muhl.
1—Seed
(Vishaya Schkolla, Moscow, 1963)

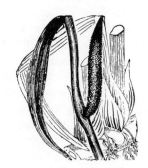

SWEET FLAG Acorus calamus, L.

SWEET FLAG Acorus calamus, L.
(N.O. : Araceae)

Common Names: CALAMUS, MYRTLE FLAG, SWEET GRASS, SWEET SEDGE, SWEET RUSH ROOT.

273

Features: Sweet flag resembles the Blue flag (Iris versicolor). It is not an Iris, however, and may be distinguished from it by its corm and the pungent taste of the leaves. This perennial herb grows on the borders of ponds and marshes where the soil is constantly moist and rich, throughout the United States.

Medical Part: Rhizome.

Solvents: Alcohol, hot water (partially).

Bodily Influence: Aromatic, Carminative, Stomachic, Stimulant, Tonic.

Uses: The first candied root was used by the Indians and Turks for dyspepsia. It is also frequently used for heart-burn, caused by distention of the stomach by gas. In many instances those suffering from stomach discomfort from some unknown reason found Calamus a remedy by chewing the root, or the use of the tea, several times a day. The uncomfortable feeling of burning water from the stomach into the throat is usually brought under control by this ancient knowledge. Useful in flatulence, wind, colic, ague, upset or sour stomach, dyspepsia, etc. Taken at regular intervals, it is a most innocent and effective stomach conditioner, the health of which more than half of our illnesses stem from. The Egyptians used Sweet flag for the legendary disease of scrofula, but it should be combined with supporting, more effective herbs for this chronic condition.

Dose: Infusion of 1 oz. of the cut or granulated herb to 1 pint of boiling water. May be taken frequently in cupful amounts. Tincture of Calamus alone, 10–40 drops in water, according to age and severity of condition.

Russian Experience: There are many insinuating names for Sweet flag (Calamus) in Russia, two of which are Mongolian poison and Bitter poison. Originally China and India were the motherland of Calamus, which was first brought to Russia in the eleventh century when the Mongolians overcame the Russian territory. Tartars (Mongolians) considered that Calamus purified the water. When they planned on settling in a new territory, Calamus was always planted near the watering place to ensure of pure drinking water for the horses. The Mongolians brought many new adaptations from China to Russia. Around this time in history China was on a very high cultural standard and medicine, particularly herbal was in great favour (Vishaya Schkolla, Moscow, 1963).

In the Ukraine, Baltic area and Poland, Calamus has been well known since the thirteenth century. In the seventeenth century sugared rhizomes of Calamus were imported to Germany from Constantinople (Istanbul), Turkey, but the Calamus plant was not known to them at this time. Angerius von Busback, Austrian ambassador in Constantinople, became aware of the tonic properties of this medical plant from Turkey and sent the fresh rhizomes to Praga in 1565. The fresh stock was sent to Vienna Botanic Garden in 1574, where a famous botanist, Clausius, took great pride and gave much attention to its cultivation. It was here that the first, and one of the most complete, botanical descriptions was made and proudly displayed to everyone interested. A Polish doctor came to see the Garden and disparaged the famous scientist for his attention to such a common weed as Tartar poison, bitterly known in Russia and Poland since the Mongolian invasion. This ridicule was so discouraging to the famous botanist that he gave Calamus to anybody who wanted a plant and soon the whole country was alive with Calamus. To this day botanist Clausius is remembered for his sincere devotion to Calamus, but the name of the merciless doctor is gone with the wind.

Folk Medicine soon discovered Calamus was everything but Mongolian poison and praised it highly as a healing agent. Decoction or tea for stomach condition, liver, gall-bladder, kidney and bladder, stones in the kidney and bladder, malaria. Nastoika (with vodka) as a gargle for mouth irritations and toothache. The country people kept the fresh leaves in the house as aromatic, disinfectant and insecticide. The roots were burned to clear the air when sickness from cholera, typhus, flu, etc., were present. It is used as aromatic bitter to improve appetite and the digestive system, to relieve the central nervous system, in decoctions, Nastoika and extracts. Decoctions and tea for kidney and bladder, liver, gall-bladder and general tonic. Powder used internally and externally (Atlas, Moscow, 1963).

Externally: Nastoika (with vodka) is used for bathing wounds, infected ulcers, shingles, scurvy, children with rickets, scrofula and various skin conditions. Powder for wounds and ulcers. A hair decoction of Calamus, Burdock and Hops is a preventive for falling hair and improves the hair and scalp if application is massaged regularly.

Veterinary: For stomach, liver and various internal ailments. The powder for external wounds, ulcers, etc.

Industrial and Commercial: 1 ton of raw rhizomes when dry yields about 500 lb. (Naukova Dumca, Academy of Science, Ukraine, Kiev, 1963). Sweet flag oil is used medicinally, in the food industry and as a wine aromatic.

India and Pakistan Experience: Known in this country as Bacha or Vacha. Their ancient history and experience has generations of expressed approval.

Bodily Influence: Aromatic, Antispasmodic, Aphrodisiac, Bitter tonic, Carminative, Diuretic, Expectorant, Emetic, Emmenagogue, Laxative, Nauseant, Stimulant.

Uses: Diarrhoea, dysentery, bronchitis and chest affections. Infusion for epilepsy of children. In small doses for flatulence, colic, chronic diarrhoea and dysentery, loss of appetite, bronchitis and catarrh, fevers, ague, haemorrhage. As an emetic, 30 grains is effective, used instead of Ipecacuanha. For asthma, 10 grains every 3 hr.

275

Externally: The burnt root mixed with some bland oil is used as a poultice for flatulence and colic. Also for paralysed limbs and rheumatic swellings. Dry powdered root is dusted over foul and indolent ulcers and wounds.

The above mentioned is the most popular, but use varies individually and by location (Medical Plants, India, Pakistan, J. F. Dastur, Bombay, 1962).

SWEET GUM Liquidambar styraciflua, L.
(N.O.: Hamamelidaceæ)

Common Name: RED GUM, STAR-LEAVED GUM.

Features: Sweet gum, a tree of the Witch hazel family (Hamamelidaceae), native of the eastern United States, also Mexico and Central America. Along the rivers of the south-eastern United States, Sweet gums exceed 125 ft. in height and 4 ft. in diameter. The deeply cut grey or brownish-grey bark forms winged projections on the twigs. The alternate, palmate, shiny leaves have usually five pointed, finely toothed lobes, and are fragrant when bruised. In the autumn the star-shaped leaves turn brilliant red to purple, making a valuable ornamental tree. The staminate flowers are inconspicuous, the pistillate in spherical heads maturing into long-stalked, globose masses of spiky-tipped capsules. The wood is fine-grained, moderately hard and fairly strong; the heart wood is known as red gum and hazelwood, is variously coloured red and brown, the sapwood is paler. From incisions made in the tree a gum exudes which is resinous (storax) and adhesive, and somewhat like white turpentine in appearance, which finally hardens.

Medicinal Parts: The bark and concrete juice.

Solvents: Boiling water (bark, partially), warm alcohol (more completely).

Bodily Influence: Stimulant, Expectorant, Diuretic, Antiseptic, Disinfectant.

Uses: As a remedy for catarrhs of genito-urinary passages, coughs of pulmonary affection generally, gonorrhoea, gleet, amenorrhoea, leucorrhoea, phthisis (wasting disease, tuberculosis of the lung, consumption) and asthma. Also excellent for bloody flux, dysentery and all bowel complaints of children.

Dose: 1 teaspoonful of the cut or granulated bark to 1 cupful of boiling water; drink 1 or 2 cupfuls a mouthful at a time during the day; adjust to condition and age.

Externally: The balsamic juice may be melted with equal parts of olive oil or tallow as a detergent ointment when conditions of indolent ulcers, frost-bite, scabies, itch, ringworm, fistula, scrofula, fever sores and haemorrhoids are present.

TACAMAHAC   Populus balsamifera, L,
(N.O.: Salicaceae)

Common Name: BALSAM POPLAR.

Features: The name of various oleoresins allied to elemi; balsam is exuded by different species of trees found in East India, Africa, Brazil and Siberia. Our Balsam poplar is found in northern parts of the United States and Canada.

This tree attains a height of 50–70 ft., with a trunk about 18 in. in diameter. The branches are smooth, round and deep brown. The leaves are ovate, gradually tapering and dentate, deep-green above and smooth on both sides. In America the leaf buds are in bloom in April, and this is the official part and time for collection. They have an agreeable, incense-like odour and an unpleasant, bitterish taste. The balsamic juice is collected in Canada in shells and sent to Europe under the name of Tacamahaea.

The Populus balsamifera is generally confused with the Populus canadensis, from whose buds we get the virtues known as the Balm of Gilead; but it is much the superior tree for medical purposes.

Medicinal Part: The buds.

Solvent: Alcohol.

Bodily Influence: Stimulant, Expectorant, Tonic, Diuretic. Antiscorbutic.

Uses: The buds are used as a stimulating expectorant for all conditions affecting the respiratory functions when congested. In tincture they have been beneficially employed in affections of the stomach and kidneys and in scurvy and rheumatism, also for chest complaints. The bark is known to be tonic and cathartic and will prove of service in gout and rheumatism.

Dose: Tincture of the buds, 1–4 fl. drams in water as needed. As a tea, 1 teaspoonful of the buds to 1 cupful of boiling water.

Externally: The buds are chiefly used in the form of ointments and plasters for counter-irritant purposes.

TAMARACK   Larix americana, Mill.
(N.O.: Pinaceae)

Common Names: AMERICAN LARCH, BLACK LARCH, HACKMETACK, SALISB.

Features: Larch, the common name of a small genus (Larix) of medium-sized coniferous trees of the pine family (Pinaceae). They differ from other genera in being deciduous and in bearing short, green needle-like leaves on dwarf and long shoots. The spruce-like, erect cones with thin, persistent scales and long, accuminate bracts mature in one season. Most species are 40–80 ft. high except when growing near the timber-line. Of the ten species now recognized, American larch (L. americana), also known as Black larch, or Tamarack, is the most common in the eastern United States and Canada extending west to the Rocky Mountains and north-west to the Yukon River in Alaska, where it is sometimes called L. alaskensis: growing in the southern parts of this area in swamps and sphagnum bogs. The gummy sap that seeps from the tree has a very good flavour when chewed.

Medicinal Part: The inner bark.

Solvent: Boiling water.

Bodily Influence: Alterative, Diuretic, Laxative.

Uses: Because of its astringent and gently stimulating qualities the inner bark is especially useful for melancholy, often caused by the en-larged, sluggish, hardened, condition of the liver and spleen with in-activates various other functions of the metabolism. For domestic use in emergencies, or long-standing bleeding of any kind, in lungs, stomach, bowels, or too profuse menstruation. Also for diarrhoea, rheumatism, bronchitis, asthma and poisonous insect bites. J. Kloss in "Back to Eden", recommends the weak tea as an eye wash and the warm tea dropped in the ear to relieve earache. A decoction of the bark, com-bined with Spearmint (Mentha viridis), Juniper (Juniperus communis), Horse radish (Cochlearia armoracia), and taken in wineglassful doses has proven valuable in dropsy.

Dose: As a tea, 1 teaspoonful of the inner bark to 1 cupful of boiling water; steep 30 min.

Externally: As a wash used to cleanse ulcerated sores of long standing, if the condition has progressed to the bone, combine with Comfrey (Symphytum officinale) fresh or dried (taken internally too). As a poultice, dress often and continue until new skin seals the areas. Also used for haemorrhoids as a salve, or sitz-bath.

Russian Experience: Listvennitza Sibirsky, Larix siberia (Tamarack), grows 150 ft. tall in Siberia and the far east. The very wide branching tree is one of the most beautiful and magnificent to adorn their country-side. Turpentine of Larix, known in Russia as venetian terpentain, is one of the by-products.

Externally: The oil in compound is used for rheumatism, neuralgia, gout; new twigs and bark made into an antibiotic and antiseptic is used as an inhalant steam for catarrh of the lungs, abscesses, gangrene of the lungs, throat, bronchitis. Also of help to kidney and bladder.

Clinically: As oil of turpentine.

TANSY Tanacetum vulgare, L.
(N.O.: Compositae)

Greek Name: Alhanasia, "immortality".

Features: Tansy, of a perennial creeping root, was introduced into America from the northern Old World. The tough, slightly ribbed stems reach a height of 2–3 ft., terminating in flat, button-like, gold-coloured heads of rayless florets. The plant may be easily recognized in July and August as the flower heads look as if all the petals have been pulled off, leaving only the central florets. It is a handsome plant, with dark-green, deeply cleft and pinnatifid, fernlike leaves, being 6–8 in. long and 4 in. broad. A familiar herb of waste lands and roadsides. The crushed leaves and flowers give a pronounced aromatic smell and have a bitter taste.

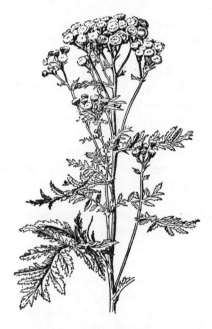

TANSY Tanacetum vulgare, L.
(Vishaya Schkolla, Moscow, 1963)

It contains volatile oil, wax, stearine, chlorophyll, bitter resin, yellow colouring matter, tannin with gallic acid, bitter extractive gum and tanacetic acid, which is chrystallizable, and precipitate lime, baryta and oxide of lead.

Medicinal Part: The herb.

Solvent: Alcohol, water.

Bodily Influence: Tonic, Emmenagogue, Diaphoretic, Stimulant.

Uses: Large doses cause vomiting, convulsions, coma, feeble respiration and pulse. In small doses the cold infusion will be found useful in convalescence from exhausting diseases, dyspepsia and jaundice. The warm infusion is diaphoretic and emmenagogue and is used for colds, fevers, la grippe and agues. The herb is also used for treatment of hysteria and certain other of the nervous disorders of women. For this purpose take 1 tablespoonful of the infusion frequently, when needed.

Tansy seeds are vermifuge and should be steeped, $\frac{1}{4}$ oz. to 1 pint of boiling water, and taken after night and morning fast, previously cleansing the alimentary tract with a herbal laxative. You may like to know the creatures respond more favourably when the moon is full.

A good remedy to promote menstruation, but should be used only when the suppression is due to conditions other than pregnancy. Tansy is a capable and useful herb in the hands of the experienced when prescribed for daily use.

Dose: Of the tincture, 5–10 drops, the larger dose only in extreme cases of hysteria and suppression of the menses due to causes other than pregnancy. Of the infusion, 1 teaspoonful of Tansy steeped in 1 pint of boiling water of $\frac{1}{2}$ hr.; 1 teaspoonful every 3 hr.

Externally: Hot fomentations wrung out of Tansy tea are excellent for swellings, tumours, inflammations, sciatica, bruises, freckles and sunburn, and will check palpitation of the heart in a very short time, (J. L. Kloss, "Back to Eden").

Homoeopathic Clinical: Tincture of the fresh plant in flower; attenuations of the oil—Abortion, Amenorrhoea, Chorea, Dysmenorrhoea, Epilepsy, Eyes (sclerotica inflamed), Hydrophobia, Labia (abscess of), Paralysis, Strabismus (right inward), Worms.

Russian Experience: Riabinka obiknovennaya, or (close to the sound of) Pishma, grows everywhere in Russia except the extreme north.

Folk Medicine: Used as a tea and powder with honey or sugar for worms; decoction in stomach sickness, diarrhoea, nervous disorders, liver, headache, TB of the lungs. Children are bathed in a solution when frightened (Bello-Russ. Academy of Science, Minsk, 1965); 5 per cent of the flowers with vodka (Nastoika) for stomach and duodenal ulcers (Moscow University, Moscow, 1965).

Clinically: Flowers, and in some cases the whole plant, are used. Oil for worms is very effective but toxic. Powder, decoction, oil for ascaris and various other worms, diarrhoea, liver and stomach (Atlas, Moscow, 1963).

Commercial: Powder used as insecticide (Moscow University, 1965).

THUJA   Thuja occidentalis, L.
(N.O.: Coniferæ)

Common Names: ARBOR-VITAE, YELLOW CEDAR, TREE OF LIFE, FALSE WHITE CEDAR.

Features: The name White cedar is often applied to the Arbor-vitae (Thuja occidentalis), a well-known, handsome ornamental American evergreen. It atttains heights of 70–80 ft., with a trunk diameter of 2–6 ft., which is sometimes distorted. The erect spreading branches have thin and flat pendulous twigs, fragrant green leaves, and tiny bluish-purple cones covered with bloom, turning reddish-brown with six to twelve pointless thin oblong scales. Found growing in wet ground from New Hampshire to Florida. There are various species of Cedar found in Africa, India, Australia and Alaska.

Medicinal Parts: Branchlets and leaves.

Solvents: Alcohol, water.

Bodily Influence: Stimulant, Diuretic, Irritant, Expectorant, Emmenagogue, Anthelmintic.

Uses: Thuja is useful as a counter-irritant in the relief of muscular aches and pains, chronic coughs with association of shortness of breath, fevers, the sudden attacks of acute pain in the joints that may last for a few days or weeks, the associated gout (uric acid retention). The pain of menstruation due to the cessation of flow is relieved by the hot tea taken frequently.

Dose: Infusion of 1 teaspoonful to 1 pint of boling water taken in teaspoonful to wineglassful amounts.

Externally: The leaves and twigs boiled with oil make an excellent salve. Also for removal of warts and fungoid growths.

Homoeopathic Clinical: Tincture of the fresh green twigs—Abdomen (distended), Abortion, Angina pectoris, Anus (fistula in; fissure of), Asthma, Balanitis, Cancer, Catalepsy, Chorea, Clavus, Condylomata, Constipation, Convulsions, Coxalgia, Diarrhoea, Disparunia, Dysmenorrhoea, Ear (polypus of), Enuresis, Epilepsy, Epulis, Eyes (tumours of; granular inflammation of), Fatty tumours, Feet (fetid) Flatus (incarcerated), Frontal sinuses (catarrh of), Ganglion, Gleet, Gonorrhoea, Haemorrhage, Haemorrhoids, Hair (affections of), Headache, Hernia, Herpes zoster, Ichthyosis, Intussusception, Jaw (growth on), Joints (cracking in), Levitation, Morvan's disease, Mucus patches, Muscae volitantes, Myopia, Naevus, Neck (chronic catarrh of; polypus of), Paralysis, Pemphigus, Polypus, Post-nasal catarrh, Pregnancy (imaginary), Prostate (disease of), Ptosis, Ranula, Rheumatism (gonorrhoeal), Rickets, Sciatica, Seminal emissions, Nocturnal Sycosis, Syphilis, Tea (effects of), Teeth (caries of), Tongue (ulcers of; biting of), Toothache, Tumours, Vaccination, Vaccinosis, Vaginismus, Warts, Whooping cough.

281

THYME   Thymus vulgaris L.
(N.O.: Labiatae)

Common Names: GARDEN or COMMON THYME, TOMILLO, MOTHER OF THYME, SERPYLLUM.

Features: Originating from the Old World, Thyme is recognized around the world as an aromatic, flavouring herb, or for ornamental decor. The small, shrubby perennial herb T. vulgaris is an erect or somewhat decumbent plant, 1–3 ft. high, has sessile linear lanceolate leaves with revolute margins. The pale-lilac flowers are small and in interrupted whorled, spikes at the end of the branches. It has a strong, pungent,

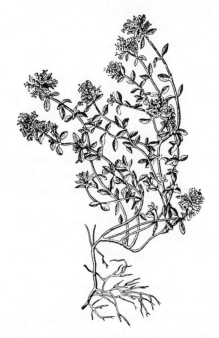

THYME   Thymus vulgaris, L.
(G. N. Kotukov, Lekarstevennye, Naukowa Dumka, Kiev, 1964)

spicy taste and odour. In preparing the herb for out-of-season use, it should be collected in the summer when in blossom and thoroughly dried in the shade. Thyme is favoured by the bees, and the honey is a superior replacement for sugar.

Medicinal Part: The herb.

Solvents: Boiling water, alcohol.

Bodily Influence: Tonic, Carminative, Emmenagogue, Antispasmodic.

Uses: Culpeper states: "It is under the dominion of Venus and under the sign of Aries and therefore chiefly appropriated to the head", Astrology or not, we agree with Culpeper, as we use Thyme for hysteria, headache, nervous disorders of giddiness and weakening nightmares. This unsuspecting herb is admirable for strengthening the lungs and children's colic, colds, irritable stomach, dyspepsia, flatulence and ill-disposition. To sooth the throat of bronchial irritation and in spasms of whooping cough, thyme has been most reliable; it induces free perspiration, important to the beginning of a cold and in ordinary fever. (Make sure the person is free from draught and is kept warm.) Also of use in suppressed menstruation. Use the cold tea freely in small amounts for stomach complaints.

Dose: Infusion of 1 teaspoonful of thyme to 1 cupful of boiling water; steep ½ hr. Of the tincture, 20–50 drops in hot water.

Externally: The oil of Thyme is used for toothache, neuralgia and painful swellings.

Russian Experience: This plant's name is easily recognizable in three languages: Thymus is Latin, Timian Russian and Thyme English. The extreme north is too cold for this herb but it grows elsewhere in Russia.

Clinically: In a Pharmacopoeial preparation, Thymol, volatile oil is extracted and used as antiseptic and disinfectant. Combined with other herbs for congested chest, bronchitis, whooping cough, worms and skin conditions (Atlas, Moscow, 1963).

Commercially: Plantations in Ukraine, Moldavia, Don River regions have been assisted by Agro-Technic. They seed 4–5 lb. per acre and collect 1–2 tons of dry herb. Once seeded, plantations can be harvested for three or four years (Medicine, Moscow, 1965).

TURKEY CORN   Corydalis canadensis, Goldb.
(N.O.: Papaveraceae)

Common Names: WILD TURKEY CORN, STAGGER WEED, CHOICE DIELYTRA, SQUIRREL CORN.

Features: This indigenous perennial plant is a beautiful little herb that grows in North America, Canada to Kentucky, in rich soil, on hills, among rocks and old decayed timber. The plant grows 6 to 12 in. high. It has small, tender stalk and small fine leaves of bluish-green colour, round bulbous root, about the size of a large pea; from two to four of these peas to a stalk, attached to small roots which are hard, and of yellowish colour; quite bitter, and nearly odourless. The six to ten small, reddish-purple, nodding flowers are seen very early in the spring and the root should be gathered while the plant is in flower. The fruit is a pod-shaped, many-seeded capsule. The alkaloid, Corydalia, is the active principle.

Medicinal Part: The root.

Solvents: Alcohol, boiling water.

Bodily Influence: Tonic, Diuretic, Alterative.

Uses: Do not disregard the action of this herb by the barnyard sound of the common name (the root growth resembles a corn kernel). Turkey corn is one of the best alterative agents in the herbal kingdom. It is usually combined with other remedies such as Burdock (Lappa), Queen's delight (Stillingia), or Prickly ash (Xanthoxylum fraxineum). A Philadelphia professor has this to say about the small root: "There is no fact better established than that this medicine, judiciously administered, has the power to remove syphilis from the system." The tincture should be prepared from the fresh herb and given in doses of 20–30 drops, three times a day. Also admirable for scrofula and all skin diseases. Recommended in menstrual complaints, as its tonic properties render it as an alterative in all enfeebled conditions.

Dose: Infusion of 1 teaspoonful of the root, cut small or granulated, to 1 cupful of boiling water; steep $\frac{1}{2}$ hr.; drink cold a wineglassful three or four times a day. Of the powder, 5–10 grains. Of the tincture, 20–30 drops three or four times a day.

Homoeopathic Clinical: Tincture of bulbous root gathered when plant is in flower; trituration of dried root; triturations of Corydalia—Gastric catarrh, Scrofula, Syphilis, Ulcerations.

Russian Experience: The most interesting Russian literature is given to one kind of Turkey corn, Corydalis, commonly called "Chochlatka", which means in folk language hens or chickens cackling indiscriminately. The shadowy bush or brush growth of central and south Russia is an ideal setting for survival. Indication of past Folk Medicine is not mentioned, only Atlas (1963) giving botanical description and medical details.

Clinically: As extracts of Corydil and in combinations, for trembling, nerve paralysis and nerve disorders: it stimulates and increases muscle tone. Experiments on animals show positive effect on the central nervous system. Physiologically Iscoriaodine is calming to the central nervous system. As there is no other information from available books, interested readers will get the best scientific information about chemical, botanical and clinical properties from Atlas, Moscow, 1963.

This brief information is given with the thought that the local knowledge of the Indians and Folk Medicine in North America has been confirmed scientifically and clinically by scientists in other countries.

VALERIAN   Valerian officinalis, L.
(N.O.: Valerianaceae)

Common Names: GREAT WILD VALERIAN, SETWELL, CAPON'S TAIL.

Features: Valerian type genus incorporate many species of herbs or shrubs growing in Africa, Britain, Greece, U.S.A., etc. The flowers have five parted perianths and funnel-shaped, short-spurred corollas which are generally of a pale rose colour, flowering June to August. The Calyx, which is rudimentary, when in flower becomes a feathery pappus at the top of the fruit. The plant is often cultivated in gardens for its flowers and its root. It has an erect, round, pale greenish stem, 2–5 ft. long. The leaves are simple or pinnate, without stipules; ascending rhizome, with many fibrous roots. Has a warm, camphoraceous, slightly bitter, somewhat acrid and nauseous taste growing stronger with age. Cats are very fond of the odour of Valerian and tear the plant to pieces and roll in it. They are said even to dig up the roots and devour them. The root as trap bait attracts rats if you don't have a cat around to catch them.

Found in many damp places, low-lying meadows and woods, along banks of rivers and lakes and in marshy, swampy ground generally. The carrot-like roots of V. edulis, a tall glabrous plant of the western U.S.A. with undivided stem leaves, and yellowish-white flowers in elongated panicles, are eaten by the Indians either raw or dried. The Piutes even grind them into flour and use in the form of bread or mush. To this day in northern England the dried root is used in broths, pottage or physical meats as a counter-poison and medicinal preservative against pestilence, as are treacles, mithridates, etc. Besides valerianic acid the root contains starch, albumen, valerian yellow extractive matter, balsamic resin, mucilage, valerianate of potash, malates of potash, lime, phosphate of lime and silica.

Medicinal Part: The root.

Solvent: Water.

Bodily Influence: Antispasmodic, Calmative, Stimulating Tonic, Nervine.

Uses: Valerian is used by Herbalists today as a nerve tonic. Is best combined with Skull cap (Scutellaria), Blue vervain (Verbena hastata), and Mistletoe (Viscum album). Gentian (Gentiana lutea) and Peppermint (Mentha piperita) increase the promptness of its action, which is more effective than when combined with bromide. Employed in epileptic fits, St. Vitus dance, nervous derangement or irritations, debility, hysterical affections (especially female), restlessness, and in wakefulness

285

during fever. Valerian excites the cerebro-spinal system. In medicinal doses it acts as a stimulating tonic, antispasmodic and calmative. In large doses it causes headaches, mental excitement, visual illusions, giddiness, restlessness, agitation and even spasmodic movement.

Dose: Of the tincture, 1–2 teaspoonfuls three times a day; of the infusion, a wineglassful; of the extract, 3–6 grains; of the oil, 5 drops.

Externally: An infusion of ½ cupful of the root can be used in the bath to relieve nervous exhaustion.

Russian Experience: Valeriana is known to Folk Medicine as having a general calming and sedative effect on the central nervous system, to induce sleep and rest, spasms of the stomach, intestines and blood vessels, nervous heart conditions. Further acknowledgement as appetizer, headache relief, hysteria, epilepsy, tape worm, diarrhoea, lose stomach, fever.

Externally: Vapour baths given to children will quieten and encourage restful sleep (Bello-Russ. Academy of Science, Minsk, 1965).

Clinically: Extracts of Valerian are used in compounds of tablets, tinctures, etc.

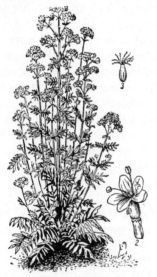

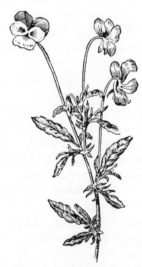

VALERIAN Valerian officinalis, L.
1—General 2—Flower 3—Seed pod
(Naukova Dumka, Kiev, USSR, 1964)

VIOLET Viola odorata, L.
(Vishaya Schkolla, Moscow, 1963)

VIOLET Viola odorata, L.
(N.O.: Violaceae)

Features: The Violets have a large family tree of some 400 species, predominantly perennial herbs but with a few annuals. Violets are found in damp woods and other shady places and are among the best-known wild

286

plants, with characteristically scented and coloured flowers. They are highly adapted to cross-pollination by insects. Some species are indigenous to North America, however V. odorata is native to Europe but has been naturalized in the United States. Violet leaves contain certain glucosidal principles of distant antiseptic properties and the flowers are expectorant and have been used for generations in syrup form for coughs, colds, etc.

Medicinal Parts: Leaves and flowers.

Solvent: Boiling water.

Bodily influence: Antiseptic, Expectorant.

Uses: Violets are mostly thought of as decorative, or in memory of a tender occasion. Their admirable qualities as a herb are never realized by the "out of touch with nature" modern society.

Violet has been recommended and used with benefit to allay pain in cancerous growths, some even say "to cure cancer". In 1902, "Potters New Cyclopaedia", page 313, claims that Lady Margaret Marsham, of Maidstone, was cured from cancer of the throat by infusion of Violet leaves. The following are extracted from the publication: "In a week the external hard swelling had gone, and in a fortnight the cancer on the tonsil had disappeared." "Pour a pint of boiling water over a handful of fresh Violet leaves and let stand for 2 hours. Strain, when required, apply to the affected part and cover with a piece of oilskin, change when dry or cold."

The influence of the dissolving properties seem to have intricate inward skill, reaching places only the blood and lymphatic fluids penetrate. For difficulty in breathing when conditions are caused from a morbid accumulation of material in the stomach and bowels causing gas, distention and pressure, Violet tea taken daily for some time will make you feel that the beauty of the plant is of secondary importance. It is cooling to any high temperature of the body, internally or externally. Of service in headaches and heat to the head; a specific for ear disturbances, having a soothing and healing effect on inflamed mucal surfaces. Colds, sore throat, inflammation of lungs, hoarseness, whooping cough, etc., of children and adults is greatly controlled by a handful of dried or fresh violet leaves and flowers in $\frac{1}{2}$ pint of water, steeped for $\frac{1}{2}$ hr., administer 2–3 tablespoonfuls (more for adults) every 2–3 hr., and a mouthful to gargle (make sure the bowels eliminate properly).

Dose: As a tea 1 teaspoonful of the herb to 1 cupful of boiling water.

Externally: Crushed Violet bound as compress on inflamed tumours, sore throat, swollen breasts, to the back of the neck for headache, or the cloth saturated in Violet tea will often give unbelievable results, if applied assiduously. Keep a supply of the dried leaves and flowers for out-of-season use.

Homoeopathic Clinical: Tincture of fresh plant in flower—Cancer,

287

Choroiditis, Cough (spasmodic; by day), Hoarseness, Hysteria, Neuralgia (supra-orbital), Otorrhoea (suppressed), Rheumatism, Seminal emissions, Styes, Whooping cough, Wrist (rheumatism of).

Russian Experience: Fialka Polevaya, Violet, is a popular all-the-year-round decoration—in the fields in the summer time and as a house plant in winter. Tri-colour Violets are formally and tenderly called Anutini Glazki, "Eyes of Annie", but much sentiment is lost in the English translation. The country folk are less illuminating in speech and use Ivan and Mary, Ivan da Maria. Medical properties and uses are carried over from ancient history (Vishaya Schkolla, Moscow, 1963).

Folk Medicine use decoctions, tea, Nastoika (with vodka), internally and externally, as diuretic, diaphoretic, blood purifier. For diathesis, coughs, eczema, TB of the skin and other skin conditions (Bello-Russia). Decoction for female condition, toothache, chest pain of cold (Bello-Russ. Academy of Science, Minsk, 1965).

Externally: Decoction to drink and as poultices, or for complete bath immersion, for chronic and persisting skin conditions, scrofula, eruptions, children's eczema (Bello-Russ. Academy of Science, 1965).

Medically: Special preparations of the whole plant are administered for lung and chest trouble as expectorant in chronic catarrhal accumulation (Atlas, Moscow, 1963).

India and Pakistan: Known as Banaf Shah, the flowers are emollient, demulcent, astringent, diaphoretic, diuretic, laxative. Used in cases of prolapsus of the uterus and rectum, nervous disorders, biliousness, epilepsy, inflamed swellings. For diaphoretic use when needed for colds, coughs, kidney and bladder disorders. In large doses the flowers are emetic; 2 oz. of stem will act as purgative, emetic; juice will cause nausea, vomiting and nervous conditions. The underground stem is emetic and purgative and is valuable if used instead of Ipecacuanha. Their use goes further still, antipyretic and febrifuge. From "Medical Plants of India", page 175, (by J. F. Dastur, Bombay, India, 1962) credit is given to the control of cancer in the following way: "The fresh leaves are a reputed drug for the treatment of Cancer: they relieve pain of cancerous growths, especially in the throat; two and a half ounces of the fresh leaves are infused in a pint of boiling water in a covered stone jar for 12 hours; the strained liquid is taken in the course of a day, in doses of a wineglassful at a time; for treatment of cancer of the tongue only half the quantity is taken in a day; the other half is used to foment the tongue; a liquid extract of the fresh leaves, in teaspoonful doses, is equally efficacious. On cancerous growths either the hot infusion or an extract of the fresh leaves is applied as a compress."

Dose: 1 part of flower to 100 parts of water, or a syrup; 30–50 g. doses. As emetic, dose 40–50 grains.

Externally: For Eczema.

VIRGINIA SNAKEROOT   Aristolochia serpentaria, L.
(N.O.: Aristolochiaceae)

Common Names: RED RIVER SNAKE ROOT, TEXAS SNAKE ROOT, SANGREL, SANGREE ROOT, BIRTHWORT, SERPENTARIA.

Features: Virginia snakeroot is a perennial plant found in hilly woods of Pennsylvania, Virginia, Ohio, Indiana and Kentucky, and the southwest states, Louisiana to Texas, of the U.S.A. The root is fibrous and of a brown colour, has numerous stem scars and bears a dense tress of branching roots about 3 in. long, with a gingery, aromatic, identifiable fragrance; bitter taste. The one or more erect, zigzag jointed stems are 1–2 ft. high, with a purplish colour near the plants base. The leaves are oblong and about 3 in. long and 1 in. wide. June and July finds the few purple or dull-brown flowers in bloom, attached to short stems which come from the root.

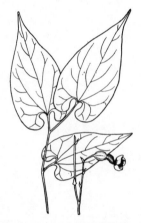

VIRGINIA SNAKEROOT   Aristolochia serpentaria, L.
(U.S. Agricultural Department, Appalachia, 1971)

Solvents: Alcohol, boiling water.
Bodily Influence: Stimulant, Diaphoretic, Anodyne, Antispasmodic, Tonic, Nervine.
Uses: The action of Virginia snakeroot is so prompt that it has a great reputation for snake bites, hence its name. This is a pure stimulant whose action is mainly employed in diverting the flow of blood outward; and for this reason it is largely employed in eruptive diseases before the appearance of outward manifestations are noticed. It rids the system of any offending matter by producing perspiration and supporting the vital forces. As a nerve stimulant it acts very promptly and is much used in depressed or exhausted conditions of the nervous system, especially in the latter stages of smallpox, scarlet fever and pneumonia. The influence

289

on the circulation will also be felt by the whole arterial system as the heart's impulse becomes stronger and fuller. The often suppressed menstruation due to colds will be brought about by 5–10 drops of V. snakeroot tincture in Pennyroyal tea. Also for cold extremities of hands and feet due to general receding of blood from the surface. The cold infusion is used for strengthening purposes and it may be drunk freely and is often employed with good effect in dyspepsia, croup, throat and kidney congestion and renal torpor. In proper doses it stimulates appetite and digestion in indicated conditions. In large doses, however, it is irritant, causing vomiting, vertigo, purging, etc.

Dose: Of the tincture, 5–20 drops three times daily. As an infusion, 1 teaspoonful of the granulated root to 1 cupful of boiling water, steeped 30 min. Take in tablespoonful amounts three to six times a day.

Homoeopathic Clinical: Trituration of dried roots—Dyspepsia, Flatulence.

WAFER ASH Ptelea trifoliata, L.
(N.O.: Rutaceae)

Common Names: WINGSEED, HOPTREE, SHRUBBY TREFOIL, SWAMP DOGWOOD.

Features: Wafer ash is a shrub common to America, growing most abundantly west of the Alleghenies in sandy moist places and edges of woods and also in rocky places. This handsome shrub is 6–8 ft. high with dark brown branches; the leaves are downy beneath when young; trifoliate and marked with pellucid dots. The June flowers are polygamous, greenish-white, nearly $\frac{1}{2}$ in. in diameter, and of a disagreeable odour; usually four stamens; short styles and the fruit a two-celled samara. The light-brown root bark is wrinkled with a thin epidermis, internally yellowish-white, darkens with exposure; odour peculiar, aromatic; taste bitter. Petelein is its active principle.

Medicinal Part: Root bark.

Solvents: Boiling water (partially), alcohol (more completely).

Bodily Influence: Tonic, Antiperiodic, Stomachic, Stimulant.

Uses: It is used for the same purpose as Quinine and may be tolerated by the stomach when other tonics are rejected. Useful for low fever with gastro-intestinal irritation and typhoid conditions. It has a soothing influence upon the mucous membrane in all cases of debility and during intermittent and remittent chills and fever and febrile diseases where a tonic is indicated. Regarded as a remedy for asthma when tinctured with whisky and taken in doses of 1–2 tablespoonfuls every 2–3 hr. It is very useful as a promoter of the appetite. The leaves and young shoots are anthelmintic and the fruit (samara) aromatic, bitter and a good substitute for Hops. 1 teaspoonful of the root bark, cut small, to 1 cupful of boiling water. Drink 1 cupful throughout the day a mouthful at a time. Of the powder, 10–30 grains. Of the tincture, 1–2 drams.

Homoeopathic Clinical: Tincture of root bark—Asthma, Constipation, Dysentery, Dyspepsia, Erysipelas, Gall-stones, Gastralgia, Headache (gastric; bilious), Intermittents, Jaundice, Liver (congestion of), Nightmare, Phosphaturia, Rheumatism, Spleen (affections of), Worms.

WAHOO   Euonymus atropurpureus, Jack.
(N.O.: Celastraceae)

Common Names: INDIAN ARROWROOT, BURNING BUSH, SPINDLE TREE, EUONYMUS, PEGWOOD, BITTER ASH.

Features: Wahoo in botany is a name of American Indian origin, most commonly applied to a large shrub, or small tree, 6–25 ft. tall native to North America. (The name Wahoo is also given to an Elm (Ulmus alata) and another variety, Euonymus americanus.)

E. atropurpureus has obtusely four-angled twigs; leaves, 2–5 in. long, oval in shape, with finely toothed margins and covered below with fine hairs. The purple flowers, appearing in May or June, are about $\frac{1}{2}$ in. across are borne in groups of seven to fifteen on a short stalk. The fruit is a deeply four-lobed purple capsule bearing brown seeds covered with

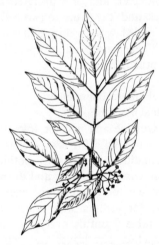

WAHOO
Euonymus atropurpureus, Jack.
(U.S. Agricultural Department,
Appalachia, 1971)

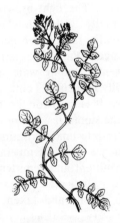

WATER CRESS
Nasturtium officinale, R. Br.
(U.S. Agricultural Department,
Appalachia, 1971)

a scarlet aril. The plant grows in many sections of the United States, in woods and thickets and river bottoms. The bark of the root has a bitter and unpleasant taste.

Medicinal Part: Root bark.

Solvents: Water, alcohol.

Bodily Influence: Tonic, Alterative, Cholagogue, Laxative, Expectorant.

Uses: Valued in liver disorders especially those following or accompanied by fever. For constipation due to inactivity of liver it may be given with every confidence, especially as its action is mild and non-

292

irritant. The influence is not restricted to the liver alone, the pancreas and spleen are also assisted by its properties. An effective agent for dropsy and dyspepsia, having cathartic effect. Euonymus is often used in combinations of other tonics, laxatives, etc., in pill form.

Doses: 1 small teaspoonful to 2 cupfuls of boiling water, simmered 30 min., 2–3 cupfuls a day 1 hr. before meals.

Homoeopathic Clinical: Tincture of fresh bark and root—Albuminuria, Bilious fever, Biliousness, Cholera morbus, Gall-stones, Levitation, Liver (affection of), Vertigo.

WATER CRESS   Nasturtium officinale, R.Br.
(N.O.: Cruciferae)

Common Names: TALL NASTURTIUM, WATER CRESS.

Features: Water cress is of the mustard family native to Europe, but has migrated to most of North America and is found in moist banks and running waters below 8,000 ft. The branching stems are 1–3 ft. long and generally extended with leaves above the water. The leaves are somewhat fleshy, elliptic and in pairs of three to seven with small white flowers in enlongated racemes; pods $\frac{1}{2}$–1 in. long. Water cress is most popular as a garnish only; the mineral-rich plant is an excellent addition to daily salads. Has been in use as this by people since ancient times.

Medicinal Parts: Leaves, root.

Solvent: Water.

Bodily Influence: Tonic, Stimulant, Blood purifying.

Uses: The American Indians used the herb for liver and kidney trouble and to dissolve kidney stones. Parkinson, in 1640, says: "The leaves of juice applied to the face or other parts troubled with freckles, pimples, spots or the like at night and washed away in the morning. The juice mixed with vinegar to the forehead is good for lethargy or drowsy feeling." For the above use the fresh herb daily for skin improvement. The high content of the vitamin and mineral part is a preventive for scurvy, and a blood builder in every sense of the word. The Romans considered it as excellent food for those who have deranged minds.

J. E. Meyers, Botanical Gardens of Hammond, Indiana. U.S.A., informs us that Water cress is one of the best sources of Vitamin E. This is the fertility vitamin (it was discovered by Prof. Herbert Evans of the University of California), helping the body use oxygen, which increase physical endurance and stamina and improves heart response. Tests and research by professors of science show that dried Water cress contains three times as much Vitamin E as do dried lettuce leaves. (Researches Mendel and Vickery worked with Dr. Karl E. Mason, of Vanderbilt University, U.S.A.)

Dose: Infusion of the fresh or dried herb, 1 teaspoonful to 1 cupful of boiling water then steeped. Drink 3–4 cupfuls daily.

Be sure to wash Water cress carefully if there is possible drainage from farmyards. Also be cautious of polluted water.

WATER PEPPER   Polygonum punctatum, Ell.
(N.O.: Polygonaceae)

Common Names: SMART WEED, AMERICAN WATER SMART WEED, ARSESMART, PEPPERWORT.

Features: This annual plant is a member of the buckwheat family growing in England and America in ditches, low lands, among rubbish and around brooks and water courses.

The herb has a smooth stem, 1–2 ft., with a reddish- or greenish-brown colour, of the often decumbent base. The leaves are alternate, lanceolate, petiolate, with dots of thin skin throughout the leaves. The small greenish-white or greenish-pink flowers are loose, slender and drooping with erect spikes. It flowers in August and September. The taste is bitter, pungent and acrid. Water pepper should be collected and made into tincture or tea while fresh, as age decreases its properties and results.

Medicinal Part: The whole herb.

Solvents: Alcohol, water.

Bodily Influence: Antiseptic, Diuretic, Diaphoretic, Emmenagogue.

Uses: The infusion in cold water has been found serviceable in gravel, colds and coughs and in milk sickness. For the pain of suppressed menstruation, taken internally and fomentations wrung from the hot tea and applied to the lower back, where there is usually pain, will soon bring relief. Of use in female obstruction as a feminine douche when in pain, itching or leucorrhoea. In cholera, if the patient is wrapped in a sheet moistened with a hot decoction it will aid recovery; also taken internally but making sure the bowels are active. The infusion in cold water forms an excellent local application in the sore mouth of nursing mothers and in mercurial salivation.

Dose: 1 teaspoonful of the herb, cut small, to 1 cupful of warm water; taken in wineglassful, or teacupful, amounts. The decoction or infusion in hot water is not so active as when prepared in cold or warm water. Of the tincture, 30–60 min.

Externally: The fresh leaves bruised with the leaves of Plantain (Plantago lanceolate), and moistened with oil of turpentine and applied to the skin will speedily relieve chronic erysipelatous inflammations.

Homoeopathic Clinical: Tincture of whole fresh plant—Amenorrhoea, Antrum (pain in), Blepharitis, Colic (flatulent), Cough, Diarrhoea,

Dysentery, Dysuria, Eczema, Epilepsy, Gonorrhoea, Gravel, Haemorrhoids, Heart (affections of), Hysteria, Laryngitis, Nephritis, Neuralgia, Orchitis, Prostatitis, Sciatica, Spermatic cord (pain in), Spleen (affections of), Strangury, Ulcers.

Russian Experience: Vodianoy Peretz, Water pepper, grows in Siberia and other parts of Russia, but more abundantly in European Russia. Russian literature credit for medical, commercial and industrial properties are prominent. The fresh leaves when used as food are bitter, burning and spicy (Vishaya Schkolla, Moscow, 1965). The whole plant is used and collected in late autumn when in full flower. They cut 10–20 cm. from the ground with attention given to proper species, as it is easily mistaken with other Polygonum with less benefit.

Folk Medicine: As a tea for bleeding of the stomach, female complaints, haemorrhoids.

Externally: The fresh leaves slightly bruised and applied to the back of the neck instead of mustard poultice for headaches. Simmer, covered, ½ lb. of leaves 1 hr. and add to sitz-bath for bleeding haemorrhoids.

Clinically: Strong warning is given about using the extract—recommended for use by medical practitioners only. Extracts, Nastoika (with vodka) and in preparations with other ingredients for female bleeding, bleeding haemorrhoids and to stop pain (Atlas, Moscow, 1963). Recent study and experiment show that the plant is a rich source of Vitamin K (coagulating substance), Vitamin P, Vitamin C and rutin.

Industrial: For textile dye, Polygonum can be collected from spring to autumn for beautiful shades of golden-green, gold, steel and camouflage shading of green.

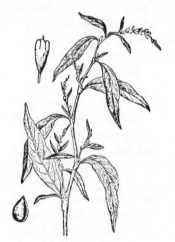

WATER PEPPER
Polygonam punctatum, Ell.
(Medicina, Moscow, 1965)

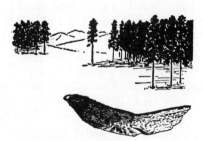

WHITE PINE   Pinus strobus, L.

295

WHITE PINE   Pinus strobus, L.
(N.O.: Pinaceae)

Common Names: SOFT PINE, DEAL PINE.

Features: Pine is the common name of the largest and economically most important genus (Pinus) of the pine family (Pinaceae) of the conifers (cone-bearing trees) in general. Of the ninety or more species of pines, thirty are native to North America, distributed from north of Mexico, eastern, northern and the western states.

The outstanding characteristics of the genus are mostly erect, much branched, twigs with long shoots with scaled leaves and dwarf branches bearing long needles surrounded by scaled leaves at the base; the leaves are either primary, solitary, scale-like, spirally arranged, and usually deciduous some weeks after their appearance. The unisexual flowers (cones, strobile) appear in the spring on the same tree. Conifers often produce twin trees resulting from the presence of more than one embryo in a single ovule. Traditionally the genus Pinus is subdivided into two main groups: (1) the soft pine, or white pines, and (2) the hard or yellow pines.

Medical Parts: Inner bark or sprigs.

Solvent: Boiling water.

Bodily Influence: Expectorant.

Uses: The pine trees play an important part in the domestic life of the Indian. They use pine needles for sewing, resins as cement, and the nuts as food and decoration. The appealing use as medicine and food is, to us, the most outstanding. Pine nuts were made into a paste consistency and added to soups for infants and adults. They chewed the gum resin for sore throats; the same was also dried, powdered and applied to the throat with a swab. The resin and parts of some other plants such as small twigs of Juniper (Juniperus osteosperma) were used as a tea for colds, rheumatism, tuberculosis, influenza and chronic indigestion, kidney trouble, etc. The bark and new sprigs are useful as an expectorant, to modify quality and quantity of the mucus secretions and to favour its removal in bronchial and catarrhal trouble, rheumatism, scurvy, all chest affections, tonsilitis, laryngitis, croup and the like.

It is best to combine 1 teaspoonful of each of the following with 1 pint of water: Wild cherry bark (Prunus serotina), Sassafras (Laurus) and Spikenard (Aralia racemosa); steep $\frac{1}{2}$ hr.; administer $\frac{1}{2}$ teaspoonful to a mouthful every hour, depending on age and condition. Of use in diabetes with Uva ursi (Arctostaphylos), Marshmallow (Avthea) and Poplar bark (Populuas tremuloides). Prepare as above and take 3–4 cupfuls daily of the tincture, $\frac{1}{2}$–1 fl dram.

Externally: The heated resin is used as a dressing to draw out imbedded splinters or to bring boils to a head; sores, cuts, swellings and insect

296

bites also respond favourably. The hot resin can be spread on a hot cloth and applied as you would a mustard plaster for treating pneumonia, sciatic pains and any general muscular soreness.

WHITE POND LILY   Nymphaea odorata, Solond.
(N.O.: Nymphaeaceae)

Common Names: WATER NYMPH, WATER CABBAGE, SWEET SCENTED POND LILY, COW LILY.

Features: The Lily family embraces many economically important genera, including sources of fibres, food (Onion, Garlic), spices, resins, medicines, soap, poisons and essential oils. However the so-called water lily (Nymphaea) and Calla lily (Calla palustris) are not members of the Lily family. White pond lily grows in ponds, with large, round, dark-green leaves, floating in the water, bearing a large white flower, that looks like a large Gardenia in shape. Growing from Canada to Florida and Louisiana.

Medicinal Part: The root.

Solvents: Water.

Bodily Influence: Antiseptic, Astringent, Demulcent, Discutient.

Uses: An old-fashioned home remedy brought into use by the Indians, the knowledge of which has been passed down for generations. There

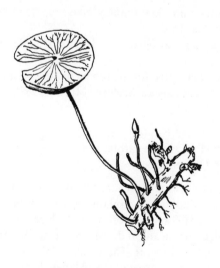

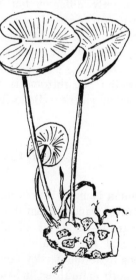

WHITE POND LILY
Nymphaea odorata, Soland.
(Ontario Department of Agriculture,
Toronto, Canada, 1967)

YELLOW WATER LILY
Nuphar advena, Ait.
(Ontario Department of Agriculture,
Toronto, Canada, 1967)

297

are few remedies which act more promptly than this in old cases of leucorrhoea, where there is chronic inflammation of the womb or abrasion of the vagina, and for ulceration of the womb it has proven efficacious, having completely cured the disease after all other available means have failed. It should be used locally, by injection of the infusion to the neck of the womb, and taken internally. Very accommodating in cases of dropsy and kidney trouble, catarrh of the bladder, irritation of the prostate. Has been used largely for diarrhoea and bowel complaints, excellent for infant diarrhoea, scrofula and diseases of the lungs. The infusion is healing to sores, ulcerated mouth, inflamed gum, canker, sore throat.

Dose: 1 oz. of the root boiled in 1 pint of water for 20 min., taken from wineglassful to teacupful amounts two or three times a day. Of the fluid extract, 10–15 drops, morning and night.

Externally: The fresh juice of the root mixed with lemon juice is excellent for removing freckles, pimples and dark discolorations of the skin. Make a strong tea for use as a local application applied with Turkish towels, or white cotton, for painful swellings, boils, ulcers, etc. The bruised leaves are healing to wounds and cuts applied as poultice.

Homoeopathic Clinical: Tincture of the root—Back (pain in), Coryza, Diarrhoea, Throat (sore).

Russian Experience: In Russian literature mention is made of two kinds of Pond lily—Kuvshinka Nymphaea alba and Nymphaea candida. They are slightly different but used medically the same way. In some undisturbed areas of ponds, lakes and slow-running water up to 6 ft. deep, Lily's will cover the peaceful surface.

Folk Medicine use both species as astringent for female trouble of amenorrhoea.

Clinically: The rhizome is used medically for palilloma of the kidney and acidic gastritis (Bello-Russ. Academy of Science, Minsk, 1965).

WILD CARROT Daucus carota, L.
(N.O.: Umbelliferae)

Common Names: BIRD'S NEST, QUEEN ANNE'S LACE, DEVIL'S PLAGUE.

Features: Daucus, from the Greek daukos, or daukon—a kind of carrot or parsnip—a genus of about sixty species of annual, biennial or perennial herbs mainly of Mediterranean and African distribution, belonging to the parsley family (Umbelliferae). The biennial Wild carrot is a herb naturalized in America, found growing in old meadows and pastures.

The fleshy root tapers, is yellowish-white, sweetish and faintly aromatic. Its erect, branching, bristly-hairy stem is usually 1–5 ft. high.

The leaves are basal or alternate and pinnately compounded. The flowers are usually white or roseate to purplish and arranged in flat-topped compound umbels, with the central flower, usually dark red or deep purple, blooming in June or July. The seeds are of a dull brown colour, flat on one side and convex on the other. The Wild carrot cannot be transplanted to gardens to produce an edible product. It taints milk with a bitter flavour if cattle eat too much of it, although it is not poisonous.

Medicinal Part: The whole plant.

Solvent: Water.

Bodily Influence: Diuretic, Deobstruent, Stimulant.

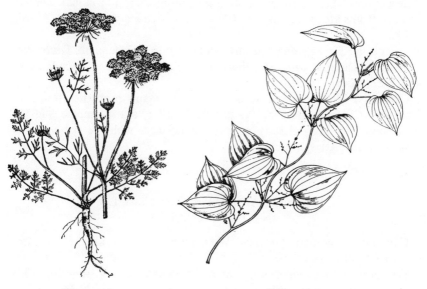

WILD CARROT
Daucus carota, L.
(Ontario Department of Agriculture,
Toronto, Canada, 1966)

WILD YAM
Dioscorea villosa, L.
(U.S. Agricultural Department,
Appalachia, 1971)

Uses: Culpeper comments "Wild Carrot belongs to Mercury, and therefore breaketh wind, and removeth stitches in the sides, provoketh urine and women's courses, and helpeth to break and expel the stones." Wild carrot blossoms are used as a tea and are effective as a remedy for dropsy when all other treatment fails. The root and seeds are often ground and used for colic, liver, kidney and bladder, painful urination, to increase the menstrual flow, and in expelling worms from the bowels. Some physicians believe that the bruised seeds steeped (not boiled) are more effective in kidney diseases, dropsy, inflammation of

299

the bladder and in gravel. You will find that improvement in some of the above conditions will relieve rheumatic pain.

Dose: Infusion of seeds and/or herb, 1 teaspoonful to 1 pint of boiling water, steeped 30 min., 3–4 cupfuls daily.

Externally: Grated carrots made into a poultice is recommended for ulcers, abscesses, carbuncles, scrofulous, cancerous sores and bad wounds. The leaves bruised and applied with honey are also cleansing to running sores or ulcers. Apply according to severity, fresh with each application.

Russian Experience: Morkov, Wild carrot, grows everywhere in Russia except the extreme north; it is cultivated domestically everywhere.

Folk Medicine: Decoctions of the plant for worms and as laxative; decoction of the whole plant for liver, gall-bladder and jaundice conditions. Roots alone for anaemia (Bello-Russ. Academy of Science, Minsk, 1965).

Externally: For swelling and abscesses crush the whole plant. Decoctions to bathe children when skin becomes yellow (Bello-Russ. Academy of Science, Minsk, 1965).

Clinically: Doucorin extract is one of the many properties found in carrots. Clinically prepared as a mild laxative, antispasmodic and for avitaminosis, arterisclerosis, coronary deficiences with the symptoms of stenocardia (Atlas, Moscow, 1963).

WILD JALAP   Convolvulus jalapa, LN.
(N.O.: Convolvulaceae)

Common Names: MECHAMECK, WILD POTATO, MAN ROOT, MAN OF THE EARTH, MAN IN THE GROUND.

Features: Mechameck belongs to the United States of America. This is a climbing perennial herb of the Morning glory family. The root is very large and tapering from which arise several long, round, slender, purplish stems, 4–8 ft. high. The leaves are cordate at the base, alternate and acuminate and about 2–3 in. long. The large white flower opens in the forenoon; flowering from June to August, followed by a two-celled fruit capsule. Thrives in light, sandy soil, seldom found in the northern latitudes. The roots can be dug when young shoots appear but it is best to wait until autumn, after aerial stems have decayed, then wash, peel and dry (if necessary over fire).

Medicinal Part: The root.

Solvents: Diluted alcohol (completely), Water, or alcohol alone (partially).

Bodily Influence: Hydragogue, Cathartic, Diuretic.

Uses: The influence seems to be especially useful for lungs, liver and

300

kidney. Equal parts of root and Skunk cabbage (Symplocarpus foetidus) made into a syrup is very effective in consumption, cough and asthma. An infusion, taken in wineglassful doses every hour, is useful in dropsy and calculous affections. The milky juice of the root is said to be a protection against the bite of the rattlesnake.

Dose: Of the infusion, wineglassful or less every 3 hr. Of the tincture, 2 teaspoonfuls.

WILD YAM   Dioscorea villosa, L.
(N.O.: Dioscoreaceae)

Common Names: COLIC ROOT, CHINA ROOT, RHEUMATISM ROOT.

Features: Yam is the common name for plants of the genus Dioscorea of the family Dioscoreaceae (called the Yam family) or for their tubers. Yams are herbaceous vines whose stems twine consistently to the right or left, depending on the species, of which about 600 are known; four are native to the United States and Canada. Yams are among the most important tropical root crops, some kinds being baked, boiled, fried, used in soup or dried and ground into meal. Most species are nutritious. The variety differs greatly in shape, colour and size of tubers.

Dioscorea is thought to have sixty-seven species in Mexico alone. The complicating resemblance of the leaves is misleading. This delicate, twining vine grows in thickets and hedges of Canada and the United States, more prolific in the south. The vine and leaves resemble a Philodendron, with a reddish-brown stem. You will have to be very observant to find the small greenish-white flowers in June and July. Botanically the potato is long, branched, crooked and the weight about 4 lb., the average size collected. The flesh inside is moist, fibrous and faintly rose coloured. Referred to as a rhizome, or underground stem, as is the Iris. From this a preparation of Diosorein, or Dioscorein, is prepared containing its active qualities.

Medicinal Part: The root.

Solvent: Water.

Bodily Influence: Antispasmodic, Antibilious, Diaphoretic.

Uses: Aztec records show that Chipahuacxihuitl, or "The Graceful Plant" known to us as Dioscorea, was used for skin treatment of scabies and poultice for boils. Mexican yam is a source of male sex hormone testosterone and is used for rejuvenating effects. The Chinese use the Wild yam to brighten the eyes and as an elixir. North American Herbalists employ its properties for bilious colic and spasm of the bowels. To relieve the nauseous symptoms of pregnancy, Dioscorein is the very best and is prompt in action. Given in small, frequent doses during and until the wife is a mother.

J. Kloss, in "Back to Eden:" "Combined with Ginger (Tussilago farfara) will greatly help to prevent miscarriage." Can be combined with Squaw vine (Mitchella repens) and Raspberry leaves (Rubus strigosus) for the above mentioned—given every ½ hr. or a mouthful of the tea as needed throughout the day.

Herbalists of the past and present combine the root in many formulas for a variety of ailments. It stimulates the removal of accumulated wastes and congestions in the system, relieving pain and joint stiffness. "Natures Healing Agent," by C. Clymer, recommends the following:

> Tincture of Burdock root (Arctium lappa), 10–40 drops.
> Tincture of Black cohosh (Cimicifuga racemosa), 2–15 drops
> Tincture of Motherwort (Lonurus cardiaca), 10–20 drops
> Tincture of Rheumatism root (Dioscorea villosa), 20–40 drops

in water three or four times a day.

In large doses Wild yam is regarded as diuretic and to act as an expectorant. For this, it is always best to combine with other material of a similarly excellent character. Valued in hepatic congestion and rheumatic pains.

Dose: Of the decoction, 2–4 oz.; of the tincture, 20–60 drops; dioscorein, 1–4 grains.

Homoeopathic Clinical: Tincture of fresh root, or trituration of resinoid, dioscorein—Abdomen (distended), Acne, Angina pectoris, Biliousness, Cholerine, Chorea, Colds, Colic, Constipation, Cough, Cramps, Diarrhoea, Dysentery, Dysmenorrhoea, Dyspepsia, Enteralgia, Flatulence, Gall-bladder (affection of), Gastralgia, Haemorrhoids, Headache, Knee (pain in), Legs (pain in), Liver (disorders of), Lumbago, Mind (affection of), Neuralgia, Paronychia, Parotitis, Pregnancy (pyrosis of), Renal colic, Rheumatism, Sciatica, Side (pain in), Spinal irritation, Spleen (pain in), Smell (disordered), Spermatorrhoea, Tea (effect of), Toothache, Whitlow.

WILLOW, BLACK, AMERICAN   Salix nigra, Marsh.
(N.O.: Salicaceae)

Common Names: BLACK WILLOW, PUSSYWILLOW, CATKIN WILLOW.

Features: Willow, of the family Salicaceae and genus Salix, has many trees and shrubs; 300 species vary from less than 1 in. in height to trees of 100 ft. or more, depending on local and climatic conditions. In North America we can claim over 100 of the species variety. Largest of the Willows of eastern North America is the Black willow S. Nigra. It has dark-brown, ridged bark, reddish to orange twigs, and long, narrow leaves that are taper-pointed. The flowers are in elongated clusters,

302

aments or catkins, of two different types; however, in rare instances, the flowers are bisexual. The "precocious" catkins are ornamental, and among flowering plants Willow is ancient, fossils extending back to the Cretaceous.

Medicinal Part: The bark.

Solvent: Boiling water.

Bodily Influence: Aphrodisiac, Tonic, Astringent, Detergent, Antiperiodic.

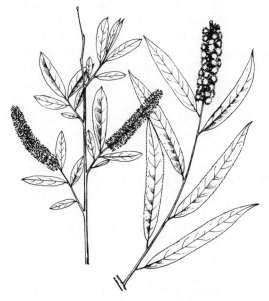

WILLOW, BLACK, AMERICAN   Salix nigra, Marsh.
(U.S. Agricultural Department, Appalachia, 1971)

Uses: Willow is very similar in action to quinine; the active principle is Salicin and is believed to be far more valuable for ague and low grades of fever. These salicylic acids are found in a number of herbal remedies used throughout the world, some dating as far back as the Stone Age. We cannot trace the discovery of how the Willow first became known to the American Indians, we can only tell you that when they were in need of a fever-reducing agent Willow bark tea was given.

In 1763 the Rev. Edward Stone applied an old-fashioned theory. Three things were obvious—low, marshy regions; rheumatism; Willow trees. He tried a decoction of Willow bark on sufferers of rheumatic complaints and thus rediscovered the effectiveness of salicylic acid (Salix is Latin for Willow). It wasn't long before experimentally inclined chemists began synthesizing this substance from common coal tar and petroleum derivatives, according to a standard recipe given in many

303

elementary chemistry text books. Today it is known as common aspirin. The amount swallowed to date in the U.S.A. is approaching an annual 35 million lb., or five tablets a week for every man, woman and child. The contents of modern aspirin is from man's integrity rather than from God's goodness. Is highly recommended and largely used in the treatment of spermatorrhoea, nocturnal emissions, etc. Also relieves ovarian pain.

Dose: Combine 3 grains Willow (S. nigra) and $\frac{1}{2}$ grain Capsicum (Cayenne) when there is great prostration. Add $\frac{1}{2}$ grain Golden seal (Hydrastis canadensis) when the heart as well as the nervous system needs sustaining. To be given in gelatin capsule three times daily before meals. Of the infusion, 1 oz. of bark to 1 pint of boiling water, steeped 15 min., taken in wineglassful amounts three or four times daily.

Externally: A poultice made by simmering the powdered bark in cream is most effective in gangrene and indolent ulcers, etc.

Homoeopathic Clinical: Tincture of fresh bark—Diarrhoea, Emissions, Fever, Gonorrhoea, Impotence, Masturbation, Night sweat, Nymphomania, Prostatitis, Satyriasis, Spermatorrhoea.

Russian Experience: There are several kinds of Willow in Russia, Eva, Salix alba, S. capra, S. fragilis and others. The Willow, especially Weeping willow, so artistically portrayed in melancholy expressions of poetry and music, is extremely popular in parks and private gardens.

Folk Medicine: No preference is shown as to the species used for medical purposes. A decoction is prepared for fevers, rheumatism, worms and to stop bleeding (Bello-Russ. Academy of Science, Minsk, 1965).

Commercially: The Willow is not capricious as to soil conditions and is used to control eroding soil, as it is fast growing (Moscow University, Moscow, 1963). The wood is used in many farm implements and household items. The bark is used in the leather tanning industry.

WINTERGREEN   Gaultheria procumbens, L.
(N.O.: Ericaceae)

Common Names: TEABERRY, BOXBERRY, CHICKERBERRY.

Features: Wintergreen is a name applied to several plants of the family Ericaceae which retain their foliage during winter. In eastern North America the aromatic little Gaultheria procumbens is the one most often referred to. This low-growing barley, 6 in. high, has glossy, leathery, broad leaves with creeping stems from which arise erect reddish branches. They bear solitary white flowers, usually below the leaves, followed by the rather generous fruit, considering the size of the plant, which has enclosed the seed capsules and assumed the form of a

304

bright scarlet, edible, mealy and spicy berry. The whole plant is pungent in taste the spiciness being due to the volatile oil. Collection is somewhat difficult in its scattered wild state. Cultivation requires specially constructed shade such as Golden seal and Ginseng. Wild plants may be used for propagation; divisions of these may be set in the autumn or spring, about 6 in. apart each way in permanent beds. The soil, which should be thoroughly mixed with a 4-in. depth of leaf mould, will give a fairly good growth. Collection is usually at the end of the growth season, around October.

Medicinal Part: The whole plant.

Solvent: Water.

Bodily Influence: Astringent, Stimulant, Anodyne.

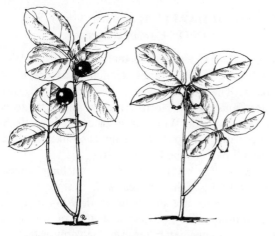

WINTERGREEN   Gaultheria procumbens, L.
(U.S. Agricultural Department, Appalachia, 1971)

Uses: Distilled Wintergreen oil is chiefly used for flavouring confectionery or pharmaceutical preparations. Our Indians employed the plant for rheumatic conditions, internally and externally. Compared to the size of Willow (Salix nigra) or Birch (Betula lenta), Wintergreen is a very small plant, but they all have a common agent, salicylate, which is most useful in relieving pains of rheumatism and as a stimulating nervine. May be employed in diarrhoea and as an infant's carminative. Adjust does according to age.

Dose: 1 teaspoonful of the plant, cut small or granulated, to 1 cupful of boiling water; drink 1 cupful, cold or hot, during the day, a large mouthful at a time. Of the tincture, 5–20 min. Too large an amount can cause vomiting.

Externally: Oil of Wintergreen may be added to the bath or steam cabinet. The fresh or dried herb put into a white cotton bag and

305

simmered in a large vessel, adding liquid and container bag to the bath water, is effective for joint pains and swellings. Do not immerse the whole body, just waist high; if the shoulders and neck have the same condition, squeeze the simmered bag over this area. If you feel drowsy, too relaxed or have heart palpitations, get out. Continue once or twice a week for thirty times consecutively. Other suitable herbs can also be used and combined in this type of bath. It is wise to drink a herbal diuretic tea mixture during this period so that the uric acid, or deposits, will not re-locate.

Homoeopathic Clinical: Tincture of fresh leaves—Gastritis, Neuralgia, Pleurodynia, Rheumatism, Sciatica.

WITCH HAZEL   Hamamelis virginica, L.
(N.O.: Hamamelidaceae)

Common Names: SPOTTED ALDER, SNAPPING HAZEL NUT, WINTER BLOOM.

Features: Witch hazel is of the family Hamamelidaceae, or of the extract of H. virginiana. The genus includes five species, of which two are native to eastern and central North America and three to eastern Asia. H. virginiana, the common Witch hazel of eastern North America, is a shrub or small tree found growing in bunches like the Alder in damp woods in nearly all parts of the United States.

In appearance it has several crooked branching stems, 2–6 in. in diameter and 10–12 ft. high, covered with a smooth grey bark, with brown spots. The leaves are alternate, oval, wavy-margined and turn yellow in the autumn. They possess a degree of fragrance and when chewed are at first somewhat bitter, very sensibly astringent, and then leave a pungent sweetish taste which remains for a considerable time. Its flowers have four yellow, strap-shaped petals, four fertile stamens and four staminoid, blooming mostly in November and December after the leaves have fallen off. The fruit, ripening the next autumn, is a nut-like capsule or pod. Witch hazel is unusual, especially among trees and shrubs, in its time of flowering. Twigs and crotches of H. virginiana have been used as divining rods.

Medicinal Parts: Bark and leaves.

Solvent: Boiling water.

Bodily Influence: Astringent, Tonic, Sedative.

Uses: Another medicinal tree used by the Indians for various irritations and is still best known as a non-alcoholic preparation. To check internal bleeding it is among the best, especially for excessive menstruation, haemorrhages from the lung, stomach, uterus, bowels, etc. There is hardly an inflamed condition, internally or externally, that does not respond to the properties of this product. It is useful for weakening and pain of diarrhoea, dysentery, excessive mucus, and is seldom surpassed for haemorrhoids. If bleeding, inject $\frac{1}{2}$ oz. solution into the rectum and retain as long as possible; repeat after every bloody discharge. Make the ointment from the boiled leaves, bark and coconut oil; chill and make into suppostories. Can be used also as enema in diarrhoea, dysentery, leucorrhoea, simple vaginitis and falling of the womb. Has been valued in incipient tuberculosis and painful tumours. A mouth wash is useful for bleeding gums and inflamed conditions of the mouth and throat; also as a cotton application for inflamed eyes. The leaves, twigs and bark may be made into an infusion and are stronger than the distilled extract.

Dose: Simmer 10 min. 1 oz. of the leaves or bark to 1 pint of water. Take in wineglassful doses three or four times daily. Of the tincture, 5–20 drops. Children according to age.

Externally: The Indians used Witch hazel in poultice form for all external irritations of broken or unbroken skin conditions. Has been mixed with flax seed for inflamed swelling and tumours of a painful character. For varicose veins an extract of the fresh leaves and young twigs of Witch hazel is applied on a loosely woven white cotton cloth and kept constantly moist, for relief and to arouse circulation.

Homoeopathic Clinical: Tincture of fresh bark of twigs and root (A resinoid, Hamamelin, is also prepared)—Abortion (threatened), Ankles (weak), Black eye, Bruises, Burns, Cancer, Chilblains, Constipation, Enteric fever, Gastric ulcer, Haematemesis, Haematuria, Haemorrhages, Haemorrhagic diathesis, Haemorrhoids, Leucorrhoea, Menstruation (disorders of; vicarious), Nipples (sore), Noises in the head, Nose (bleeding from), Ovaries (affections of), Pelvic haematocele, Phimosis, Phlegmasea alba dolens, Purpura, Rheumatism, Scapula (rheumatism of), Scurvy, Smallpox, Testicles (inflamed), Ulcers, Uterus (affections of), Vagina (spasm of), Varicocele, Veins (varicose), Wounds.

Russian Experience: In Russian literature close attention is given to Witch hazel; they use the same Latin name with a Russian accent. Witch hazel does not grow wild in their country. Hamamelis virginica, native of North America, and Japanica, of Japan, is cultivated commercially.

Folk Medicine: Is not indicated.

Clinically: Extracts used in unwanted, excessive, bleeding; bleeding haemorrhoids; and other similar cases (Atlas, Moscow, 1963).

307

WORMSEED Chenopodium anthelminticum, A. Gray.
(N.O.: Chenopodiaceae)

Common Names: AMERICAN WORMSEED, JERUSALEM OAK, CHENO-
PODIUM, MEXICAN TEA.

Features: Wormseed is the common name given to various plants and
their derivatives. American Wormseed, C. anthelminticum, also known
as C. ambrosioides, is in the goosefoot family chenopodiaceae, which is
a native of the American tropics but has widely escaped to waste places
in almost all parts of the United States (cultivated in Maryland).

The plant grows 2–4 ft. high and has yellowish-green flowers, which
are oval and gland-dotted on the underside; they flower from July to
September. The glossy black seeds ripen in the autumn, at which time
they should be collected. The whole plant and seeds are distinguished by
a peculiar disagreeable smell. The oil is the best form of administration.

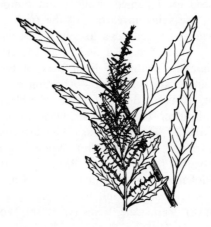

WORMSEED Chenopodium anthelminticum, A. Gray; Chenopodium
ambrosioides, L.
(U.S. Agricultural Department, Appalachia, 1971)

Medicinal Parts: Seeds and top.
Solvents: Distilling with water or super-heated steam; alcohol, 70%
proof.
Bodily Influence: Anthelmintic, Antispasmodic.
Uses: Chiefly used to expel intestinal worms, the cause of many mis-
treated symptoms. The infusion of the plant is often employed to
promote menstruation, and to overcome uterine colic and cases of
hysteria, if used in small amounts daily.
Dose: Of the oil, 4–20 drops with honey, or molasses, for children

according to age. The infusion of the tops and pulverized seeds, 1 teaspoonful to 1 cupful of boiling water; steep 15 min. administer in wineglassful amounts. To expel worms with more success plan to give the above during a full moon, as the tenants are more active at this time. Omit the evening meal, give the prescribed dose and again in the morning before breakfast, followed by a herbal cathartic; repeat for three days to make sure the larva is expelled.

Homoeopathic Clinical: Tincture of fresh plant; solution of oil seed— Aphasia, Apoplexy, Asthma, Cerebral deafness, Convulsions, Dropsy, Epilepsy, Headache, Hemicrania, Hemiplegia, Leucorrhoea, Menses (suppressed), Paralysis, Scapula (pain in), Tinnitus, Tonsilitis.

Russian Experience: Two kinds of Mar (Wormseed), Chenopodium anthelminticum and Chenopodium ambrosioides, are cultivated. Russian literature objectively clings to the properties of healing as well as a prophylactic agent for several types of worms. There is no indication of it being used as Folk Medicine from personal available books.

Clinical: Chenopodium oil is used for worms; ascaridiasis, ankylostoma (hook worms) and others. For children the oil is prepared with castor oil (laxative) and given occasionally in small doses; it has no side effect in this amount. Usually after expelling the worms most persons are relieved of the sometimes visible worm eggs and larvae as well. They do warn that an overdose can cause headache, vomiting, stomach pain, dizziness, etc. May also affect the liver, kidney, bladder, blood pressure, breathing.

Commercially: Russian Agro-Technic literature instructions may get you off to a faster start. Since the seeds are slow growing (14–16 days) they mix them with seeds of some fast-growing plant like lettuce, about 15–20 lb. per acre. Wormseed harvest is from $\frac{1}{2}$–1 ton per acre. For industrial oil extraction, cutting machines are set to harvest the plant just to the lower stem, which does not have leaves. This is done when the plant becomes brownish and seeds are mostly ripened, which is the maximum content for volatile oil, Chenopodium and Ascaridol. Seed harvest alone is by a selected method.

WORMWOOD Artemisia absinthium, L.
(N.O.: Compositae)

Common Names: ABSINTH, AJENJO, OLD WOMEN.

Features: Wormwood is native to Eurasia and has been introduced into North America, where it occurs as a casual weed in waste places in the northern United States and southern Canada. Michigan, Wisconsin and Oregon grow this herb commercially. There are various other species of Artemisia, Common wormwood, Sea wormwood and Roman wormwood, similar in appearance but different in properties. A. absinthium, of the compositae family, is a perennial, commonly 2–4 ft. tall, with clustered stems and silvery-grey herbage. The leaf blades are up to about 4 in. long and are divided into numerous blunt or rounded small segments, the basal leaves being long-stalked and larger than those of the stem. The numerous flower heads, which are scattered along branches that have reduced leaves, are small, yellowish and individually

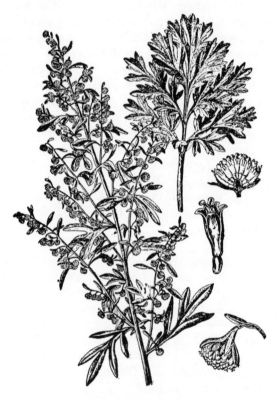

WORMWOOD   Artemisia absinthium, L.
1—Flower head;   2—Flower head vertical section;   3—Single flower
(Vishaya Schkolla, Moscow, 1963)

rather inconspicuous, being hardly $\frac{1}{4}$ in. wide, flowering from June to September. Odour aromatic; taste very bitter. It yields what is known to druggists as absinthine.

Medicinal Parts: The tops and leaves.

Solvents: Diluted alcohol, water (partially).

Bodily Influence: Tonic, Stomachic, Stimulant, Febrifuge, Anthelmintic, Narcotic.

310

Uses: Without a doubt Wormwood ranks first for conditions of enfeebled digestion and debility. Often melancholy is due to liver inactivity and it is impious for a good man to be sad. A small amount of Wormwood daily will decrease the yellowness of the skin, revealing the improvement of the gall-bladder.

This herb is used for the following diseases: intermittent fever, jaundice, worms, want of appetite, amenorrhoea, chronic leucorrhoea, diabetes, obstinate diarrhoea, swelling of the tonsils and quinsy. Travellers who are much troubled with indigestion and nausea should never forget to take with them as a faithful companion their little bottle of Wormwood, in tincture form mixed with enough alcohol to ensure that it will last as a travelling companion for a long time. Taken too strong and too often it will irritate the stomach and dangerously increase the action of the heart and arteries.

Dose: 1 teaspoonful of the tops and leaves, cut small or granulated, to 1 cupful of boiling water; take in wineglassful amounts three or four times a day. Of the tincture, 5–30 drops three or four times a day, according to age and condition. Of the powder, 3–4 grains twice a day.

Externally: The oil of Wormwood is an effective ingredient in liniment for sprains, bruises, lumbago, etc. Fomentations from the hot tea is excellent for application to rheumatism, swellings, sprains and local inflammations.

Homoeopathic Clinical: Tincture of fresh root—Catalepsy, Chorea, Convulsions, Epilepsy, Hydrocephalus, Hysteria, Somnambulism, Worms.

Russian Experience: Wormwood, known in Russia as Polin, is considered the most bitter plant in the world; 10,000 parts water to 1 part Wormwood will still have a bitter taste. It used to be thought that the bitter taste of Wormwood was supposedly due to the plant's absorption of bitter human sufferings and dissolution of mankind, therefore its properties would drive sickness from the body and restore peace and calmness to the soul (Similia Similibus Curantur). In the eighteenth century a toast to joy, happiness and pleasure was accompanied by a drop of Wormwood in a cup.

It is written by the most ancient that Wormwood had many healing properties. Today all we can do is to confirm this belief by our scientific, sophisticated ways, and tell you it contains absentine and anabsentin, Vitamin C and Volatile oil. Lonicerius wrote: "The herb, leaves and flowers added to food and beverage is useful for the stomach, promotes bile, warms the body and expels poison."

Folk Medicine use the medicine straight or in compound with Sage, Mint, Sunflower leaves, etc., depending on conditions being treated. Nastoika (with vodka), tea, decoctions for indigestion, appetiser, gastritis, stomach ulcers, dysentery, TB of the lungs, liver and spleen

311

conditions, kidney and bladder, headache, purifying poisoned blood, fever, bleeding etc. Decoction of 1 teaspoonful to 1 cupful of water, steeped and cooled, used as an enema, will kill intestinal worms.

Externally: Many centuries ago Pliny wrote: "If pedestrians keep some Wormwood on his body, especially the feet, he will not be tired." Russians in the seventeenth century used the juice for wounds and foul ulcers. (Vishaya Schkolla, Moscow, 1963). Can be used as compresses and poultices for bruises, injuries or insect bites. Green bruised leaves for corns. Flowers and leaves scattered on the floor and furniture will discourage unwanted house insects (Bello-Russ. Academy of Science, Minsk, 1965).

Clinically: Extract for spasm, bronchial asthma, rheumatism, eczema, burns (X-ray or otherwise) (Atlas, Moscow, 1963).

India and Pakistan: Called Afsantin or Vilayati Afsantin, the plant is used much as in the U.S.A. and Russia. They use the whole herb but prefer the leaves, and consider the fresh plant more effective than the dried. As tonic, aromatic, anthelmintic.

Uses: It is praised highly for round and tape worms; powder, from 10–60 grains. Small doses are used for dispersing the yellow bile of jaundice from the skin, and for liver and spleen conditions. A tonic for the stomach, digestive system, anaemia, female complaints, amenorrhoea, general debility, wasting diseases. A decoction as an enema for intestinal worms, which will kill them instantly. The oil is anthelmintic and they mix it with Olive oil, 1:8 proportion, and give it in 50–100 gram doses.

YARROW   Achillea millefolium, L.
(N.O.: Compositae)

Features: A perennial plant of the composite family (Compositae), Yarrow inhabits Europe and North America. It is found in pastures, meadows and along roadsides, flowering from May to October. Yarrow has a rough angular stem and grows to heights of 3 ft.; the alternate leaves are 1–6 in. long, pinnatified, clasp the stem at the base, are slightly woolly and are cut into very fine segments. The flowers are white (if you are lucky you may find pin Yarrow) borne in flat-top daisy-like clusters up to 1 ft. across. The plant possesses a faint, pleasant, peculiar fragrance, and an ether sharp, rough astringent taste, which properties are due to tannic and achilleic acid, essential oil and bitter extractive achilleic. The genus to which Yarrow belongs was named after Achilles, who supposedly discovered the medicinal virtues of the plant.

Medicinal Part: The herb.

Solvents: Water, alcohol.

Bodily Influence: Astringent, Alterative, Diuretic, Tonic.

Uses: The awareness of Yarrow as a useful agent was known to our Indians as a tonic for run-down conditions and indigestion. Achilles informs us the juice put in the eye will take away redness. Herbalists know that Yarrow, together with Plantain (Plantago lanceolate) and Comfrey (Symphytum), will stop haemorrhages of the lungs, bowels, haemorrhoids and other internal bleeding. Yarrow is most useful in colds, influenza, measles, smallpox, chickenpox, fevers and acute catarrhs of the respiratory tract. The properties have the ability to keep up the strength and act as a blood cleanser, at the same time opening the pores to permit free perspiration, taking along with it unwanted waste and relieving the kidneys; more effective than quinine for the above mentioned when combined with Elder flowers (Sambucus canadensis) and Peppermint (Menth piperita).

Yarrow exercises influence over many ailments, including incontinence of urine and where there are mucus discharges from the bladder. dyspepsia, amenorrhoea, suppressed or restrained menses and in menorrhagia or profuse continued menstruation; as a feminine solution for administration for leucorrhoea (whites) and internal decoction of Yarrow boiled with white wine is used to stop the running of the reins in men and discharge of women. Chewing the leaves when troubled by toothache will frequently ease the pain.

Dose: Infusion of 1 teaspoonful to 1 cupful of boiling water is given in wineglassful to cupful amounts, three or four times a day. The essential oil, from 5–20 drops three or four times a day.

Externally: The Indians used the leaves as a poultice for skin rash. We, too, have found merit for treatment of skin wounds, ulcers and fistulas in an ointment or poultice application; both are soothing for haemorrhoids. The oil or decoction will prevent the hair from falling out, if taken internally and applied to the scalp.

Russian Experience: Tisiachelistnik or Krovavnik means one thousand leaves, or Blood plant. Achillea millefolium, also translated as one thousand leaves in Russia, along with A. asiatica and A. setacea are

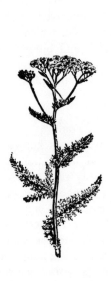

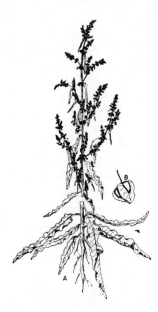

YELLOW DOCK   Rumex crispus, L.
A—Curled dock   B—Fruit
(Ontario Department of Agriculture,
Toronto, Canada, 1966)

YARROW   Achillea millefolium, L.
(Dr. A. J. Thut, Guelph, Canada)

only three of the species of Yarrow to be found there. The leaves, flowers and unseparated tops are usually called Yarrow, as known in North America.

Folk Medicine: Since the fifteenth century Russian Herbalists have used and recommended Yarrow. As tea, decoction, Nastoika (with vodka) for bleeding, stomach sickness, gastritis, ulcers, dysentery, diarrhoea, female bleeding, inflamed processes, cold, cough, liver, anaemia, headache, TB of the lungs, shortness of breath, nervousness, high blood pressure, tabes of spinal marrow.

314

Externally: Decoctions and poultice for surface or subcutaneous skin conditions.

Clinically: Recently recognition has been given to extracts and decoctions for stomach sickness, especially ulcers, and for bleeding and gastritis. Also as an appetiser and externally as styptic (Atlas, Moscow, 1963).

YELLOW DOCK   Rumex crispus, L.
(N.O.: Polygonaceae)

Common Names: CURLED DOCK, NARROW DOCK, SOUR DOCK, RUMEX, GARDEN PATIENCE.

Features: The Docks are members of the buckwheat family, native to Europe, except the blunt-leaved, which is indigenous. However, they have all been introduced into the United States. There are four varieties of Dock which may be used in medicine: the Rumex aquaticus (Great water dock), Rumex britannica (Water dock), Rumex abtusifolius (Blunt-leaved dock), and the Rumex crispus (Yellow dock). They all possess similar medicinal qualities, but the Yellow dock is the only one entitled to extensive consideration. The yellowish spindle-shaped root has scarcely any odour, but has astringent, bitter taste.

It grows 2–3 ft. high with slender, crisped-edged leaves, which are lanceolate, acute and of a light-green colour; the leaves and stalk have a sour taste. The flowers are numerous, pale green, drooping and interspersed with leaves below; can be seen in June and July.

Medicinal Part: The root.

Solvents: Water, alcohol.

Bodily Influence: Alterative, Astringent, Laxative, Antiscorbutic, Tonic.

Uses: A favourite herb of the ancient Indians, old time doctors, early settlers and herbal practitioners. For some conditions it has no equal, especially if compounded with other supporting herbs. The rich and easily digested plant iron is one of the main contents of Yellow dock, so essential for man, animal and plant life. This common herb has valuable ingredients for conditions of the blood and glandular system and is indicated in scrofula, eruptive diseases, especially when discharges are experienced, as in running of the ears, ulcerated eyelids and skin conditions, itch, scurvy, etc.

When accumulation of waste matters progress to swelling or tumours, Yellow dock is of service both internally and externally. Many Herbalists use the mineral-rich plant for cancer, leprosy, bleeding of the lungs and bowels and for rheumatic conditions. It also has much merit in dyspepsia, chronic bronchitis, ulcers and conditions affected by the spleen and lymphatic glands; also for female weakness when due to iron deficiency.

315

Dose: 1 teaspoonful of the grated or crushed root to 1 cupful of boiling water; drink 3–4 cupfuls daily. A syrup may be made by boiling ½ lb. of the crushed root in 1 pint of syrup; taken in teaspoonful doses three or four times a day.

Externally: Ulcers, hard tumours, eruptive skin diseases, etc., have been removed by the application of the bruised root in poultice form. An ointment made with the root simmered in oil (coconut oil will harden when cold and can be used for rectal suppositories) is also used for the above external care.

Homoeopathic Clinical: Tincture of fresh root—Abortion, Aphonia, Asthma, Borborygmi, Bronchitis, Catarrh, Corns, Coryza, Cough, Diarrhoea, Dyspepsia Epistaxis, Feet (tender), Gastralgia, Heart (pain in; affections of), Indigestion, Irritation, Lichen, Mouth (ulceration of), Phimosis, Phthisis, Prurigo, Rheumatism, Throat (sore; ulcerated), Trachea (affections of), Urticaria.

Russian Experience: Several species of Rumex can be found in Russia. In literature most attention is given to Rumex rumicis or Konsky Shavel, which means Horse dock.

Folk Medicine: Use the roots and fruit as astringent to check bleeding of lungs, female, haemorrhoids, bleeding diarrhoea, also for tubercular lungs and skin conditions. In Bello-Russia they use a decoction of the flowers for diarrhoea, dysentery, kidney and bladder, stomach sickness and a decoction of the root for pain after heavy lifting.

Externally: Decoctions used for ulcers, burns and skin diseases. Fresh leaves for foul wounds and ulcers, shingles or itching skin (Bello-Russ. Academy of Science, Minsk, 1966).

YELLOW PARILLA Menispermum canadense, L.
(N.O.: Menispermaceae)

Common Names: VINE-MAPLE, MOONSEED, CANADIAN MOONSEED, TEXAS SARSAPARILLA, YELLOW SARSAPARILLA.

Features: A perennial member of the moonseed family, Yellow parilla grows from Canada to Carolina, and west to the Mississippi. The horizontal, very long woody root, of a beautiful yellow colour, thrives in moist woods, hedges and near streams. The taste is bitter and it is nearly odorousless.

The stem is round and climbing and about 1 ft. in length, with roundish smooth leaves, 4–5 in. in diameter, green above, paler beneath. The small yellow flowers are in clusters in the month of July followed by one seeded fruit which is thick, black and resembles grapes. Its active principle is menispermin, and is sometimes used as a substitute for sarsaparilla.

Medicinal Part: The root.

Solvents: Alcohol, water.

Bodily Influence: Tonic, Alterative, Diuretic, Laxative.

Uses: Dr. O. P. Brown (1875): "Yellow Parilla seems to possess one virtue which is paramount to all others, it is essentially and particular antisyphilitic, anti-scrofulous, anti-mercurial." Achieving this, it is of much merit for all diseases arising from either hereditary or acquired impurities of the system. It exerts its influence principally on the gastric and salivary glands and is found expressly beneficial in cases of adhesive inflammation and where it is found necessary to break up organized deposits and hasten disintegration of unwanted tissue. It is believed by some to be superior to Sarsaparilla as a blood purifier for scrofula, blood disorders, gout, rheumatism and cutaneous skin diseases generally. Also acts as a tonic and nervine and may be given in all cases of debility and dyspepsia.

Dose: 1 teaspoonful to 1 cupful of boiling water, steeped 15 min.; take 1–4 cupfuls a day. Of the tincture, 5–20 min. Of the powder, 1–4 grains. If it produces vomiting, reduce the dosage.

Homoeopathic Clinical: Tincture of the root; trituration of menisperminum—Back ache, Headache, Itching, Tongue (swelling of).

YERBA SANTA   Eriodictyon californicum, Benth.
(N.O.: Hydrophyllaceae)

Common Names: MOUNTAIN BALM, BEAR'S WEED, CONSUMPTIVE'S WEED, TARWEED, GUM BUSH.

Features: This evergreen shrub is a member of the water leaf family (Eriodictyon), of which many species are known. It is somewhat branching and attains a height of 2–4 ft. The stems are smooth and exude a gummy substance. Leaves are 3–4 in. in length, distinctively woolly on the undersides, containing a network of prominent veins, and the resinous substance appears as if the woolly fibres have been varnished; upper surface is smooth with depressed veins. The flowers are terminal, appearing in shades of dark lavender through pale shades of lavender to white; forming funnel-shaped clusters at the top of the plant. Yerba santa honey is amber, with a slightly spicy flavour. If we follow the bees to this plant we will find them growing on dry mountain slopes and ridges throughout the coastal ranges and up into the foothills of the Sierra Nevada from Monterey and Tulare countries northward. The capsule fruit is oval, greyish-brown and contains small brown shrivelled seeds.

Medicinal Part: The leaves.

Solvents: Boiling water, alcohol.

Bodily Influence: Aromatic, Tonic, Stimulant, Expectorant.

Uses: The name "Yerba santa" (Holy weed) was given by the Spanish fathers who became aware of this corrective substance through the native Indians. They boiled the fresh or dried leaves for colds, coughs, sore throat, catarrh, stomach aches, vomiting and diarrhoea. Yerba santa is known to physicians as a leading agent for all respiratory conditions and has a reputation for healing haemorrhoids when other sources fail. Also used in kidney conditions and rheumatic pain. For more effective results some physicians recommend that Gum plant (Grindelia robusta) be combined with Yerba santa in syrup form. It should be used in small amounts as too large doses of G. robusta will irritate the kidneys. Make a 3:1 mixture and take in fluid extract, 10–30 drops, three or four times a day.

Dose: Infusion of 1 teaspoonful of crushed leaves to 1 cupful of boiling water, steeped $\frac{1}{2}$ hr. Take 1–4 cupfuls daily. Of the solid extract, 3–6 grains. Fluid extract, $\frac{1}{2}$–1 teaspoonful three to four times daily.

Externally: The Indians used the fresh or dried leaves as a poultice for broken and unbroken skin of both man and animal when in pain from rheumatism, fatigued limbs, swelling, sores, etc.

Homoeopathic Clinical: Tincture of whole plant—Asthma, Bronchitis, Catarrh, Influenza, Phthisis.

BIBLIOGRAPHY

GENERAL AND REFERENCE PUBLICATIONS

ANDREWS, RALPH W., **Curtis' Western Indians** (Life and works of Edward S. Curtis). Size 8½ × 10½ in., 176 pp., Index. Library of Congress Catalog Card Number 62–14491. Publisher: Bonanza Books, New York, N.Y., U.S.A. 1962.

Contains 199 black and white photographs taken with accuracy and a true-to-fact love of work about the vanishing Indian race. His profession and interest has seen him through conditions similar to those which our own race passed so many ages ago so that not a vestige of its natural pride and nobility remains.

ANDREWS, RALPH W., **Indian Primitive**. Size 8½ × 10 in., 175 pp., Bibliography, Index. Library of Congress Catalog Card Number 60–14425. Publisher: Bonanza Books, subsidiary of Crown Publishers, Inc., New York, N.Y., U.S.A. 1960.

The author is best known for his photo-histories of the West Coast. This book is a collection of 193 black and white photographs of Indian life as seen by Edward S. Curtis and some from the collections of the early white man. Contains information about the culture of the north-west coast Indians in Alaska, Canada and U.S.A.: totem carving, sea hunting, slave trading, ceremonial dancing, etc. Modern literature presents the American Indian as a weak, sick, miserable part of our society. As a contrast, all pre-Columbus American material and evidence portray the Indians as a very strong, handsome, alert, dignified and, as a rule, exceptionally friendly and hospitable people. From this point, it is very interesting to read historical and ethnographical works on Indian life and habits. We know of no special books on Indian medicine, but some travellers and missionaries give information about their health and sickness and how it was treated.

BENDER, GEORGE A., painted by ROBERT A. THOM., **Great Moments in Medicine: A History of Medicine in Pictures**. Size 9 × 7 in., 277 pp., original paintings illustrated in colour, Bibliography, 196 books and monographs. Publisher: Parke Davis, Detroit, Michigan, U.S.A. 1961.

A most original history of medicine in colour pictures of artistic documentary information. Several chapters devoted to Indian medicine, which is the best opportunity to comparatively study medical history.

319

Over 100 years of experience and a history devoted to research, especially herbal medicine in the American continent, has kept the Parke Davis Co. spirit young and strong. Being an industrial and commercial concern their service is widely available to the public through research and pictorial review. Book has great national success, sold by leading book dealers and department stores.

BOGORAD, B. B., NECHLUDOVA, A. C., **Dictionary of Biological Terms**. 236 pp. Published by the Ministry of Education, Moscow, U.S.S.R. 1963.

Highly recommended for reference.

CARLSON, RACHEL, **Silent Spring**. Size $8\frac{1}{2} \times 6$ in., 368 pp., Index, Index of principle source. Library of Congress Catalog Card Number 60–5148. The Riverside Press, Cambridge, Massachusetts, U.S.A. 1962.

Our hearts should overflow with thankfulness to Rachel Carlson, Biologist. The truth about destruction through supposedly controlled chemical insecticides is re-evaluated, revealing the frightening loss of every environmental surrounding, including human life. The contents are a disturbing backlash of our ingeniousness.

DE-VRIES, ARNOLD, **Primitive Man and his Food**. Size 9×6 in., 151 pp., Bibliography, Index. Chandler Book Co., Chicago, U.S.A. 1952.

Interesting collection of material about the food and health of primitive man around the world. First chapter devoted to American Indians, very informative. Interesting to Herbalists as comparative material on health and food. Unknown to most libraries but some health food and book stores carry publications. Effort to find will be rewarded.

DUELL, SLOAN, PEARCE, **The New World**. Edited and annotated by STEFAN LORANT. Size 9×12 in., Bibliography, Index. Publisher: Beck Engraving Co., Inc., Philadelphia, Pennsylvania, U.S.A. First revised edition, 1965.

The attempt of the French and English to settle in North America seventy years after Columbus, 1562–90, p. 292. Vivid portrayal of 161 sketches, water colours, engravings, some in colour, of the French and English artists of the time. Acquaint your thoughts to how man's existence in every way came from one source, nature as it exists. Many words are spoken from the pictures alone.

HICKERSON, HAROLD, **The Chippewa and Their Neighbour: A study in Ethnohistory**. Size 6×9 in., 133 pp., some illustrations and sketches. Publishers: Holt, Rinehart and Winston, Inc., New York., N.Y., U.S.A. 1970.

There are many new studies on American Indian problems. This book will be of general interest for the student of Herbalogy.

JOSEPHY, ALVIN M. (Editor-in-charge), **The American Heritage Book of**

Indians. Narrative by WILLIAM BRANDO; Introduction by JOHN F. KENNEDY, U.S. President, 1961–3. Size 11½ × 8¾ in., 424 pp., Index, price $15. Almost 500 pictures, more than 100 reproduced in full colour, from public and private collections throughout the world. Publisher: American Heritage Publishing Co., Inc. 1961.

For too many people the story of the Indian has long been distorted and fragmented, a hodge-podge of names and tribes that begins in 1492 and ends with the era of television westerns. But for more than 20,000 years Indians were the sole inhabitants of the New World "Garden of Eden" of the Western Hemisphere. J. F. Kennedy stated: "American Indians defy any single description, they were and are far too individualistic. They shared no common language and few common customs." The book covers the period from the time before the earliest white man entered the New World to the present day. The study of numerous Indian dwelling places and the climate and conditions under which the different tribes lived reveals how varied the supply of natural resources were, yet in each location they survived because of their knowledge of plant and animal needs.

LAFARGE, OLIVER, **A Pictorial History of the American Indian**. Size 9½ × 12½ in., 350 illustrations (some colour plates), Bibliography. Library of Congress Catalog Card Number 56–11375. Crown Publishers, Inc., New York, N.Y., U.S.A. 1956.

An inspiring account of the many different Indians and their varied dwelling-places in mountains, deserts, plains and sea shore. Includes details of food, medicine, religion, ceremonies, crafts, war, etc.

HERBALOGY

ALLSHORN, GEORGE EDWARD, M.D., **Domestic Homoeopathic Practice**. Edited by ADOLF HAHNEMANN ALLSHORN, M.D. XVI & 208 pp. Publisher: Houlston and Write, London, England. Fourth Edition, 1871.

A book written as a result of the life' work of the author as a prominent physician. Material on herbal use is exceptional and is still in use after 100 years. A collector's item, but of practical use to practitioners and students. Very concentrated, small book. Not available.

Aquatic Plant and Algae Control. Size 9 × 6 in., 20 pp., illustrations. Publisher: Ontario Water Resources Commission, Toronto, Ontario, Canada. No date.

Many little books and brochures are compiled and published by the Canadian and U.S. Governments, Provincial, State and Federal. It is easy to obtain their very useful material for research and study. There is practically nothing on Herbalism, but as a source of botany and flora they are very reliable.

BAILEY, L. H., **How Plants get their Names**. Size $8\frac{1}{2}$ × $5\frac{1}{2}$ in., 181 pp., Some illustrations. Publisher: Dover Publications, Inc., New York, N.Y., U.S.A. 1965.

After thirty years the book was reprinted and would be very useful to beginners as a reference book. Many pages can be read with great interest, dealing with the plants and the history of their names. As the original Latin or medical names are rather confusing, the book will be helpful to Herbalists and as a general reference source.

BALLS, EDWARD K., **Early use of California Plants**. Size $7\frac{1}{2}$ × $4\frac{1}{2}$ in., illustrated beautifully in colour and black and white, Bibliography, Index, Price $1.50. Publisher: University of California Press, Los Angeles, California, U.S.A. 1962.

The University of California has published many small but original facts on California's · natural history. Herbalists will find this book useful, as mention is made of 163 plants used by the Californian Indians for medicine, food, clothing, etc. Difficult to get the book outside of California, but possession of the work would be rewarding. Not usually in libraries.

BARKER, EILLIS J., **New Lives for Old**. How to cure the incurable, with Introduction by Sir Herbert Barker, 357 pp. The Homoeopathic Publishing Co. Ltd., London. Second Edition, 1949.

E. J. Barker is editor of the "Homoeopathic World", and author of many well-known books on homoeopathy. "New Lives for Old" 'is rich in material, theoretical and practical in character.

BENJAMIN, HARRY, **Unorthodox Healing Versus Medical Science**. Size $7\frac{1}{2}$ × 5 in., 192 pp. Publisher: Health for All Publishing Co., London, England. 1951.

This is a theoretical work on natural treatments, Herbalism included. Valuable as an introductory book to compare the stature of herbalogy in general medical science.

BERNARD, RAYMOND, **Herbal Elixir of Life**. Size 11 × $8\frac{1}{2}$ in., 29 pp. Publisher: Health Research, Mokelumne Hill, California, U.S.A. 1959.

This company reprints many rare and old books, either by photostatic or mimeographic methods. This is a compilation from various well-known authors on the subject of "Mystery Herbs of the Far East, believed by Orientals to rejuvenate and prolong life". Not in libraries, only private mailing, as limited numbers are printed.

BROWN, PHELPS O., DR., **The Complete Herbalist**. Size $7\frac{1}{2}$ × 5 in. 502 pp., Illustrations, General Index, Herbal, Petit type, Price $2. Published by author, Jersey City, N.Y. 1875.

Many publications of a "one book author' are scattered through-

322

out the country. This one has the sub-title "The people their own Physician, the great curative properties found in the herbal kingdom". The Author was a medical doctor and for many years practised as taught professionally. After grievous defeat he became a self-trained Herbalist. The book is about his professional experience. The first part is theoretical, with his own conceptions and philosophy, and could be of interest to students and researchers. The second part describes herbs and their properties, then sickness and treatment. In international literature it is rare to find the well-trained doctor employing the natural treatment of herbs. They have the most categorical and convincing arguments supported by their fifty to sixty years of medical practice. A hundred years have almost passed since "The Complete Herbalist" was published. Originally priced at $2, on today's market it would be very much more. Collector's item.

BRYANT, GEORGE, **Gathering Medicinal Berries**. Size 11 × 8½ in., 4pp. R. R., 2 Lawrenceburg, Kentucky, U.S.A. 1957.

This is a mimeographic pamphlet. Editorials give valuable information on how to gather, how to sell, and addresses of the buyers, etc. Publishers of the American book market print fancy items in colour about flowers and scientific botany books, but nothing on Herbalogy. The authors of such information are in the "do it yourself" category.

BUDD, ARCHIBALD C., BEST, KEITH F., **Wild Plants of the Canadian Prairies**. Size 10 × 16½ in., 519 pp., Illustrations, Index, price $3. Published by Research Branch, Canada Department of Agriculture, Ottawa. 1964.

Of all the books published by the Canadian Government, this is one of the best. Actually it belongs to a "one book writer", Archibald Charles Budd (1889–1960). Without formal training, but a devoted Botanist, A. C. Budd created a work that will live for generations. About 1,200 species of plants are described. Excellent, full-page drawings in black and white. Very detailed cross index. There is nothing on the medicinal properties of plant life, only practical information for reference and study. Can be obtained directly or for use in libraries.

CHOPRA, R. N., NAYAR, S. L., CHOPRA, I. C., **Glossary of Indian Medicinal Plants**. Size 10 × 6½ in., XX & 328 pp. Published by Council of Scientific & Industrial Research, New Delhi, India. 1956.

The book is very good in many respects if the common names and uses can be translated into English. The work consists of articles of a rather technical nature, which appeared in 357 magazines and periodicals in Germany, England, China, France, Belgium, Japan, the Philippines, Italy, America and Canada. Included is a Latin alphabet with Indian common names. There is indicated properties of the plant with reference to the sources; Index of 130 pp.; Common Vernacular names (pp. 263–318) which gives over 7,200 local names; Editorial; and Index of Chemical Constituents (pp. 319–30). Of the few Indian medical botanics on hand this is possibly the most condensed material.

CLARKE, JOHN HENERY, M.D., **A Dictionary of Practical Materia Medica.** In three volumes. Size 9 × 6 in. Volume I: Abies canadensis, Hypericum, XVI & 951; Volumes II & III; Ibers, Zizia, XII & 1,635 through 1,900. Publisher: Health Science Press, Rustington, Sussex, England. 1962.

First edition took over thirty years of practice and fortitude. Highly specialized, but excellent book for daily use and to study. One of the classic books on Homoeopathy, it gives the most wide and reliable knowledge on their use of medicine in general and on medical botanics in particular. Many Indian herbal remedies incorporated as official medicine. In the text of our work we followed "Clarke's Dictionary", but only as a general guide for certain herbs, so professional practitioners can make a study of Clarke's work for details of symptoms and use. Homoeopaths cannot name anything of more service than this work; four generations have already gained from this type of specialization.

COLBY, BENJAMIN, **Guide to Health, Thomsonian System of Practice.** Size 7 × 4½ in., VIII & 181 pp., Petit type, very compact pages. Published by Health Research, Mokelumne Hills, California, U.S.A. 1965.

Samuel Thomson (1767–1839) was one of America's pioneers in the subject of Herbalogy. His gift of nature and Indian folk medicine by far surpassed his formal education. Self-determination under criticism, prosecution and many handicaps did not alter his ability and faith in his work. Again and again his name received credit as a wonderful healer. In his lifetime more than 2,000,000 people were unquestionably saved, or had their life prolonged, due to his methods. His original works are not often found. Libraries and encyclopaedias do not mention the Thomsonian system among the numerous Thomson names of less prominence. In his lifetime he was able to put into practice some rather strong, but accepted, theories which became known as the Thomsonian System. Samuel Thomson gave much to the practice of treatment through Herbalogy. Present-day medicine is indebted to him for the introduction of Lobelia, Golden seal, and others, herbs which for centuries were used by the North American Indians. Students and practitioners may not agree completely, but it is one of the products of North America that you cannot bypass.

This book may be a decisive factor in your way of thinking as you learn from his followers. The total title is rather lengthy, "Guide to Health" being the exposition of the principle of the Thomsonian system and its mode of application in the cure of every form of disease. First published in 1845 with the third edition appearing in 1846. Latest on hand to the author is a reprint from 1965. Because the book was unobtainable for so many years the reprint was done at the request of the public.

CULBRETH, DAVID M. R., PH.G., M.D., **A Manual of Materia Medica and Pharmacology.** VII & 627 pp. and 32 pp. of Index not marked. Publisher: Lea & Febiger, Philadelphia, U.S.A. Seventh edition, thoroughly revised, 1927.

Pharmacopoeia comprising the organic drugs which are or have been recognized by the United States Pharmacopoeia and National Formulary together with important allied species. Especially designed for doctors, druggists, pharmacists and physicians. Contains 497 illustrations. Difficult to get, but very informative and useful to all concerned with medical practice. Rather technical for the beginner, but excellent for reference. Many Indian Materia Medica included as accepted in official Pharmacopoeia. Beautiful illustrations, now fading laborious gravures.

Culpeper's Complete Herbal. Size $7\frac{1}{2} \times 5$ in., XII & 430 pp., illustrations in colour, Index of Diseases and Herbs that cure, Petit type, very compact pages. Publisher: W. Foulsham and Co., London (England), New York (U.S.A.), Toronto (Canada), Sydney (Australia) and Cape Town (South Africa).

There are descriptions of 398 herbs, which includes plants of North America as they were adopted in Anglo-American medical practice. Full title, "Culpeper's Complete Herbal", consisting of comprehensive descriptions of nearly all herbs with their medical properties and directions for compounding the medicines extracted from them. The history of the popular herbs as medicine are not so many that mankind has forgotten them in centuries and millenniums.

Nicholas Culpeper (1616–54) lived only 38 years, but left to us a name and practice which has lasted for over 300 years. Many original manuscripts on astrology and herbalism are treasures mankind has enjoyed and profited by from his short but impressive works. What Culpeper's popularity represents in terms of dollars no one can estimate today. Due to public demand the book is in libraries, and its sales in leading department stores tops that of many of the so-called best sellers. It has a steady, unseasonable, unpromoted demand.

DANA, W. S., MRS. Illustrated by MARION SATTERLEE, **How to know The Wild Flowers.** Size $8\frac{1}{2} \times 5\frac{1}{2}$ in., XLI & 418 pp., Illustrations in black and white graphics. Publisher: Dover Publications, Inc., New York, N.Y., U.S.A. 1962.

This book was written by Mrs. William Starr Dana and dedicated to the same person. First published in 1895, it was later revised by

325

Clarence J. Hylander. One of the best illustrated books as a guide to the names, haunts and habits of our common wild flowers. The botanical descriptions that are useful for students working in the field, and it contains excellent graphical drawings. Easily available, as it is published in both London, England, and the U.S.A. Today (1973) it is seventy-eight years old, comparatively young for a herbal book as most are of service and going strong after 300–400 years of use.

DASTUR, J. F., **F. N. I. Medical Plants of India and Pakistan.** Size 7½ × 5 in. Publisher: Taraporevala Sons and Co., Bombay, India. 1962.

A compact book with detailed and very valuable information on Indian and Pakistan Herbalogy. Contains description and details of use of 249 plants. Wide use of herbs, leaves, seeds, roots, teas, powder, extract and compound is expressed by many centuries of experience. In North America the book is very rare, not being available in libraries at present. Not available in India. Contains a classification of plants according to their medical properties and use and a glossary of some technical terms used in the text. Also a very valuable bibliography listing sixty-four publications in English, thirteen of which were published between 1826 and 1900 and fifty-one between 1901 and 1950; also nineteen additional periodicals in English giving latest information.

DOOLE, LOUISE EVANS, **Herbs and Garden Ideas.** Size 8 × 5½ in., 128 pp., Index, black and white illustrations by Shizu Matsuda and Deitra Carpenter, price $2.95. Publisher: Sterling Publishing Co., Inc., New York, N.Y., U.S.A. 1964

Sterling Publishers have several books about Herbalism on the market, including reprints of "Culpeper's Complete Herbal". This book will appeal especially to the very young, for stimulating interest of immediate and future ideas. Easily available in leading department stores if not in the libraries.

FERRANDEZ, Dr. V. L., **Guia de Medicina Vegetal.** 6 × 9 in., 399 pp., Illustrations, Index. Publisher: J. Impentor, Bilbeny-San-Celoni, Spain. 1967.

Dr. Ferrandez is an international authority on medical botanics and Folk Medicine at Del Colegio Oficialde Medicos de Barcelona, Spain. This work gives a short description of the plants, their properties and uses. Names are given in Latin, Spanish, English and French. The book is artistically produced with excellent original drawings. For Spanish-speaking students in South and North America it is a most valuable book.

FOX, WILLIAM, M.D., **Family Botanic Guide.** Size 8½ × 6 in., 304 and 5 pp., Illustrations. Publisher: Health Research, Mokelumne Hill, California, U.S.A. Reprinted 1963.

This book is in the "one book author" category. Being of advanced years when first published, the life experiences of Dr. Fox will be mentioned and referred to many times in Herbal treatment. The Fox edition of 1904 was revised by his two sons, A. R. Fox and W. C. Fox. Seventeen previous editions of 90,000 copies were rapidly sold. Both publications will outlive father and sons, as this type of material and experience will always assist thoughts and facts of knowledge. There are descriptions of 129 herbs and uses, herbal preparations, and many formulas. Contains many of the practised North American Indian herbals. Trained as a medical doctor, Dr. Fox achieved his success by following the Thomsonian System.

FRANKTON, CLARENCE, **Weeds of Canada**. Illustrations by W. H. WRITE. Size 10 × 6½ in., 196 pp. Publisher: Canada Department of Agriculture, Ottawa, Ontario. Publication No. 948, 1967.

There are several books highly valued by Herbalists published by the Federal and Provincial Governments of Canada. The book under review is for field workers and deals with collection and cultivation. There are good botanical descriptions, excellent drawings in black and white and an Index of over 600 names. First edition in 1955, reprinted 1961, 1963 and 1967. Priced very low and easily available in Canadian libraries, or directly from the Government agencies.

Gerards's Herbal, Introduction by MARCUS WOODWARD. Size 10 × 8½ in., XIX & 303 pp., Illustrations (wood cuts from the original). Publisher: Spring Book, London, England. 1964.

There is public demand for books on Herbalogy and health in general. It is a sign of our times to reprint and revise our opinion of the old Herbalists. This book has an introduction or "the essence thereof, distilled by Marcus Woodward" from the edition of Th. Johnson, 1936, first edition 1927, latest 1964. It is a common thing to buy Gerard, Culpeper and Kneip in leading department stores and book dealers. Usually published very fancy for collector's item. Still very valuable for students and practitioners.

GIBBONS, EUELL, **Stalking The Healthful Herbs.** Size 6 × 8 in., XIV & 303 pp., drawings by RAYMOND W. ROSE. Publisher: David McKay Co., Inc., New York, N.Y., U.S.A. 1966.

This is one of the books produced in response to public demand for information on herbs. Descriptions of about fifty herbs, giving information commonly known by the herbalist and beginner. In some cases information uncritical and not dependable. Widely promoted with publicity. Drawings very good.

GREER, J. H., M.D., **A Physician in the House (for Family and Individual Consultation)**. Size 8 × 5½ in., XXVIII & 890 pp. with 42 pp Appendix and Index, 28 pp. Illustrations. Publisher: The Model Publishing Co., Chicago, U.S.A. 1958.

The book was first published in 1915, reprinted 1921, latest on hand 1958. For fifty years the book has enjoyed steady interest and success. Herbalist will be interested in the 110 herbs described, with formulas and their uses. Text refers to Indian herbs as the plants were already accepted in Anglo-American literature. If not in libraries, health food supply houses usually distribute this book.

HAHNEMANN, SAMUEL, **Organon of Medicine**. Translated with Preface by WILLIAM BOERICKE, M.D.; Introduction by JAMES KRAUSS, M.D. Size 7½ × 5 in., 314 pp., portrait of S. Hahnemann, compact, Petit type. Sixth edition. First Indian edition.

There are only a few outstanding personalities in medical history who will be with us for centuries, if not for ever. These personalities were first of all gifted people and with their outstanding talent they created their own conception, theory or school. You may accept or dispute their conception, but you may never be indifferent. One of these outstanding names, with creative influence around the world, will be Samuel Hahnemann, creator of the school of Homoeopaths. His works are translated into many languages. He has both followers and opponents, but he stands in the world very strong. Herbalists will find many good indications for using herbs and proof of many properties of herbs which recently have been discovered by modern medical science. This book is a must, regardless, for the student of Herbalogy. This is the original sixth edition which orthodox Homoeopaths use as their testimony.

HARDING, A. R. **Ginseng and other Medicinal Plants**. Size 6½ × 5 in., 367 pp., Illustrations (drawings and half-tones). Published by the author, Columbus, Ohio, U.S.A. 1908.

The book gives much factual material about the personal experience of the author. The trend of prevailing literature and official reports about Ginseng being a corrective herbal has often been denied in the civilized U.S.A., despite Chinese knowledge of the past and present, and strong professional and public opinion. The book encourages cultivation and collection of Ginseng as a most profitable commercial item. The book was reprinted several times by the author himself, in 1967 by request. One of his latest editions gives statistical data since 1913. At one time copies of this book were scarce and therefore expensive but the reprints are more reasonable.

HARDY, GEORGE A., HARDY, WINIFRED V., **Wild Flowers in the Rockies**. Illustrations by FRANK L. BEEBE, Size 10 × 7 in., Bibliography, Index, Glossary. Publisher: H. R. Larson Publishing Co., Hamilton, Saskatoon, Vancouver, Canada. 1949.

A rare publication covering 200 wild flowers of the Rockies. Lithographic reproductions are copies of full water colour originals. Each illustration described botanically; no medical properties. A useful guide to Herbalists for wild flower identification. Bibliography of ten works, all original and very valuable, on wild flowers of certain areas. Publications from 1906 to 1936, seldom found in libraries; sometimes in museums or long-established educational institutes. Possession rewarded for beauty and usefulness to every nature lover.

HARPER, LT.-COL. SHOVE, **Prescriber and Clinical Repertory of Medicinal Herbs.** Size 7½ × 5 in., XII & 228 pp. Publisher: Health Science Press, Bognor Regis, Sussex, England. Second revised edition, 1938.

In the history of medicine and Herbalogy we can find many exceptional and valuable contributions from non-professionals. In our bibliographical review there are many books contributed by devoted persons, as in this case by Lt.-Col. Harper. The book under review is exceptionally treasured by professional practitioners and students. It is technical in character; 542 plants are classified by botanical names, and then classified by sickness, their property, and dosage. Prescriptions are given precisely, for example, for thirty-seven different conditions of constipation, sixty-four conditions of diarrhoeas, etc. All English health publications are priced very low; the value received surpasses the payment.

HOUSE, HARRY C., HOUSE, AUDREY M., **The Practical Herbalist.** Size 9 × 6 in., VIII & 144 pp. Published by the authors, Seattle, Washington, U.S.A. No date.

Those interested in Herbalogy and herbal astrology will find this book priceless. Besides astrological interpretations of herbalism there is practical information on herbal treatments and 262 herbs listed with their properties and use; also herbal compounds and formulas.

HUNTER, KATHLEEN, **Health Foods and Herbs.** Size 6 × 4 in., 156 pp. Publisher: Collins, London and Glasgow, U.K. 1962.

Contains general information on health foods, organic gardening and Herbs; also formulas and recipes. Included is an Index and a Bibliography of forty-seven titles only.

JAMES, CLAUDIA V., **Herbs and the Fountain of Youth.** Size 8 × 5½ in., 79 pp., Illustrations. Publisher: Armita Books, Edmonton, Alberta, Canada.

Small booklet, but good concentrated information on 341 herbs, Indian included; short introductory. Very popular in Canada and U.S.A. First edition in 1949, since then renewed every year until 1963 when editions jumped to seventeen. Quick and useful for home reference.

JARVIS, D. C., M.D., **Folk Medicine.** Size 7 × 4½ in., VI & 192 pp. Publisher: Fawcett Publications, Inc., Greenwich, Connecticut, U.S.A. 1962.

The author, a general practitioner from Barre, Vermount, U.S.A., after a lifetime of practice, prepared a book on Folk Medicine. Its beginning was met with much scepticism, but accidentally a columnist read and tried some of the fresh knowledge and was convinced that Folk Medicine had its merits. In 1962 it had already sold 500,000 copies in hard covers to libraries and institutes, and many millions of the sixteen paperback editions were also sold. Can be found in all department stores, news-stands and railway stations, selling at a price of about 50 cents. Now over eighty, the famous doctor has a best-seller of ten years standing.

KADANS, JOSEPH M., M.D., PH.D., **Modern Encyclopedia of Herbs**. Size $5\frac{1}{2}$ × $8\frac{1}{2}$ in., 256 pp.; Herb-o-matic locator index, Price $6.95. Publisher: Parker Publishing Co., West Nyack, New York, N.Y., U.S.A. 1970.

Professor Kadans is the founder and President of Bernadean University, which conducts home-study courses in Herbalogy and Naturopathy. The book gives names and properties of the plants, 600 in total. It is a good reference book for herbal dealers, herbalists and doctors. Quick condensed information with special classified indexes.

KENT J. T., A.M.M.D., **Repertory of Homoeopathic Materia Medica**. Size 7 × $9\frac{1}{4}$ in. 1,423 pp., Index, plus XXI pp. containing table of contents of names and abbreviations of 583 frequently used remedies, 1,422 indexing symptoms. Publisher: Sett Day and Co., 40A Strand Road, Calcutta, India. First Indian edition, 1961. Distributor: American Foundation for Homoeopathy Inc., 2726 Quebec Street, N.W. Washington, D.C. 20008.

To give the reader a satisfactory grasp of the value of Kent's compilation, let it be noted that, as in all Homoeopathic prescribing, the greatest importance is given to the mental symptoms; found on pp. 1–95. The book also incorporates Dr. Boenninghausen's chapter "The sides of the body and drug affinities" and Dr. Miller's "Relationship of Remedies".

KINGSBURY, JOHN M., **Poisonous Plants of the United States and Canada**. Size 6 × 9 in., 626 pp., Bibliography of 1,715 articles from periodicals and books, price $15. Publisher: Prentice-Hall, Inc., Englewood Cliffs, New Jersey, U.S.A.

John M. Kingsbury, Professor of Botany, New York State College of Agriculture, has in this book collected and classified 700 species of poisonous plants of North America, with descriptions, poisonous principles, toxicity, symptoms, lesions and conditions of poisoning. The listed Bibliography can only be covered by research institutes, Some illustrations in black and white. Useful reference book for students of Herbalogy.

KNEIPP, SEBASTIAN, **My Water Cure**. Size $8\frac{1}{2}$ × $5\frac{1}{2}$ in., XXII & 396 pp.,

25 pp., Illustrations. Publisher: Joseph Koesel, Kempten, Bavaria, Germany.

In world health literature, Father Kneipp (1821–97) is among the perennials, as each new generation intelligently searches unorthodox therapy. His one and only book, first published in 1888 while in his sixties, after forty years of experience, has kept a firm hold in international health literature. Our on-hand edition, 1956, is translated from the sixty-second German edition with 100 illustrations and a portrait of the Father. Our German edition is from 626–635 thousand. Russian and Polish editions are very brief, but popular in their own countries. Kneipp's work can be obtained from libraries and department stores anywhere and is always one of the popular sellers. It is difficult to estimate either the number of translations made of this work or the total sales. Father Kneipp used and highly recommended more than 100 herbs, many of them familiar Indian Herbs adopted in Europe. All practitioners and students know, or have heard of, his methods.

KORTH, LESLIE O., D.O.M.R.O., **Some Unusual Healing Methods**. 135 pp. Health Science Press, Wayside, Grayshott, Hindhead, Surrey, England. 1960.

Short articles about different methods of therapy. Good reference book for information about new and forgotten methods of medications.

KROCHMAL, ARNOLD, ALKER, RUSSEL S., DOUGHTY, RICHARD M., **A Guide to Medicine Plants of Appalachia**. Size 6 × 9 in., 290 pp., Illustrations, Index, price $1.70. Publisher: U.S. Department of Agriculture, Washington D.C., U.S.A. 1971.

Reference book for field workers with good pictures, botanical descriptions and condensed information on properties and uses of the plants of the Appalachia. It is aimed at the collectors of herbs, dealers and processors. The book states: "Out of 328 million prescriptions in the U.S.A. for 1962, 25 per cent of the drugs came from natural plant products."

For practical purpose a list of U.S.A. herbal importers, exporters, processors and dealers is included.

KUTS, CHERAUX A. W., B.S., M.D., N.D. (Editor-in-chief), **Naturae Medicina and Naturopathic Dispensatory**. Size $9\frac{1}{2}$ × $6\frac{1}{2}$ in., IX & 430 pp., Indexes: General, Therapeutic uses, Synonyms. Publisher: American Naturopathic Physician and Surgeon Association, Yellow Spring, Ohio, U.S.A. 1953.

A collective work of the Council of Natural Medicine and Naturopathic Dispensary of the American Naturopathic Physicians and Surgeons Association and professors of natural medicine and physiotherapy of the approved Naturopathic Colleges. The book covers a wide field of Naturopathic practice. General information on Naturopathic Botanics and remedies, Schuesslers mineral nutrition (cell-salts), vitamins and others. Of 430 pages, 294 are dedicated to herbs. General therapeutic use, Botanical synonyms index. Bibliography is not indicated, but from the contents of 299 herbs described our latest Anglo-American literature on herbs was, to our knowledge, absorbed. A division of all medical arts of healing in North America is an exclusive practice. This work represents official statements and position of the Naturopathic practitioners as formulated up to 1953 and will, along with reviewed works, help students of Herbalogy to clarify their own position, as one cannot adopt or deny what one does not know.

LEMMON, ROBERT S., JOHNSON, CHARLES C., **Wildflowers of North America in Full Colour.** Size 9½ × 6½ in., VIII & 280 pp. Publisher: Hanover House, Garden City, New York, N.Y., U.S.A. 1961.

Photographs in full colour of beautiful wild flowers. Brief botanical descriptions, no properties indicated. Helpful reference for field study and guide. Twenty useful bibliography references on wild flowers in North America, by regions.

LEYEL, C. F. (1880–1957), **Cinquifoil—Herbs to Quicken the Five Senses.** Drawings by MILDRED E. ELDRIDGE. Size 9 × 6 in., 368 pp., Indexes: General, Botanical, Familiar names, German, Italian, Spanish, Turkish, Arabian, Persian, Indian, Chinese, Malayan, Sanscrit. Publisher: Faber and Faber Ltd., London, England.

The sixth of Mrs. Leyel's books deals with herbs to quicken the five senses (sight, hearing, smell, touch, taste), and so increase perception and intuition. Each herb is classified in the contents and listed in chapters—I: Herbs for the eyes; II: Herbs for the sense of smell; III: Herbs for the sense of hearing; IV: Herbs for the sense of taste; V: Herbs for the sense of touch. Also herbs for the extremities, pages 311–345.

LEYEL, C. F. (1880–1957). **Green Medicine.** Drawings by MILDRED E. ELDRIDGE. Size 9 × 6 in., 324 pp., Indexes: General, Botanical, Familiar names, German, Italian, Spanish, Turkish, Arabian, Persian, Indian, Chinese, Malayan, Sanscrit. Publisher: Faber and Faber Ltd., London.

This is the fifth of Mrs. C. F. Leyel's "Culpeper Herbs". It shows the importance of chlorophyll for general health and gives descriptions of herbs containing chlorophyll that can be used in the form of teas and salads to overcome every ailment. Also discusses the drug arthritis, composit E or cortizone, and points out the danger of using hormones and alkaloids extracted from herb instead of using the herbs in their entirety. Each herb is classified in the contents and listed in chapters— I: Herbs for the circulation of the blood; II: Herbs for the throat; III: Herbs for the lungs; IV: Herbs for the digestive organs;

V: Herbs for the liver; VI: Herbs for the organs of Reproduction; VII: Herbs for the bladder and kidney; VIII: Herbs for the brain.

LEYEL, C. F. (1880–1957), **Heart-Easy—Herbs for the Heart**. Illustrations by MILDRED E. ELDRIDGE. Size 9 × 6 in., 333 pp., Indexes: General, Familiar names, German, Italian, Spanish, Turkish, Arabian, Persian, Indian, Chinese, Malayan, Sanscrit; price £1.05 net. Publisher: Faber and Faber, London, England. 1949.

This Herbal, the fourth of Mrs. Leyel's series, is concerned with herbs used in the treatment of the ductless glands and the heart, which is controlled to some extent by particular glands. Each herb is classified in the contents and listed in chapters—I: Herbs for the heart; II: Herbs for the glands; III: Alternative herbs; IV: Herbs for the viscera and the nerves; V: Herbs for viscera; VI: Herbs for the brain.

LEYEL, C. F. (1880–1957), **The Truth About Herbs**. Size 7½ × 5 in., 106 pp. Publisher:—Culpeper House, London, England. 1954.

Sceptics will not have a false opinion after reading the unbroken tradition of herbal medicine. The unplanned interest in the subject was brought about when, as a medical student, Mrs. Leyel's research touched on the history of the oldest healing art in the world, Herbalism. She did not complete her orthodox medical course due to circumstances and confidence gained through the use of herbs. At this time her knowledge was on the history of Herbalogy and she became interested only in how to sell herbs. Public interest in the almost forgotten, former use of plants soon came alive again. This encouraged the first of six books on herbs as corrective medication, and a new service for the public as a consulting Herbalist. A decision of a number of well established social workers encouraged the opening of her first Culpeper House Limited. At the same time, 1927, at the age of forty-seven, Mrs. Leyel also established a Herbalist society which eventually rose to be a powerful organization of 10,000 enthusiastic members of social prominency. After thirty years of study, faith and and success, mixed with prosecution and ridicule from some orthodox associations, she became a healer and Herbalist. Of 50,000 personal cases, she never took the professional title of doctor. As an authoress of international prominency, the powers of personal ambitions and promotions did not occur to her, only the knowledge of the healing power of herbs as a corrective service, through books, editorials and devotion.

All of Mrs. Leyel's intellect and accomplishments hold common sense in an uncommon degree for students of Herbalogy, doctors, researchers or general readers. The history, use and acts of parliament to protect Herbalists are all clearly and genuinely revealed.

LIGHTHALL, J. I., **The Indian Household Medic Guide**. Size 8½ × 5½ in.,

142 pp. First edition, Peoria, Illinois, U.S.A.; Second edition, Health Research, Mokelumne Hill, California, U.S.A. 1966.

General information on Indian Folk Medicine, their principles and beliefs. Sixty-nine descriptions of the most common herbs used by the Indians. Some formulas for men and horses. Few available in library, but ownership will help the layman, students and medical practitioners. Was re-published by demand of public.

LOVERING, A. T., M.D., **The Household Physician, A Twentieth-Century Medica**. Size 7 × 10 in., two volumes: Vol. I, 680 pp. and Vol. II, 681–1,444 pp., fully illustrated with natural coloured manikin, graphic and half-tone plates. Publisher: Brown-Flynn Co., Buffalo, U.S.A. New edition, 1926.

Exceptionally valuable publication almost unavailable. First published in 1905, five times repeated until 1926. Published strictly as a subscription book and was sold as such. There are sixty-three listed medical authorities in many fields of medicine. Eminent authority consulted. The book is very much valued as such. Vol. II especially for Herbalists and Homoeopaths. General index, pages 1,409–30; Index of herbs, roots and salt remedies, 1431–6; Index of Homoeopathic Department, 1,437–46, and other indexes. For Herbalists, the most valuable pages of Materia Medica, pages 982–1064, are a classification by their property and use of over 700 varieties of herbs, plants and roots. Obtained from special antique stores or collectors. Students will benefit in many ways from these volumes.

MARTIN, ALEXANDER C., ZIM, HERBERT S., NELSON, ARNOLD L., **American Wild Life and Plants**. Size 8½ × 5½ in., 500 pp., illustrations. Publisher: Dover Publications, Inc., New York, N.Y., U.S.A. 1961.

First unabridged publication, 1951, contained many good illustrations in black and white, seldom done as artistically in our day. The book will be studied by future Herbalists in close association and dependence on plant life for survival. Easily obtained, at the extremely low price of $2.50. No book of this standard containing such valuable information, can remain available at the present price.

MAUSERT, DR. OTTO, **Herbs For Health**. A concise treatise on Medicine. Herbs, their usefulness and correct combination in the treatment of diseases. A guide to health by natural means. Size 5¼ × 8 in., 205 pp. Publisher: Dr. O. Mausert, San Francisco, California, U.S.A. First edition 1932; Third edition 1940.

Many illustrations, black and white and colour, eighty-eight in total. Symptoms and what they may mean. Diseases, their symptoms and suggested remedies. 324 Formulas. Materia Medica Index by their properties. Materia Medica, description of eighty-five plants with illustrations. Materia Medica, Index of 1,130 plants, their properties and doses. General Index. Cultivation of the plants. Vitamins and Organic

Minerals in the plants. Very rare book to buy, not in libraries to our knowledge. If it could be obtained, would be valuable help for the student and medical practitioner.

MEDSGER, PROF. OLIVE PERRY, **Edible Wild Plants.** Size 8 × 5½ in., XI & 323 pp., illustrations, Indexes, Publisher: The Macmillan Co., New York, N.Y., U.S.A. 1963.

First published in 1939, thirteenth in 1963; a book in which the content matter is hardly altered by time. Written by Prof. Medsger after thirty years of experience and study. A careful and interesting work of about 600 available wild American plants as herbal food. Herbalists know that herbs alone are not the answer; proper food and harmonious conditions are also as important. From the new books we cannot point to anything as adequate; mostly old material deluded generously with stories and fine pleasure reading. Eighty excellent pen and ink drawings in the old, gracious gravure style with nineteen photographs artistically presented. The book is presented to revive public awareness of wild plant life.

MEYER, JOSEPH E., **The Herbalist.** Size 6 × 7½ in., 204 pp., illustrations, Index. Published by the author in the U.S.A. (Presume Hammond, Indiana). 1960.

First edition of pocket size, 1918. Three additional editions with latest in 1960. There are over 470 plants described in alphabetical order, then given index and supplements. Coloured illustrations. Classification of botanics by their property; spices and flavouring herbs; herbs used in wines, teas, etc. After fifty years the book still maintains memorial impressions for North America, just as "Potter's Botanical Encyclopedia" has served the Commonwealth since 1907. Herbalists, students and practitioners will find much valuable information on the often unrevealed Indian herbal medicine. Available in many libraries and still going strong in book stores and health food distributors.

New, Old, and Forgotten Remedies. Papers by many writers. Collected, arranged and edited by DR. EDWARD POLLACK ANSHUTZ Size 9½ × 6 in., VIII & 440 pp. Publisher: Roy Publishing House, Calcutta, India. Indian edition, 1966.

Rich on Materia Medica information. Easy to work remedies, therapeutic and clinical index. Needed by, and will benefit, students and practitioners in all fields of medicine.

NIELSEN, HAROLD (Author), SUSAN, EBBE (Artist), KEHLER, STEPHAN (Editor). Laegeplanter og trolddomsurter. Size 4½ × 7 in.; 400 pp., illustrations, Bibliography, Indexes, hard cover. Publisher: Politician Forlag a/s, Nygards Plads, Denmark. First edition 1965; Second edition 1969.

Compact book with highly concentrated information on medical botanics. Highly recommended for large Danish population in North America, of whom both general readers and the medical professions will find enrichment in a comparison of Anglo-American literature with that of their motherland.

OLIVER, J. H., **Proven Remedies**. Foreword by CYRIL SCOTT. Size $7\frac{1}{2}$ × 5 in., 92 pp. Publisher: Thorsons Publishers Ltd., London, England. 1962.

Thorsons Publishers have for generations performed a public service by their steady flow of publications on this subject. This little, concentrated prescriber has grown in popularity since 1949, with nine publications up to 1962. It gives prescription formulas for the treatment of common ailments by Homoeopathic, herbal and biochemical methods.

Ontario Weeds, Publication 505. Size 6 × 9 in., 116 pp., excellent graphic illustrations and photographs. Published by Ontario Department of Agriculture: Hon. WM. A. STEWARD, Minister; EVERETT M BIGGS, Deputy Minister. Composed by F. H. MONTGOMERY, PROF; Botany; C. M. SWITZER, Ass. Prof. Botany; C. H. KINGSBURY, Soil and Crop Branch.

Very useful for study in the field. Gives detailed descriptions, botanical locations with local names and botanical classifications. Information given for identification and how to destroy the weeds. Herbalists can use this as a field handbook for medical, commercial, and industrial purposes, and as a more positive approach than mere destruction for weed control. Index of 452 plants in the province of Ontario. Available on request.

PELIKAN, WILHELM, **Heilpflanzenkunde Der Mensch Und Die Heilpflanzen**. Size $9\frac{1}{2}$ × 7 in., 370 pp., illustrations. Publisher: Philosophisch–Anthroposophischer Verlag, Dornach, Switzerland. 1958.

Swiss herbs and Herbalists are well known on the North American market. German books can be found in many stores and libraries on the subject. This book describes sickness and herbal treatment. Well-known facts and information; not too much on new research. Illustrated in wood-cut style. Cross reference index.

PHILLIPS, CHARLES D. F., M.D., **Materia Medica and Therapeutics— Vegetable Kingdom**. Size 9 × 6 in., 323 pp., Index. Publisher: William Wood and Co., New York, N.Y., U.S.A. 1897.

Because this book is almost 100 years old, it will possibly only be found in universities and libraries that were in existence before its publication. All students of Herbalogy who have a chance to study in such a library or obtain the book will be rewarded greatly. As with our modern knowledge of herbs, the old books give a new light. In many cases recent scientific discovery has already been recorded in the yellowed pages of the oldest books. Our copy came to us from our friend Darrel Markel of Toronto, Canada.

POWELL, ERIC F., PH.D., N.D., **The Modern Botanical Prescriber**. Size 7½ × 5 in., 136 pp. Publisher: L. N. Fowler, London, England. 1965.

One of the latest books of well-known herbal authority. The book is condensed in the form of the prescriber; the author has forty years' experience. There are 111 medical botanics given, in many different combinations. Written in uncomplicated language, it is suitable for both the medical profession and the general reading public. Not in North American libraries but easily obtainable from England and Commonwealth.

ROBERTS, CAPTAIN FRANK, **The Encyclopedia of Digestive Disorders**. Size 8½ × 5¼ in., 168 pp. Publisher: Thorsons Publishers Ltd., London, England. No date.

Credit must be given to many publishers for the public service they perform. One of these is Thorsons Publishers, England. Capt. Roberts' books are very popular, not only in England but in the Commonwealth as well. In this book, students and practitioners will find many original and stimulating ideas. The author is in favour of many well-known Indian herbs and formulas. It is limited to digestive diseases and disorders, common and uncommon, as accepted by modern practical herbalism.

The Simmonite-Culpeper Herbal Remedies. Size 8 × 5½ in., 124 pp., illustrations, Index. Publisher: W. Foulsham & Co. Ltd., New York, U.S.A.; Toronto, Canada; Cape Town, South Africa; Sydney, Australia. 1957.

There are many compilations, digests, extracts and translations of Culpeper's works. This work is ideal for reference and study. William Joseph Simmonite, A.M. Professor of Medicine and Mathematics, was a prominent Herbalist in the early part of the century. From his own experience and practical knowledge of Herbalogy, Prof. Simmonite revised and re-classified Culpeper's material. Although it is over sixty-five years old, this book is the most recent revision of Culpeper's work.

SMITH, A. W., **A Gardener's Book of Plant Names**. Size 5½ × 8¼ in., XIX & 428 pp. Publisher: Harper & Row, New York and Evanston, U.S.A.; and London, England. 1963.

This handbook of derivations, meanings and uses includes over 4,000 botanical names, with a cross-reference of common names and a variety of enlightening information on plants in our history. A valuable book for students of botany and herbalism for use as a reliable reference in the classification of plants. The book has three parts: introduction; botanical definitions, meanings and origin of plant names; and index of common names.

SWEET, MURIEL, **Common Edible and Useful Plants of the West**. Size 9 × 6 in. 65 pp., illustrations. Publisher: Naturegraph Company, Healdsburg, California, U.S.A. 1962.

A small but useful booklet on the West's useful plants: ferns, vines, trees, shrubs, herbs. Contains about 120 references and some good drawings in black and white. It is uncommon in the libraries, but will be handy for students and practitioners.

THUT, DR. A. J., **Health from Herbs.** Size 9 × 6 in., 69 pp., 413 herbs listed, illustrations, Index. price £1.05. Publisher: Swiss Alp Herb Remedies, Guelph, Ontario, Canada. 1941.

Herbal remedies are spoken of in regard to sickness. Not obtainable.

TOBE, JOHN H., **Proven Herbal Remedies**. Size 6 × 9 in., XVI & 304 pp., indexes, no Bibliography, no illustrations, Price $7.95. Publisher: Provoker, St Catherines, Ontario, Canada. 1969.

Brief description of herbs with some indication of how to use them. A statement in one of the prospectuses for this publication stated that over 50,000 books were sold in a short period of time. An indication of how the general public in North America is turning their interest to the use of herbs.

TRETCHIKOFF, NICHOLAS GREGORY, **Herbalist—Material on Herbalogy**. Typed manuscript. Size 8½ × 11 in., 20,000 pp., 28 volumes, 2 copies only. Windsor, Ontario, Canada. 1967.

Collection of material started in China (1924–51) after experiencing the life-saving wisdom of a Chinese Herbalist. Herbal literature has been systematically classified for the last ten years on Anglo-American European, Indian, Oriental and Russian research. Regularly compiled with additional Bibliography, illustrations and pictures. The original is on hand for daily use in the office of Metro Herbalist, Windsor, Ontario, Canada. The second complete copy was presented to the authoress for study, reference and as an encouragement to write this book on North American Indian Herbalogy.

VOGEL, VIRGIL J., **American Indian Medicine**. Size 6 × 9 in., illustrations, XX & 583 pp., footnotes to Appendix, Bibliography, Indexes: botanical and general, Price $15. Publisher: University of Oklahoma, Oklahoma, U.S.A. 1970.

An academic work thoroughly analysed. Total of fourty-four pages of bibliography on unpublished material, books, pamphlets and articles. It is a good book for general readers and could provide some fresh ideas for professionals. Deals with controversial problems like herbal birth control for Indian women, but only in general terms without being specific about the use. A growing interest in Indian problems— their culture and medicine is discussed daily in the American press, on television and radio—encouraged the University of Oklahoma to publish this book. All in all it is an informative book about American

338

Indians. We did not see a single review about this book, but it deserves attention.

WARD, HAROLD, **Herbal Manual.** Size $7\frac{1}{2}$ × 5 in. Publisher: L. N. Fowler & Co. Ltd., London, England. 1962.

This is a small but informative book, useful for general reading and daily references. Author gives information on 130 of the most common herbs for medical, cosmetic, culinary and other uses. General index of herbs and their properties; some Indian herbs included as they are absorbed in English literature.

WASHBURN, HOMER C., ph.c., BLOME, WALTER H., ph.c., with a chapter on Vitamins and Insulin by WALTER PITZ M.S., **Pharmacognosy and Materia Medica.** Size $9\frac{1}{2}$ × 6 in., XIII & 586 pp., illustrations, Index. Publisher: John Wiley and Sons, London, England. 1927.

Old publications similar to this are very useful for study and reference, especially on pharmacognosy and Materia Medica—devoting attention to medical plants. Excellent book, very technical, but possession of the work will be rewarded by handy references.

WOOD, GEORGE P., M.D., RUDDOCK, E. H., M.D., **Vitalogy, or Encyclopedia of Health and Home.** Size 10 × 7 in., 974 pp., illustrations, Indexes: General; Remedies prescribed. Publisher: Vitalogy Association, Chicago, U.S.A. 1925.

Most families who are fortunate enough to have a copy of this book regard it as a highly treasured possession and hand it down from generation to generation. First published in 1904, then reprinted in 1913 and 1925. We are not able to locate it in the libraries and it is sold by subscription only. Very good information in general and over 300 herbs in Materia Medica section, with descriptions, properties and use. Contains many old Folk Medicine formulas adopted from the Indians of North America. Students and practitioners will find the book exceptionally good and informative. Over 500,000 copies were published but it is still difficult to get; once you have it, keep it!

WREN, R. C., **Potter's New Cyclopedia of Botanical Drugs and Preparations.** Size 9 × 6 in., 400 pp., Appendixes, Index of botanical and common names of the plant, Plant family, glossary, Herbal compounds, etc. Publisher: Potter & Clarke Ltd., London, England. Seventh edition, 1956.

This book is considered a classic in herbal literature, serving England and the Commonwealth from the first edition in 1907 to the seventh edition in 1956. Gives good, reliable descriptions of over 700 plants common to England and North America. Illustrations in the text, but not for all plants, some in colour. First editions were pocket-size with less information but fifty years of additional work has improved the book. Usually found in libraries and sells in book stores; very popular in Commonwealth and North America. All students and practitioners will find this a valuable daily reference in their practice. Many Indian herbs are adapted in English Herbals.

RUSSIAN PUBLICATIONS

ALEXEEV, U. E., VECHOV, V. N., GAPOCHKA, G. P., DUNDIN, R. K., PAVLOV, V. N., TICHOMIROV, V. N., FILLIN, V. P., **Herbal Plants of U.S.S.R.** Vol. 1: MISS L. M. SAMARINA, Artist. Size $5\frac{1}{2}$ × 8 in., 488 pp., 80 colour plates; Vol 2: 310 pp., 168 colour plates, black and white illustrations, Indexes: Latin and Russian names, Bibliography. Publisher: "MISL", Moscow. 1971.
Collective work of seven authors and one artist covering recent research on herbal plants in Soviet Russia; the most reliable data on the subject up to and including 1971. Literature from the whole Republic of the Soviet Union is used exclusively. Colourful illustration by the artist, L. M. Samarina, is most attractive and precisely done.
BAKULEFF, A. N., PETROFF, F. N. (Editors-in-chief), **Popularnaya Meditzinskaya Encyclopedia** (Popular Medical Encyclopaedia). Size 8 × $10\frac{1}{2}$ in., 1,039 pp. 24 illustrations, Index, 200,000 copies, price R3.50 (U.S.$3.85). Publisher: Bolshaya Soviet Encyclopedia, Moscow. Fourth revised edition, 1965.
Our encyclopaedia reference is from the latest fourth edition. The up-to-date information is on medicine and how it is accepted by the Russian medical authorities. In comparison with similar North American publications, the material is most objective and unspoiled by possible commercial and highly professional promotional influences. Herbalists and other branches of medication will observe and appreciate the clear, simple but scientific descriptions of sickness and abnormality. Methods covering Folk Medicine, herbalism and diet are given gratifyingly when known to help. This is a collective work of many hundreds of people, plus seventeen additional editorial staff members. Illustrations are of highest artistic design, with an especially good anatomical atlas in colour. An unprejudiced reference and study encyclopaedia with value beyond price.
BALASHEV, L. L., **Slovar Polesnich Rastenyi na Dvadtzati Evropeiskich Yazikach** (Dictionary of Useful Plants in Twenty European Languages), Academy of Science of the U.S.S.R., State Committee for Science and Technology Council of Ministers of U.S.S.R. Size 5 × 8 in., 366 pp. Publisher: "Nauka", Moscow. 1970.
We are in possession of many valuable reference books on medical botanics. This one is the most important for researchers and practical field workers. We have already reviewed elsewhere a dictionary in

340

seven languages, covering over 3,000 plants, but this book covers 476 cultivated plants and is aimed at botanists, biologists, agriculturalists etc., as an aid to translating works of international botanical literature.. Price is Rb1.37 (about $1.50), only 9,200 copies published. Only an academy of science with Government help can afford such a scientific, non-profitable enterprise.

BORODINA, N. A., NEKRASOV, N. S., NEKRASOVA, N. S., PETROVA, I. P., PLOTNIKOVA, L. S., SMIRNOVA, **Trees and Shrubs of U.S.S.R.** L. M. SAMARINA, artist; Size 6 × 8 in., 637 pp., 48 colour plates, black and white illustrations in text, Bibliography Index, price Rb2. Publisher: "MISL", Moscow. 1966.

Collective work of six Herbalists and one artist, all but one of them being women. It is one of many excellent works on economic botanics in U.S.S.R. A reference book for field workers, geographers, travellers and general readers. Besides perfect botanical descriptions, it contains valuable information for economical use of trees and shrubs. The original colour illustrations are most helpful.

BUNDIN, E. I., **Prirodnie Sokrovishe** (Nature's Treasures). Size 5 × 8 in. 64 pp., soft cover, 100,000 copies, price 7 kopecks (U.S.$0.08). Publisher: Medicinskaya Literatura, Moscow. 1962.

This is one of many herbal publications used in Russia. High school students are encouraged to use their vacation and spare time studying this simple but scientific booklet. A good beginning, as the booklet contains enough to make those who are really interested want more. Protection of useful wild plants, practical information, collecting, botanical characteristics and medical properties are included. Conservation is considered as national wealth.

DARABAN, E. V., **Gotovie Lekarstvennye Sredsva** (Medical Preparations). Editor: PROF. P. V. RODIONOVA. Size 5 × 8 in., 488 pp., Bibliography, Index (Russian only), 50,000 copies, price R1.35 (U.S.$1.49). Publisher: Zdorovie, Kiev. 1966.

A handbook for doctors and druggists. One of many regional publications, in this case Ukrainian. Author has compiled 1,635 (including 165 imported) prepared medications. Russian index of sickness and medical preparations. Herbals referred to are clinical and domestic. Total of fifty-five works from latest monographic and clinical literature, 1929–62.

FURSAEV, A. D., VRONINA, K. B., VOLINSKY, B. G., FREIDMAN, C. L., BENDER, K. I., KUZMINA, K. A., MARTINOFF, L. A., KUZNETZTOVA, C. G., **Lekarstvennye Rastenia I IH Primenenie V Medicine** (Medical Plants and their use as Medicine). Size 6 × 9 in., 204 pp., 25 illustrations (some in colour), Bibliography, Index (Russian and Latin), 60,000 copies, price 86 kopecks (U.S.$0.95). Publisher: Saratov University, Saratov. 1962.

This is one of the University's works for general readers, i.e., doctors, medical students, business organizations for buying, processing and cultivating; also any person interested in medical botanics. Dedicated as a regional survey mainly in the Saratov district, Volga River and Kasachstan, as prospective plant cultivating areas. Information is rich in the properties, cultivation and collection of plants. Bibliography is impressive, consisting of 365 herbal works, of which sixty-nine were published from 1872–1918. Remainder were published from 1920–62. It is noted with interest that many herbal plants have had close scientific and medical attention since the latter part of the nineteenth century, for example, Hydrastics canadensis since 1887, Lobelia inflata since 1872 and Ginseng-Panax q since 1889, to name a few.

In Russia, many universities, medical associations, research institutes, health and agriculture ministries etc., realized, even before the Revolution, the importance of the unfathomable philosophy. All evidence points to follow-up after the Revolution on a bigger and more centralized scale.

From this work we can learn much about native North American plants and confirm what effort and research have already established.

GAMMERMAN, PROF. A. F., YOURKEVITCH, I. D., Academician Editors, **Lekarstvennye Rastenia Dikorastushie** (Wild Medical Plants). Size 6 × 8½ in., 380 pp., illustrations (graphic and half-tone), Bibliography, Index (Russian and Latin), 250,000 copies, price R1.37 (U.S.$1.50). Publisher: Bello-Russ. Academy of Science, Institute of Experimental Botanics and Microbiology, Minsk, Bello-Russia. 1965.

One of Russia's most recent books on Herbalogy; a collective endeavour of the Institute of Experimental Botanics and Microbiology of the Academy of Science of Bello-Russia. A compact, very informative book on medical botanics, generally original, with historical facts of interest. Latest botanical, medical, agronomical and economical value of herbs. Many artistic half-tone illustrations and drawings.

Latin and Russian index of 500 plants; bibliography of 240 works of monographic character and books considered valuable enough to be approved by the Academy. Of 240 editions, eighteen are dated from 1781 to 1920, an average of one book every ten years over a span of 140 years. The Russian Revolution and Civil War ended about 1920. Since that time, Herbalogy and Folk Medicine has had specialized attention, which reflects in literature also. In forty-five years there were 222 books, dating from 1920–65, an average of five contributions every year. The Academy has accepted 183 formulae and valuable recipes, with North American plants used and recommended in many cases. Formulae and directions for growing, preparing and collecting are given with a calendar and map of plant geography.

These are also available in drug stores (Apteki). Preparations are listed as follows: heart 9; stomach 38; kidney and bladder 23; cancer 4; liver 12, and so on.

We are unable to name another Anglo-American book adequate to the above reviewed, where a scientific institute will uphold the findings of their academic authority. With their consent and our grateful thanks to the Academy of Bello-Russ., our book is only the smallest sample of the useful information and illustrations that can be found in their "Wild Medical Plants".

GAMMERMAN, PROF. A. F., SHUPISKAYA, M. D., YATZENKO-HMELEVSKY, A. A., **Rastenia Tzelitely-Lekarstvennye Rastenia Nashei Rodini** (Plants, Healers, Medical Plants of our Motherland). Size 6 × 8½ in., 424 pp., illustrations (traditional gravure drawings), Bibliography, Index (Russian only), 200,000 copies, price 89 kopecks (U.S. $0.95). Publisher: Vishya Schkolla, Moscow, 1963.

One of the mass editions for general readers, doctors, agronomists, universities, academies of science, research organizations, medical institutes, laboratories, experimental stations, etc. The general and historical part is excellent, with many new and original interpretations of medical botanics and medicine in general. Some 289 medical herb plants are described, including some American-Indian botanics which do not always grow in Russia. However, State purchasing organizations are very much interested in promoting cultivation of these plants. Each herb is described botanically and medically, with information on how to gather or cultivate and raw material requirements for purchasing agents.

The Russian Government encourages herbal medication, with Central Pharmacological Committees and the Ministry of Health revising and approving herbal formulae for general use by either drug dispensers (Apteki) or laymen. In this book, seventy-three formulae are selected for use as tea treatments for stomach, heart, nervousness, etc. Many combinations are indicated for more than one specific illness. All Russian literature in this field emphasizes the specific and combined malfunctions of heart, lungs, nerves, stomach and cancer, indicating how people can help themselves with the use of herbs for treating the above-mentioned drastic sicknesses of mankind.

A classified index on herbal properties is given to enable the reader to combine teas and decoctions himself. Bibliography is of forty-five works, a few from 1912–37 and the remainder from 1943–62. The work is rich in original and new material which we were unable to find in other Russian publications. Anglo-American literature contributes less up-to-date botanical knowledge.

GRUSHEVITSKY, I. B., **Genshen** (Ginseng-Panax q). A. A. FEDDROFF, Editor-in-chief. Size 7 × 10½ in., 344 pp., illustrations, Bibliography,

3,000 copies, price R1.80 (U.S.$1.98). Publisher: Academy of Science (Siberian Branch), Leningrad 1961.

One of the rare monographs outside Russia, this book contains complete information covering intent of purpose, biological, botanical, agronomical and medical, concerning the highest-priced plant in Asia. The book contains 141 drawings and half-tone illustrations plus ninety-three statistical and scientific tables. The bibliography, with annotations, is resourceful and most valuable. Monographs on Ginseng total 267, of which 170 are Russian, 85 English, French or German and 12 Chinese or Japanese. These date from 1828–1960, the most active research being within the last twenty years.

To date, the medical value of Ginseng has been denied in American publications. However, the commercial value is high, as the Chinese have always esteemed Ginseng as the most valuable of herbal plants, especially the wild variety, and have always bought all available American stock. In this case, our health resource lies in our own backyard, but to be convinced of this we need to study numerous monographs, also research and clinical data, from academies of science in other countries. With very limited facilities, our own efforts allowed classification of at least 500 works on Ginseng alone, which give full credit to the healing properties of the plant.

KAREEV, F. I., **Rastenia Primeniaemie V Bitu** (Plants for Daily Use). Size 6 × 8½ in., 243 pp., illustrations, 200,000 copies, price 90 kopecks (U.S.$1.00). Publishers: Moscow University, Moscow 1963.

One of the typical books published by universities for the general public. In this case, giving shrubs, berries and herbs useful for decoration, nutrition and medication. A collective work of well-established scientific writers and researchers under the general direction of the editor, F. I. Kareev. Good information on local and foreign plants, with close attention and prominency to North American plant life. Wide interpretation of economical use of versatile plants.

KISELEFF, G. E., **Tzvetovodstvo** (Flower Gardening). Size 7 × 10½ in., 981 pp., illustrations, Bibliography, Index (Russian and Latin), 70,000 copies, price R2.67 (U.S.$2.93). Publisher: Kolos, Moscow. Third revised edition, 1964.

This book was prepared by Kiseleff but the editorial is by nine outstanding authorities in the field. Generally for gardeners, botanists or agronomists, with no direct information on medical value of plants. Botanical information is valued for general study on herbalogy and in field work. Many photo-illustrations, with some in colour. Bibliography totals fifty-one original works, monographical in character, dated 1947–55.

KONDRATENKO, P. T., KUR, S. D., ROJOKO, F. M., **Zagotovka, Virashivanie I Obrabotka Lekarstvennich Rasteny** (Collecting, Cultivating and Processing Medical Plants). Size 6 × 9 in., 346 pp., illustrations, Bibliography, Index (Russian and Latin), 13,000 copies, price R1.12 (U.S.$1.23). Publisher: Medicina, Moscow. 1965.

A book of especial interest to state institutes and organizations collecting or processing medical plants; also for cultivators on state-owned farms, teachers and youth organizations, in general, all interested in the growing, cultivating and usage of medical plants. Authors give botanical descriptions, properties and commercial or industrial demand; also geographical and agronomical calendar. The book is divided into three parts: general information on medical plants with historical review and practical information on cultivating and processing requirements for State purchasing agents; botanical description, listed alphabetically; and information regarding processing and storing of herbs. This last part will be of interest to prospective herb gardeners and distributors.

We know of no Anglo-American publication on this subject with as much detailed and illustrated technical information. Also given useful agronomical and business information on native North American plants.

KOTUKOFF, G. N., **Lekarstvennye I Maslicnie Kulturi**—Spravochnik (Medical and Aromatic Plants). Size 5 × 8 in., 200 pp., sketched illustrations, Index (Russian and Latin), Bibliography, 8,000 copies, price 31 kopecks (U.S.$0.34). Publisher: Naukova Dumkw, Kiev. 1964.

Kiev has a long-standing reputation as one of the important cultural centres in Russia, with its University, Research Institute and Academy of Science. Ukrainians have produced many excellent works on medical botanics. This work is in the form of reference and practical material, of interest to doctors, students, agronomists, biologists, botanists, etc., and includes the economical aspect of cultivation. For those interested in Herbalogy the theoretical and practical information is very reliable and valuable. About 200 of the most popular plants are described, including many for those persons interested in promoting further use. Bibliography lists eighty-two of the latest editions from 1936–65. Many artistic graphic illustrations in black and white.

KOTUKOV, G. N., **Kultivovani I Dikorosli Likarski Roslini** (Cultivated and Wild Medical Plants). Size 5 × 8 in., 166 pp. illustrations, Indexes, 60,000 copies, price R0.63 (U.S.$0.70). Publisher: Naukova Dumka, Kiev, Ukraine. First edition, 1971.

This, the author's second book, shows progress in research since his first book in 1966. In all works on Herbalogy the general idea is to encourage people to grow, collect and experiment with what nature has provided. Not just new plants of the area, but introductions from other countries. Keen interest is shown in the North American Indian inheritance of Folk Medicine. Many researchers and writers are very persistent about new facts, and wish to check on their own findings. Those in command of the Russian Ukrainian languages will be rewarded greatly if they follow the progress and experience of the Ukrainian and Russian scientists in this field.

KOVALEVA, N. G., **Lechenie Rasteniamy** (Herbal Treatments—Outlines on Phytotherapy). Size 7 × 10 in., 352 pp., illustrations, Indexes, Bibliography, price R2.99 (U.S.$3.30). Publisher: Nauka (Academy of Science), Moscow. First edition, 1971.

In our book we made comparisons between Indian Folk Medicine and herbal practice and those of Russia and India. When the above book arrived we were pleased to find that it followed a similar pattern to our own study. The writer, Dr. Nina Georgievna Kovaleva, had the patience and devotion to analyse and classify 300 works on Austrian, Chechoslovakian, French, German, Indian, Italian, Polish and Russian literature. For instance, we learned for the first time that our common Plantain is used in Bulgaria to treat cancer of the spleen, and that in China they use Burdock to dissolve mercury in the blood. Dr. Kovaleva writes about the plants prescribed in her practice. This assurance enables her to speak with authority. The book is intended for use by doctors, researchers, students, botanists, agronomists, and pharmacologists.

MESHKOVSKY, PROF. M. D., **Lekarstvennye Sredstva**—Posobie dlia Vrachey (Medical Preparations—Reference Book for Physicians). Size 6 × 9 in., 240 pp., Bibliography, Index (Russian and Latin), 240,000 copies, price R1.19 (U.S.$1.31). Publisher: Medicina, Moscow. 1964.

The last four editions, from 1960–4, introduce many new medical preparations. A most informative book, especially for herbalists, who will find the latest research achievements help prove the theory of the importance of herbs in medicine. The book is highly technical but useful for herbalists and students requiring up-to-date information. Many familiar North American plants take on a new aspect in medical use, something yet to be found in Anglo-American publications. Bibliography is convenient for students, as medicine is itemized separately. A total of 396 monographs dating from 1960–4 indicate how dynamic medical literature is abroad.

MESHKOVSKY, PROF. M. D., **Lekarstvennye Sredstva** (Medical Preparations. Size 5½ × 8 in., 2 volumes of 708 pp., and 462 pp., respectively, compact pages, Bibliography, Index (Russian and Latin), 6 editions, 100,000 copies, price R4.50 (U.S.$5) complete. Publisher: Medicina, Moscow. 1967.

A handbook for doctors, this is the latest and most complete work on the subject. In each preparation the dose is on drugs and herbal medicines, with brief characteristic chemical formulae of clinical amounts in effect and side-effect. The most significant part is the bibliographical material. The author reviews a total of 1,424 medical publications, mostly monographs and clinical reports, from 1960–6. This sixth edition of the book is revised and improved. Herbalists will find the latest information on herbal material administered in clinical doses only. "Folk Medicine" is not mentioned. Being designed as a handbook for doctors, on a clinical and prescriptive level, this book is too technical for general reading, but the information is exceptionally good.

NOSAL, M. A., NOSAL, I. M., DROBOTKA, V. G. (Editor), **Likarski Roslini I Sposobi IH Zastosuvania V Narodi** (Ukrainian Medical Plants and Folk Medicine). Size 5 × 8 in., 300 pp., illustrations, Index (Ukrainian and Latin), 150,000 copies, price 87 kopecks (U.S.$0.95). Publisher: Zdorovie, Kiev. Second edition, 1964.

One of many books on Ukrainian Folk Medicine and medical botanics, with a detailed description of 143 plants growing either wild or under cultivation in Ukraine. The book is instructive for biologists, doctors and all interested in botanics in general. Many valuable formulae and recipes as used in Folk Medicine are officially approved for general use. With practical information on collecting and growing herbs, this book places tangible help within the reach of persons knowing and using the rich source of field and garden plants around them.

REDACTIONNAYA KOLLEGIA BELIKOFF, I. F., GRUSHEVITSKY, I. V. KOSMAKOVA, B. E., **Material K Izucheniu Jenshenia and Limonnika** (Volume IV: Material on Research of Ginseng and Limonnic). Collective work, size 7 × 10½ in., 248 pp., illustrations, Bibliography, 1,500 copies, price R10 (U.S.$11). Publisher: Academy of Science, Leningrad. 1960.

This is a limited edition, there being only 1,500 copies; in this field the usual for Soviet publications is 100,000 to 250,000 copies. The monographs, totalling twenty-nine, cover a wide field on Ginseng (Panax-Aralia family) and Chinese Limonnik (Scizandra chinensis-Turez). The book covers field, clinical and laboratory researches, supported by 186 monographic bibliographies. Numerous illustrations, statistical data, classified clinical and laboratory findings, tablet preparations, schemes, plus photographic documentary data. For today's analysis about the ancient use of Ginseng, this scientific research is a collective work of reliable information for students of herbalogy. Panax canadensis has as much extensive attention as Japanese Ginseng.

ROJKO, Y. D., **Yagodi I IH Lechebnye Svoistva** (Medical Properties of

Berries). Size 5 × 8 in., 60 pp., illustrations, Bibliography, 104,000 copies, price 8 kopecks (U.S.$0.09). Publisher: Kiev Knijnaya Fabrica, Kiev. 1966.

The idea of berries as food and medicine has stimulated many publications giving chemical analyses of the most popular domestic and wild berries. Very good information on cultivating the wild species for domestic, medical and nutritional health.

TUROVA, M. A., A.D. (Editor-in-chief), **Lekarstvennye Sredstava Iz Rastenyi** (Medical-Herbal Preparations). A collective work, size 6 × 9 in., 316 pp., diagrams and tables, Bibliography, 20,000 copies, price R1.15 (U.S.$1.26). Publisher: Medicinskaya Literatura, Moscow. 1962.

One of the monographs we would like to have in English, as there is so much valuable material on the latest research by the seventy-five scientists who prepared this volume All articles are subdivided into narrow topics, as teams of two to eight scientists prepared independent articles on their own laboratory and clinical cases. Containing a rich and valuable bilbiography of 199 monographs not available outside the U.S.S.R. The purpose of the book is limited to a scrutiny of a few plants from a medical point of view. It is satisfying to know that some familiar North American plants have been closely studied.

The book is divided into three parts: the first devoted to the heart and blood circulation; the second to the central nervous system; and the third to kidney and bladder, and diuretic problems as such. It is a very technical work with eventual conclusions for medical practitioners or students of Herbalogy. The illustrations are schemes, charts, records of cardiographs, electronic equipments, etc. The book was sold out on publication, to institutes, libraries and researchers. The value of this book is seldom duplicated in our research institutes.

TZITZIN, N. B., ANICHKOFF, C. V., ITZKOFF, N. Y., (Editors-in-chief), **Atlas Lekarstvennych Rastenia U.S.S.R.** (Atlas of Medical Plants of U.S.S.R.). Size 9 × 12 in., VIII & 704 pp., illustrations. Index (Russian and Latin) on chemical properties, 16,000 copies, price R11.57 (U.S.$12). Publisher: Gosudarstvennoe Izdetelstvo Medicinskaya Literature, Moscow. 1963.

No Anglo-American publication compares with this book our favourite, on medical herbs. While studying the illustrations a strong desire to understand the Russian language is essentially felt. Over 600 botanical, chemical, agronomical, medical and pharmaceutical plants are described, many of which are native to North America. More information is now available on American medical botanics in Russian publications than Anglo-American. As a rule, our herbal books are written, published and sold by the herbalists themselves; with some of the older books being reprinted by private companies on request.

The book reviewed, however, is the combined efforts of the State Research and Scientific Institute of Aromatic and Medical Plants. In addition to the members of the Academy of Science, twenty-eight outstanding national and international editorial board members have been associated with the book. The editorial staff was divided into sections: general plan and direction; botanic; agro-technic; chemistry; medical use; artistic illustrations. With this personalized background each group has given each plant its respectful place; many have all-round purpose throughout the book.

A team of 209 authors and artists prepared this luxurious atlas with full-page original pictures in natural water-colour showing every part of the plant in detail. The research of plants was from almost every territory—in 1960 an estimated 17,000 plants were subjected to further research. Our thanks go to those concerned with this book for consenting to our use of some of the illustrations.

The only other copy of the atlas known to be in this country was proudly displayed to us by a Mexican herbalist in California. He eagerly showed us the book and the English translations of the plant properties taken from the atlas. The book is well worth $12 for the valuable information of plant identification alone. The atlas is a wealth of knowledge with standards to match. We only wish translations were available to those interested. An understanding of the ten years' work would be a real eye-opener; a job for someone in command of both Russian and English and an expert in his field, be it agronomy, pharmacopea, botany, medicine, or whatever. In our work as herbalists we are informed as to medical use, botanical descriptions and agronomy, leaving thorough study to the experts in each respective field. As a created existence plant life is uncomplicated, but as a study it needs much explanation.

VESELOV, E. A. **General Biology**. 298 pp., illustrations. Official publication of The Ministry of Education, Moscow. 1963.

A very good textbook, handy for reference and information of new, officially-accepted educational material.

VOLKOVA, P. A., DOLGOVA, A. A., IVANOVA, C. D., LUKSHENKOVA, E. Y., LVOV, N. A., RAZDORSKAYA, L. A., RODIONOVA, V. M., **Dikorastushie Lekarstvennie Rastenia** (Wild Medical Plants R.S.F.R. Moscow Region) (Moscow Oblast). Editor: E. Y. LUKSHENKOVA, Size 5 × 8 in., 144 pp., halftone illustrations, Index (Russian and Latin), Bibliography, 20,000 copies, price 37 kopecks (U.S.$0.41). Publisher: Gosudarstevennoe Izdatelstvo Medicinskoy Literaturi, Moscow. 1963.

This particular herbal booklet is for the Moscow region only. Numerous publications of this kind are popular throughout the Soviet

Union for general guidance and practical use to regional research institutes, universities and State publishing houses. Information is given on the geography, agriculture, botany, State purchasing agents—in general, herbal know-how from the soil to the market or home including Folk Medicine and poisonous plants. Bibliography covers a total of thirty-two works, from 1925–54, books and monographs of medical plants of the Moscow region, or closely-related literature. The local publication is a concentrated source of neighbourhood herbal knowledge. Despite our bountiful Materia Medica and botanical gardens, this type of publication does not exist on the North American continent.

PERIODICAL PUBLICATIONS

Herb Collector's Manual and Marketing Guide. Size 9 × 6 in., 70 pp. Publisher: J. Kelly, Looneyville, West Virginia, U.S.A.

Very good practical material on herbal descriptions, collecting, processing, marketing, Agro-Technic, soil, etc. Published once a year on 1st January. Our copy is from 1958. Not in libraries but with some effort book and health food stores can obtain.

National Health Federation Bulletin. Official Organization of the National Health Federation, Monrovia, California, U.S.A.

Published monthly. The American crusade for better health is active nationally on the latest information in this field.

Novie Knigi USSR (New Book of U.S.S.R.). Size 6 × 8½ in., 80 pp. (average). Publisher: Mejunarodyna Kniga, Moscow.

As in all economic and social activities in the U.S.S.R., publishing matter is centralized. This is a bulletin on a few books currently being published. A weekly review of eighteen to twenty different sections of Russian books (occasionally Ukrainian, English, French, German, Spanish, etc.) Object of the subscription is to keep readers up to date in their own field—medicine, biology, Herbalogy, botany, pharmacology, etc. Each book review lists title and character with annotations, so that before ordering a book one is well informed as to its content.

The Layman Speaks—A Homoeopathic Digest. Editor: B. Green. Size 9 × 6 in., 40 pp. (average), Bibliography, price $4 per year, $4.40 foreign. Publisher: American Foundation for Homoeopathy, Inc., 2726 Quebec Street N.W. Washington, D.C. 20008.

Monthly publication reviewing rich and well-informed material, including homoeopathic use of herbalism.

The Provoker. Written and Published by John H. Tobe, St. Catharines, Ontario, Canada. Size 8 × 10½ in.; 32 pp. illustrations. Circulation 200,000. Price £3.50 yearly. Published quarterly.

J. H. Tobe, the most aggressive promoter of Health Food and Herbs. Emphasis on food mostly, distributing books and publications on Health and Natural Medicine. J. Tobe has devoted a lot of his time to travelling around the world and then using new material and information to promote his ideas through *The Provoker*, his books, lectures, special bulletins, films and slides. Many statements very provocative and controversial, but people read with great interest.

The World Forum, incorporating Health from Herbs. Published by H. H. Greaves, Ltd., London, England. Size 7 × 10 in.; *The Forum* 44 pp. + *Health from Herbs* 12 pp., illustrations. Editor of *The Forum*, J. D. Magnab; *Health from Herbs,* Frederick A. Dawes, M.N.I.M.H. Quarterly. Price £1 yearly.

The *Health from Herbs* magazine has been published by the National Institute of Medical Herbalists since 1864. The magazine serves professional Herbalists of Great Britain and Commonwealth countries, with interesting material. Materia Medica given regularly with short annotations. In many cases new Herbals are introduced of interest to both general readership and professionals.

A selected list of North American native people's periodicals

These are publications of general interest. There are many other native publications which serve as newsletters for their own tribe, area, or group, as well as governmental publications which purport to write Indian news.

Indian Voice, Editor: FERN WILLIAMS, P.O. Box 2033, Santa Clara, California 95051, U.S.A.

Warpath, Editor: LEE BRIGHTMAN, United Native Americans, P.O. Box 26149, San Francisco, California 94126, U.S.A.

Akwesasne Notes, (circulation 38,000) Editor: RARIHOKWATS, Mohawk Nation via Rooseveltown, New York 13683, U.S.A.

Americans Before Columbus, National Indian Youth Council, 3102 Central SE, Albuquerque, N.M. 87106, U.S.A.

The Blue Cloud Quarterly, Blue Cloud Abbey, Marvin, South Dakota 57271, U.S.A.

Early American, California Indian Education Association, P.O. Box 4095, Modesto, California 95352, U.S.A.

Tribal Indian News, N'Amerind Friendship Centre, 613 Wellington Street, London, Ontario, Canada.

The Indian Historian, American Indian Historical Society, 1451 Masonic Avenue, San Francisco, California 94117, U.S.A.

Kanai News, P.O. Box 432, Cardston, Alberta, Canada.

Legislative Review, Indian Legal Information Development Service, 1785 Massachusetts Avenue, N.W. Washington, D.C. 20036, U.S.A.

The Native People, Alberta Native Communications, 11427 Jasper Avenue, Edmonton 11, Alberta, Canada.

Sun Tracks, SUPO 20929, University of Arizona, Tucson, Arizona 85720, U.S.A.

Tosan, 318 North Tacoma, Indianapolis, Indiana 46201, U.S.A.

Native Times, Indian Brotherhood of NWT, P.O. Box 2338, Yellowknife, NWT, Canada.

INDEX

353

Anasarca, 133, 167, 265
Anemone, 130
Aneurism, 122
Angelica, 13; atropurpurea, 13
Angina, 59; faucium, 43; pectoris, 65, 66, 116, 132, 152, 167, 168, 180, 186, 224, 281, 302
Anise, 61, 76, 217, 246
Ankles, weak, 307
Ankylostoma, 309
Anodynes, 31, 44, 49, 50, 77, 133, 151, 153, 159, 166, 198, 203, 214, 239, 289, 305
Anorexia, 86
Anterior crural neuralgia, 135
Anthelmintics, 9, 21, 44, 54, 75, 124, 153, 155, 206, 217, 281, 291, 308, 310, 312
Anthemis nobilis, 60, 80, 174
Anti-asthmatic cigarettes, 152
Antibacterial, 56
Antibiotic, 278
Anti-catarrhal, 244
Antidote, 45, 47, 60, 147, 155, 185
Antidysenteric, 97
Antimercurial, 317
Antiperiodics, 20, 59, 134, 174, 177, 189, 206, 291, 303
Antipyretic, 288
Antiscorbutic, 1, 241, 247, 255, 277, 315
Antiscrofulous, 317
Antiseptics, 24, 30, 32, 34, 51, 77, 82, 83, 89, 114, 119, 121, 122, 127, 163, 169, 183, 188, 190, 198, 205, 206, 207, 208, 211, 219, 235, 239, 259, 266, 276, 278, 283, 287, 294, 297
Antispasmodics, 39, 46, 48, 49, 56, 59, 61, 72, 75, 80, 86, 99, 100, 101, 121, 134, 138, 147, 151, 166, 184, 198, 199, 203, 209, 214, 227, 228, 230, 235, 249, 251, 267, 268, 272, 275, 282, 285, 289, 300, 301, 308
Antisyphilitic, 54, 66, 317
Antitoxin, 113
Antivenereal, 261
Antrum, pain in, 19, 294
Antrum of Highmore, inflammation of, 74
Anus, affections of, 9; burning in, 53; fissure of, 58, 210, 224, 281; fistula in, 281; herpes of, 62; itching of, 203; prolapsus of, 120, 137, 193
Anutini glazki, 288
Anxiety, 154
Aperients, 44, 61, 89, 97, 109, 125, 212
Aphasia, 167, 309
Aphonia, 43, 55, 135, 156, 316
Aphrodisiacs, 50, 54, 72, 75, 97, 108, 138, 139, 275, 303
Aphrodite's shoe, 174
Aphthae, 71

Aphthous ulcers, 131
Apiol, 212
Apium graveolens, 75
Apocynum, 65; androsaemifolium, 39, 40, 49, 196; cannabinum, 49
Apoplexy, 17, 150, 164, 167, 309; threatened, 100
Appendicitis, 113, 139, 164
Appendix, inflammation of, 116
Appetizer, 14, 22, 38, 50, 68, 75, 242, 275, 286, 290, 291, 311, 315
Appetite, 4, 33, 77, 139, 141, 145, 149, 221, 275, 311
Apple cider, 4
Apple peru, 166
Aralia manchurian, 242, 257; nudicaulis, 240, 241; racemosa, 240, 256, 296
Arberry, 29
Arbor-vitae, 279, 281
Arbutus, 14; trailing, 14
Archangel, 13
Arctium lappa, 62, 234, 262, 302
Arctostaphylos uva ursi, 15, 29, 30, 169, 225, 296
Ardor urinea, 226, 250
Aristolochia serpentaria, 289
Armoracia rusticana, 155
Arnica, 15; chamissonic, 17; montana, 15, 16
Aromatics, 14, 37, 75, 142, 161 189, 197, 198, 239, 243, 274, 275 291, 312, 317
Arsesmart, 10, 294
Artemisia absinthium, 309, 310; vulgaris, 200, 201
Arterial sedative, 55, 149; tension, 149
Arteriosclerosis, 87, 95, 300
Arthritic pains, 5, 164; symptoms, 26
Arthritis, 20, 83, 87, 93, 223
Arum triphyllum, 112
Asarum canadense, 28, 136, 137; europeum, 137
Ascaris worm, 280, 309
Ascites, 50, 52, 75, 172, 180, 210, 246
Asclepias syriaca, 195; tuberosa, 155, 221, 222
Ash tree, 19
Aspidium filix mas, 217
Aspirin, 304
Asthenic insomnia, 214
Asthma, 3, 23, 32, 44, 47, 50, 55, 68, 71, 75, 92, 93, 101, 112, 116, 121, 122, 138, 144, 147, 149, 150, 151, 155, 157, 161, 162, 166, 168, 172, 176, 179, 185, 186, 187, 188, 189, 191, 196, 203, 222, 224, 227, 236, 240, 242, 245, 246, 251, 256, 259, 267, 275, 276, 278, 281, 291, 301, 309, 316, 318; from anger, 81; bronchial, 152, 167, 173, 180, 193, 244, 312; spasmodic, 123

354

Asthma weed, 184
Astigmatism, 135
Astringents, 3, 4, 10, 12, 15, 28, 29, 32, 34, 35, 36, 44, 45, 48, 54, 66, 75, 85, 86, 89, 92, 94, 101, 103, 107, 111, 116, 121, 122, 127, 128, 129, 131, 142, 146, 157, 159, 165, 170, 180, 183, 184, 188, 189, 195, 203, 204, 206, 207, 213, 218, 219, 228, 231, 235, 237, 239, 247, 249, 254, 258, 259, 263, 264, 266, 278, 288, 297, 298, 303, 305, 306, 313, 315, 316
Atonic dyspepsia, 110; gout, 68; intestines, 14, 211; leucorrhoea, 180
Atrophy of testes, 244
Aunee, 117
Auxiliary glands, suppuration of, 53
Avena sativa, 208, 209
Avitaminosis, 38, 100, 211, 300
Avthea, 296
Axilla, pain in, 65

Babies, teething, 59
Babunah, 82
Babuni-ke-phul, 82
Bacha, 275
Back ache, 17, 23, 62, 83, 93, 100, 118, 160, 229, 298, 317
Balanitis, 281
Baldness, 17
Baldrianic acid, 18
Balls, E. K., 57
Balm of Gilead, 22, 225, 277
Balmony, 21
BALSAM: fir, 22; poplar, 277
Balsam resin, 31, 285
Banaf shah, 288
Bania, 38
Baptisia tinctoria, 163
Barberry, 23, 24, 25, 119
Barber's itch—see Sycosis
Barley, 25; wild, 26
Barley water, 26, 27
Barosma betulina, 98, 212; crenata, 15
Barrenness, 56
Baryta, 279
Basserin, 241
Basswood, 181
Bastard agrimony, 2
Bayberry, 27, 231
Bearberry, 29, 30
Bearing down pains, 56, 96, 102
BEAR'S: foot, 31, 201; moss, 148; weed, 317
Beast killer, 259
Beaver tree, 189
Bed sores, 17, 114
Bedstraw, 89
Bed-wetting—see Enuresis
Bee-stings, 205, 240
Beechdrop, 31, 104

Beechnut tree, 32
Beech tree, 32
BEGGAR'S: buttons, 62; tick, 272
Belaya/bereza, 38
Belena chernaya, 152; vonuchaya, 152
Beleni obelsia, 152
Belladonna, 43, 132
Berberidis amerenis, 25; vulgaris, 25
Berberis vulgaris, 23, 24, 119
Beresovy venic, 38
Bernard, Dr. R., 139
Beth root, 33
Betula alba, 36, 37; lenta, 305
Bichu, 206
Bidens bipinnata, 272; connata, 272; frondosa, 272; triparita, 272, 273
Bilberry, 34, 35
Bile, 24, 41; to increase, 25; to promote, 17, 95 194, 198, 223, 311
Biliary colic, 25
Bilious attack, 25, 52, 58, 110, 164, 194, 247, 265, 288, 293, 302; colic, 53, 105, 130, 301; disease, 193; fever, 52, 61, 62, 135, 165, 222, 223, 293; headache, 81, 134, 164, 194, 236
BIRCH, 36, 37, 77, 305; broom, 38; mushroom, 76, 77
Bird's nest, 39, 298
Bird pepper, 67
Birth root, 33
Birthwort, 289
Bites, 147, 164, 172, 210, 212, 259; insect, 9, 120, 166, 219, 250, 278, 296, 312; mad dog, 40, 63, 113, 152, 159, 160, 210; snake, 20, 47, 113, 114, 120, 155, 160, 166, 183, 219, 221, 245, 246, 250, 269, 289, 301
BITTER: ash, 292; bloom, 76; clover, 76; herb, 21; poison, 274; root, 39, 40, 49, 65, 196; sweet, 42
BLACK: alder, 4; birch, 36; cohosh, 45, 46, 58, 98, 177, 223, 302; haw, 47, 48, 201, 212, 260; henbane, 152; Indian hemp, 49; larch, 277; nightshade, 133; prinos verticillatus, 4; root, 51, 105, 159, 193; Sampson, 113; snakeroot, 45, 239; walnut, 52, 53; willow, 302
Blackberry, 44, 115
Black eye, 17, 172, 307
Blackheads, 64
Bladder, 9, 30, 33, 49, 74, 99, 100, 102, 141, 203, 213, 248, 249, 259, 265, 271, 275, 278, 312, 316; affections of, 25, 43, 122, 164, 191, 242, 288; bleeding of, 34, 208; catarrh of, 34, 104, 160, 179, 182, 218, 226, 246, 298; gravel, 89, 146, 255; haemorrhage, 127; infection, 116; inflammation of, 23, 94, 133, 143, 144, 154, 179, 201, 212, 272, 300; irritation of,

Bruises, 3, 16, 17, 19, 25, 68, 81, 84, 92, 93, 97, 128, 159, 162, 166, 172, 173, 201, 230, 243, 248, 254, 258, 259, 263, 280, 307, 311, 312
Buchu, 15, 63, 89, 98, 121, 212
Buffalo herb, 7
Bugbane, 45
Bug chaser daurian, 47
Buk, 33
Bull's foot, 91
Bunions, 63, 150, 259
Burdock, 25, 62, 67, 75, 159, 234, 242, 253, 262, 265, 275, 284, 302
Burning bush, 292
Burning sensation, 69, 98, 112; fever and infections, 207, 222
Burns, 43, 63, 88, 93, 97, 100, 114, 116, 133, 159, 164, 167, 205, 208, 210, 215, 216, 219, 226, 233, 235, 259, 266, 307, 312, 316
Burnt alum, 5, 10
Burr marigold, 2
Bursting veins, 258
Buttercup, 105, 106
Butterfly weed, 221
BUTTER: nut, 64; rose, 122
Button snakeroot, 119

Cachlearia officinalis, 98
Caecum, inflammation of, 150
Calamus, 41, 273
Calcium, 7, 26, 56, 92, 110, 269; oxalate, 112
Calculus, 25, 97, 143, 146, 242; affections, 119, 301; prevention of, 205; urinary, 15
Calendula, 6, 16, 201
Calico bush, 66
Californian buckthorn, 69
Calla lily, 297; palustris, 297
Calming, 82, 111, 151, 154, 174, 200, 202, 225, 285
Calomel, 51
Canada snake root, 136
CANADIAN: golden rod, 142; moonseed, 316
Cancer, 6, 32, 43, 55, 74, 78, 79, 83, 90, 93, 132, 144, 149, 164, 194, 224, 226, 233, 234, 235, 281, 287, 288, 307, 315; of breast, 218; of lip, 144; of rectum, 224; of stomach, 83, 102, 252; of throat, 287; of tongue, 48, 288; of womb, 253
CANCER: root, 31, 32; weed, 183
Cancerillo, 43
Cancerous cachexia, 113; degeneration, 131; sores, 300
Candle berry, 27
Canker, 38, 231, 266, 298; sores, 63, 145, 236
CANKER: lettuce, 228; root, 145; wort, 109

Capillary, 68; bronchitis, 23; circulation of brain, 139
Capon's tail, 285
Capsella bursa pastoris, 247, 248
Capsicum, 28, 67, 68, 101, 126, 144, 185, 227, 250, 304; frutescens, 67; minimum, 67
Caraway, 246
Carbohydrates, metabolism, 211
CARBONATE: of lime, 68; of potash, 71
Carbon monoxide poisoning, 187
Carbuncles, 17, 29, 63, 113, 114, 122, 182, 201, 203, 242, 259, 300
Cardamon, 76
Cardiac diseases, 135; sclerosis, 41, 50, 200; stimulant, 46
Cardial asthma, 47; dropsy, 38, 40, 263
Cardialgia, 186
Carminatives, 14, 41, 67, 72, 75, 80, 82, 89, 125, 136, 142, 143, 161, 168, 197, 198, 209, 210, 211, 227, 239, 274, 275, 282, 305
Carolina pink, 216
Carotene, 99
Carotin, 54, 100
Carpinus americanus, 32
Cartilage, 53
Cascara sagrada, 4, 69
Case wort, 247
Cassia, 193, 217, 247; acutifolia, 247; angustifolia, 247; marilandica, 52, 246
Castanea dentata, 85, 86
Castor bean, 70
Castor oil, 10, 70, 71, 309
Catalepsy, 167, 201, 281, 311
Cataract, 157, 194, 218
Catarrh, 29, 33, 43, 44, 50, 55, 61, 81, 97, 104, 119, 121, 122, 137, 144, 159, 171, 182, 191, 210, 223, 241, 245, 246, 248, 263, 267, 275, 278, 313, 316, 318; of bladder, 34, 104, 160, 218, 226, 246, 298; of duodenum, 25, 71, 194; gastric, 144, 194, 284; of genito-urinary passage, 276; intestinal, 55, 144, 224; of lungs, 33, 204, 258, 278; nasal, 75; post-nasal, 75, 145, 281
Catarrhal affections, 188, 222, 252, 288, 296; conditions, 24, 117, 157, 179; diarrhoea, 28; fever, 197; inflamed bowels, 27; pneumonia, 210
Catchstraw, 89
Cathartics, 4, 21, 49, 51, 52, 57, 64, 65, 70, 74, 115, 127, 133, 136, 160, 175, 184, 193, 197, 223, 245, 246, 261, 277, 293, 300; excess, 192
Catheter fever, 212
Catkin willow, 302
Catmint, 72
Catnip, 72, 185

357

362

363

Haemoptysis, 55, 74, 152, 172
Haemorrhages, 5, 10, 34, 43, 104, 128, 134, 144, 152, 169, 180, 200, 203, 205, 206, 207, 231, 240, 248, 263, 266, 267, 275, 281, 307; of bladder, 127; of bowels, 12, 306, 313; of lungs, 28, 107, 204, 306, 313; of stomach, 28, 107, 204, 255, 306; rectal, 266; of urinary organs, 204, 306
Haemorrhagic diathesis, 307
Haemorrhoidal discharge, 186
Haemorrhoids, 9, 10, 19, 23, 29, 43, 45, 51, 55, 68, 69, 73, 74, 87, 88, 97, 116, 120, 121, 127, 133, 144, 159, 164, 194, 203, 204, 207, 219, 220, 224, 236, 253, 254, 257, 259, 261, 262, 263, 276, 278, 281, 295, 302, 307, 313, 314, 318; bleeding, 10, 107, 208, 248, 295, 307, 316; inflamed, 203; itching, 208
Haemostatic, 206, 207
Hair, affections, diseases, 44, 281; light, alive, 81; loss of, 159, 206, 208, 238, 275, 314; restoring, 71, 83; tonic, 31, 64, 154, 190, 191, 205, 269, 275
Haircap moss, 148
Hamamelis japanica, 307; virginica, 306
Hands, affections of, 56; chapped, 240, 242; pains in, 172
Hardrock, 263
Hashish, 50
Hay fever, 43, 106, 127, 135, 142, 197, 210, 225, 246, 252, 257
Hay maids, 5
Hazelwood, 276
Head, hot distempers of, 45, 99, 287; lice, 51; noise, 144, 251, 307
Headaches, 6, 9, 16, 32, 33, 47, 50, 52, 53, 55, 65, 66, 68, 74, 82, 89, 102, 112, 130, 132, 135, 137, 139, 146, 157, 171, 173, 174, 176, 182, 186, 197, 198, 206, 221, 223, 224, 225, 227, 235, 242, 251, 259, 263, 266, 267, 272, 280, 281, 283, 286, 287, 295, 302, 309, 312, 314, 317; bilious, 81, 134, 150, 164, 194, 236, 258, 291; of children, 203; chronic, 97; due to colds, 115; dull, 177; gastric, 110, 291; intermittent, 58; migraine, 47, 50, 58, 65, 100, 108, 137; numbness, 177; nervous, 41, 73, 75, 132, 134, 150, 174, 214, 250, 268; syphilitic, mercurial, catarrhal, 262; from sun, 66, 135, 167
Heal-all, 263
Healing herb, 92
Hearing, altered, 224; decayed, 6
Heart, 6, 59, 66, 68, 69, 92, 123, 141, 157, 255, 304; affections, conditions diseases, disorders, trouble, 19, 29, 41, 44, 50, 66, 89, 94, 102, 129, 130, 132, 133, 135, 137, 144, 147, 149, 150, 158,

164, 186, 200, 203, 221, 223, 224, 236, 251, 263, 271, 286, 295, 316; deficiencies, 41; failure, 95; fatty, hypertrophy of, 46, 86, 224; neurosis, 200; pains in, 194, 316; palpitations, 32, 48, 85, 137, 153, 186, 194, 199, 209, 272, 280; stimulant, 49, 197, 206; tonic, 49, 133, 190; weakness of, 17, 43, 86, 139, 200, 250
Heart-burn, 14, 24, 54, 68, 75, 130, 132, 198, 274
Heart herb, 200
Heat, effects of, 135, 187
Hectic fever, 85, 105, 164
Hedeoma, 215; pulegioides, 214, 215, 250
Hedera helex, 165
Helianthemum canadense, 131, 234
Helianthus annuus, 268
Hellebore, 148; American, 148, 150
Helleborus foetidus, 201
Hemicrania, 309
Hemiplegia, 227, 309
Hemlock, 134
Hemp agrimony, 2
Henbane, 150, 151; sticnky, 152
Henbell, 151
Hepatic, 88, 130, 193; affections, 57, 74, 262; congestion, 302; disease, 51, 125; lack of activity, 227; torpor, 117, 123
Hepatica acutiloba, 170; americana, 170; nobilis, 170
Hepatitis, 185
Herba ledu, 172
Herb peter, 99
Hernia, 68, 82, 94, 210, 242, 281; strangulated, 23
Herpes, 5, 25, 53, 54, 65, 97, 133, 253; of anus, 62; labialis pudendi, 23; neuralgia, 66, 220; of prepuce, 242; preputialis, 53; zoster, 58, 66, 106, 281
Heuchera americana, 10
Hiccoughs, 1, 62, 75, 86, 106, 150, 152, 167, 197, 242, 250
Hickory nut, 52
High blood pressure, 41, 47, 77, 95, 102, 180, 190, 200, 211, 251, 265, 314
HIGH: cranberry, 101; mallow, 191
Hindheel, 279
Hip, gout, 5; joint disease, 58, 262,
Hlopok, 96
Hmel, 154
Hoarseness, 62, 88, 112, 128, 155, 156, 165, 177, 179, 182, 191, 198, 263, 287, 288
Hog apple, 192
Hog's bean, 151
Holy weed, 318
Home-sickness, 68, 77, 146, 180
Hood-wort, 249

365

Hook worms, 309
Hop horn beam, 176
Hops, 144, 153, 275, 291
Hoptree, 291
Hordeum distichun, 25; jubatum, 26; vulgare, 25
Horehound, 91, 154, 199
HORSE: balm, 263; chestnut, 86; dock, 316; fly bush, 163; hoof, 91; mint, 203; radish, 155, 156, 278; tail, 157, 158; weed, 263
Horsetail grass, 1
Hound's tongue, 158, 159
Hren, 157
Huckleberry, 34
Humulus lupulus, 153
Hurtleberry, 34
Hvosh polevoy, 158
Hydragogue, 115, 133, 193, 300
Hydrangea, 160; arborescens, 160
Hydrastis, 4, 104, 227; canadensis, 25, 52, 95, 111, 130, 142, 143, 145, 218, 234, 236, 250, 304; kanadsky, 145
Hydrocele, 106, 165
Hydrocephaloid, 123, 194
Hydrocephalus, 50, 132, 202, 311
Hydrocyanic acid, 85
Hydrophobia, 23, 33, 113, 152, 167, 249, 250, 259, 280
Hydro-salpingitis, 135
Hydrothorax, 65
Hyoscyamus niger, 150. 151
Hypericum perforatum, 257
Hyperpyrexia, 150
Hypersensitiveness, 259
Hypnotic, 49, 151, 153
Hypochondriasis, 23, 152, 174
Hypovitaminosis, 211
Hyssop, 161
Hyssopus officinalis, 161
Hysteria, 9, 14, 19, 46, 47, 49, 53, 73, 81, 82, 101, 102, 125, 126, 135, 137, 146, 155, 164, 167, 174, 180, 185, 186, 199, 200, 202, 208, 215, 225, 227, 250, 252, 258, 261, 280, 283, 285, 286, 288, 295, 308, 311
Hysterics, to relieve, 56, 197

Ice plant, 39
Ichthyosis, 281
Ilet decidua, 29
"Imanin", 259
Impetigo, 5, 58, 147; figurata, 65
Impostumes, 110
Impotence, 63, 108, 146, 220, 224, 259, 304
Incipient nephritis, 97; structure, 144
Incontincene, 44, 75, 98, 108, 120, 146, 160, 193, 203, 313

INDIAN: apple, 192; arrowroot, 292; balm, 33; bark, 189; chamomile, 82; corn, 94; cup plant, 230; elm, 252; ginger, 136; gum, 230; hemp, 49; hyssop, 59; indigo, 164; physic, 135; pink, 216; pipe, 39; plant, 54; poke, 148; sage, 60; salt, 265; sarsaparilla, 242; senna, 247; solanum, 44; spikenard, 256; tobacco, 184
Indigestion, 14, 38, 60, 62, 68, 69, 85, 119, 125, 138, 139, 146, 169, 197, 198, 213, 236, 261, 263, 296, 311, 313, 316
Indigo–wild, 163
Indolent tumour, 90; ulcers, 4, 34, 104, 147, 165, 186, 227, 234, 276, 304
Infantile cholera, 71, 104, 123, 194, 215; colic, 247; convulsions, 80; diarrhoea, 225, 231, 298
Infant's carminative, 305
Inflammations, 1, 22, 25, 65, 66, 71, 88, 89, 94, 95, 116, 119, 126, 127, 128, 129, 133, 134, 148, 149, 168, 186, 188, 191, 202, 203, 207, 208, 229, 241, 252, 253, 255, 256, 259, 269, 280, 288, 306, 311, 314, 317; of bladder, 23, 94, 133, 143, 144, 154, 179, 201, 212, 272, 300; of bowels, 27, 88, 135; of brain, 112; of breast, 31, 71; of ears, 162, 172, 220, 287; of eyes, 77, 88, 115, 132, 176, 191, 269, 307, 313; of gall-bladder, 23, 25; of genetalis, 17, 25, 253; of gums, 298; internal, 88, 241; of intestines, 87, 219, 254; of kidneys, 94, 133, 179, 180, 201, 204, 212; of liver, 88; of lungs, 59, 88, 126, 176, 182, 198, 222, 287; of nose, 17, 29; of stomach, 88, 126, 129, 145, 221, 254; of throat, 45, 102, 203, 234, 266, 307; of urinary tract, 29, 121, 160
Inflammatory rheumatism, 149, 196
Influenza, 28, 55, 61, 62, 74, 82, 120, 135, 144, 150, 161, 163, 164, 174, 191, 197, 198, 209, 210, 222, 223, 224, 233, 246, 262, 275, 280, 296, 313, 318; intermittent, 77
Inguinal glands, swollen, 23
Injuries, 25
Inkberry, 223
Inonotus, obliquus, 76, 77
Insanity, 6, 23, 50, 73
Insect bites, 9, 120, 166, 219, 250, 278, 296, 312; stings, 34, 164
Insecticide, 151, 160, 175, 275, 280
Insomnia, 135, 154, 174, 199, 200, 209, 214, 215, 247, 249, 250, 251; during fever, 285
Insulin, 36, 211
Intermittents, 61, 68, 77, 156, 194, 205, 218, 242; chills, 291; fever, 20, 39, 59, 61, 62, 80, 111, 122, 135, 136, 146, 165,

Intermittents—*cont.*
177, 206, 208, 212, 230, 236, 239, 248, 291, 311; influenza, 77
Intemperance, 61, 165
Internal bleeding, 92, 94, 96, 206, 221, 256, 266, 306, 313; bruises, 230; inflammation, 88, 241; wounds, 3, 5. 221
Intestinal catarrh, 55. 144, 224; pains of colic, 215; conditions, 27, 116, 176, 188; malfunctions, 264; tract, 28, 48, 158, 161, 178, 222, 239
Intestine, anaemia of, 47; atony of, 14, 211; chronic constipation, 51; inflammation of, 87, 219, 254, ulceration of, 23, 219, 221; weak, 264
Intoxication, 61, 165, 172
Intramammary pain, 56
Intussusception, 281
Inula helenium, 117, 118
Inulin, 63, 99, 110, 117, 118, 125
Invigorate the blood, 141
Involuntary emission, 59
Iodine, 6, 149, 269
Ipecacuanha, 275, 288
Iridin, 57, 58,
Iris, 57; douglasiana, 57; pseudacorus, 57; versicolor, 57, 58, 75, 262, 274
Iritis, 23, 147, 246
Iron, 6, 56, 86, 110, 111, 134, 188, 245, 249, 251, 269, 315; deficiency, 315
Iron oxide, 241
IRON: weed. 164; wood, 176
Irritant, 281
Itch, 24, 71, 74, 119, 128, 147, 153, 154, 172, 224, 240, 254, 265, 276, 294, 315, 316, 317
Itch weed, 148
Itching scabs, 6
Ivan and Mary, 288
Ivy, American, 165

Jack in the pulpit, 112
James, Claudia. V., 8, 90
Jame's tea, 172
Jamestown weed, 166
Jaundice, 4, 20, 22, 23, 25, 29, 41, 52, 55, 62, 66, 71, 74, 81, 82, 97, 99, 106, 110, 111, 115, 119, 130, 133, 135, 137, 144, 154, 155, 161, 171, 194, 206, 212, 218, 236, 255, 258, 271, 280, 291, 300, 311, 312; yellow, 3, 5, 24, 74, 128, 218, 248
Jaw, growth on, 281; joint pain, 112, 227
JERUSALEM: cowslip, 187; oak, 308
Jethi madh, 179
Jimson weed, 154, 166, 167
Joe-pye weed, 146
Johnswort, 257
Joint, affections, 25, 58, 89, 172, 203, 262; cracking in Menier's disease, 172, 281;

felons, 19; jaw, pain in, 112, 227; pain, 17, 76, 205, 281, 302, 306; rheumatic, 16, 82, 133, 146; sprain, 16; swelling, 116, 204, 306
Joster, 69
Juglandin, 64, 65
Juglans cinerea, 64; nigra, 52, 53; regia, 54
Jugnog, 94
JUNIPER: 167, 168, 278, 296; berries, 157, 168; bush, 168; vulgaris, 169
Juniperus communis, 167, 168, 278; osteosperma, 163, 296
Jupiter's bean, 151

Kakmachi, 133
Kalgan, 128
Kalina, 48, 102; yagoda, 49
Kalinushka, 102
Kalmia latifolia, 66
Kansas niggerhead, 113
Kasatik, 58
Kastorka, 71
Kayansky peretz, 68
Keloed, 107
Kendir konoplevy, 41, 50
Keratitis, 55, 66
Kerotin, 188, 192
KIDNEY: liver leaf, 170; root, 146
Kidneys, 9, 30, 33, 49, 74, 83, 99, 115, 141, 163, 173, 182, 203, 213, 231, 248, 249, 252, 265, 271, 275, 278, 301, 312, 313, 316; affections of, conditions of, diseases of, trouble, 23, 24, 29, 57, 63, 88, 102, 104, 116, 119, 122, 157, 160, 164, 179, 191, 196, 199, 203, 218, 219, 221, 225, 269, 277, 288, 293, 296, 298, 299, 318; congestion of, 23, 290; gravel, 89, 146, 206, 255; haemorrhage, 206; inflammation of, 94, 133, 179, 180, 201, 204, 212; pain in, 213; palilloma of, 298; sluggish, 169; to soothe, 63; stimulant, 206; stones, 37, 38, 95, 158, 202, 209, 255, 265, 275, 293; ulcerated, 93
Killing the beast, 259
King, Prof., 148
Kinnikinnik, 29
Klamath weed, 257
Klen, 195
Klopogon daursky, 47
Kloss, J., 68, 110, 160, 196, 205, 227, 233, 239, 252, 258, 278, 280, 302
Knee, pain in, 25, 302
Knight's spur, 174
Kneip, S., 168
Knit bone, 92
Knob-root, 263
Konsky cashtan, 86; shavel, 316

367

Koopena, 255
Kopiten, 137
Koroviak visoky, 203
Kozo-Poliansky, B. M., 211
Krameria triandra, 164
Krapiva, 205
Krasny peretz, 68
Kreig, M. B., 177
Krestovnik, 180
Krovavnik, 314
Krushina, 69
Kukuruza, 95
Kupchan, Dr., 43
Kurinye lapke, 128
Kuvshinka nymphaea alba, 298

La grippe—*see* Influenza
Labia, abscess of, 96, 280
Labour, 135, 263; abnormal, false pain of, 56, 102; disorders of, 82; effect of, 259; pains, 47, 202
Labrador tea, 172, 173
Lachrymal fistula, 74
Lactation, 71, 205, 227; abnormal, 224; disorder of, 218
Lactifuge, 54
Lactogogue, 71
Lady's slipper, 173, 185, 250
Lakonos americana, 224
Lambkill, 66
Lapchatka, 128
Lappa, 62, 242, 265, 284; minor, 25, 62
Larch, 277
Larix alaskensis, 278; americana, 277; siberia, 278
LARK'S: claw, 174; heel, 174
Larkspur, 174, 175
Larrea divaricata, 82
Larynx, affections of, 262; dry, 116
Laryngismus, 224
Laryngitis, 19, 55, 74, 120, 210, 267, 272, 295, 296
Laurus sassafras, 242
Laxatives, 10, 20, 24, 31, 40, 54, 69, 70, 71, 75, 88, 97, 101, 108, 137, 143, 155, 177, 179, 199, 225, 246, 247, 275, 278, 288, 292, 300, 309, 315, 317
Lead colic, 6; poisoning, 159
Lead oxide, 279
Leafcup, 31
Ledum latifolium, 172, 173; marshland, 172; palustra, 172
Leg pain 220, 302
Lemon, 177
Lemon walnut, 64
Leontodon taraxacum, 95, 109, 218, 234
Leonurus cardiaca, 98, 198, 199
Leopard's bane, 15
Leprosy, 43, 54, 314

Laptandra, 51, 193; virginica, 51, 105
Lepthandrin, 52
Lesser celandine, 73
Lethargy, 293
Leucocythemia, 236
Leucoma, 194
Leukaemia, 83; splenica, 208
Leucorrhoea, 5, 10, 13, 25, 28, 29, 30, 34, 36, 47, 55, 56, 63, 66, 93, 104, 108, 118, 120, 121, 134, 143, 144, 157, 165, 180, 182, 205, 207, 216, 219, 224, 229, 231, 236, 240, 242, 253, 254, 257, 261, 266, 276, 294, 298, 307, 309, 311, 313
Leverwood, 176
Levitation, 215, 281, 293; sensation of, 53, 137
Lewisia rediviva, 40
Lice, 4, 51, 175
Lichen, 65, 182, 187, 224, 316; caninus, 170
Licorice, 177, 178
Lienteria, 82
Life Elixir, 111
Life for ever lasting, 141
Life root, 178, 179
Lignin, 111, 249
Ligustrum amurense, 227; vulgare, 227
Like of man, 256
Lime, 134, 233, 241, 251, 285; carbonate of, 68; potash, 111
Lime tree, 181
Linden, 181; flower, 181
Liniment, 68, 69, 271, 311
Linum, 177
LION'S: ear, 199; root, 183; tail, 199; tooth, 109
Lips, cancer of, 144; chapped, 17
Lippia, 183; dulcis, 183
Lippa, 182
Liquidambar styraciflua, 276
Listvennitza sibirsky, 278
Lithotriptic, 206
Liver, 3, 9, 22, 24, 29, 33, 38, 41, 44, 59, 61, 75, 88, 99, 105, 110, 123, 147, 170, 195, 213, 258, 259, 275, 280, 299, 300, 314; to activate, 95, 141, 149; affections, complaints, conditions, disorders, malfunctions, troubles, 25, 29, 52, 58, 60, 74, 75, 77, 88, 110, 115, 130, 135, 144, 158, 177, 180, 193, 194, 196, 199, 218, 224, 225, 227, 230, 292, 293, 300, 302, 311, 312; colic, 249; congestion of, 130, 291; cough, 55; degeneration, 10; engorged, 69; enlarged, 44, 55, 133, 164, 176, 278; feverish, 35; hardening of, 223, 278, hypertrophy of, 130; inactivity, 236, 311; inefficiency, 89; inflammation of, 88; jaundice, 55, 212; morbid, 55; obstructions of, 3, 74, 110;

368

369

371

Olive oil, 253, 258, 276, 312
Onanism, effect of, 9
One berry, 213
Onion, 139, 210, 211, 297
Operations, effect of, 259
Ophthalmia, 25, 43, 51, 55, 62, 81, 104, 131, 143, 183, 194, 223, 227, 228; chronic, 25; tarsi, 240
Opium, 39, 50, 150, 151, 166, 201; excess of, 125; habit, 209
Orange root, 143
Orchitis, 51, 128, 150, 224, 295
Orobanche virginiana, 31
Ossification, too early, 240
Ostria virginiana, 176
Os uteri, dilated, 240
Otorrhoea, 75; suppressed, 288
Ova-ova, 39
Ovaries, affections of, 307; neuralgia of, 56, 106; numbness in, 194; pain in, 23, 96, 102, 194, 304; tumour of, 194
Over-excitement, 125
Oves, 209
Oxalic acid, 255
Oxaluria, 25
Ox balm, 263
Oxymethyl-anthraquinones, 18
Oxytocic, 56, 96
Ozaena, 145, 224, 240

Paigles, 99
Palma christe, 70
Palpitations, 32, 48, 85, 137, 153, 186, 194, 199, 209, 272, 280
Palsenovaya, 44
Palsy, 99, 115, 250
Palsywort, 99
Panacea, 141
Panaritium, 210, 259
Panax, 138, 141; quinquefolium, 58, 137, 138
Pancreas, 29, 117, 156, 293; affections of, 58, 235; lack of activity, 227; weak, 119
Pannag, 138
Panophthalmitis, 224
Pappoose root, 56
Paralysis, 17, 43, 68, 102, 135, 152, 156, 158, 160, 167, 176, 256, 259, 276, 280, 281, 309; agitans, 135, 152, 284; diphtheritic, 224, facial, 210, 246; temporary, 227; of tongue and mouth, 68, 227
Paraplegia, 66, 135
Parasiticide, 175
Parkinson, 40, 132, 191, 248, 293
Parkinson's disease, 176
Paronychia, 302
Parotid glands, affection of, 58
Parotitis, 82, 132, 152, 224, 302

Paroxysmal, 86
Parsley, 169, 191, 212; breakstone, 212
Partridge berry, 213
Parturients, 56, 96, 105, 136, 213, 231
Paslen cherny, 134; dolchaty, 134; kisoladky, 44
Passiflora incarnata, 214, 250, 267
Passion flower, 214, 250, 267
Pastushya sumka, 248
Peach, 169
Peach-wort, 18
Pear leaf pyrola, 228
Pearl barley, 27
Pectic acid, 241, 245
Pectin, 68
Pectoral, 5, 34, 85, 87, 91, 124, 172, 177, 179, 180, 188, 191, 203, 204, 254; affections, 203
Pedicularis palustris, 126
Pediculosis, 172
Pegwood, 292
Pelargonium, 103
Pelvic disorders, 135, 144; haematocele, 307
Pemphigus, 43, 65, 106, 281
Pennyroyal, 250, 290; American, 214, 215
Peppermint, 41, 71, 76, 197, 285, 313
Pepperwort, 294
Pereleska blagorodnaya, 171
Pericarditis, 223
Perichondritis, 82
Periodical headache, 50, 82; pains, 166
Periostitis, 185, 262
Peritonitis, 71, 82, 132, 182, 185
Peritonium, sensitive, painful, 94
PERSIAN: bark, 69; chamomile, 82
Persicaria maculata, 18
Perspiration, 57, 61, 80, 127, 157, 209, 226, 240; to promote, 73, 105, 134, 136, 142, 149, 155, 156, 182, 215, 222, 227, 250, 283, 289, 313
Peruvian bark, 111, 225
Pervo-Tzvet, 100
Petroselinum sativum, 169, 212
Petrushka, 212
Petty morrel, 256
Pewterwort, 157
Pharyngitis, 55
Pharynx, affections, 29
Phimosis, 307, 316
Phlegmasea alba dolens, 307
Phlegm, 85; in chest, 155, 258; in head, 258; in lungs, 204, 258; in stomach, 88, 204
Phlegmasia dolens, 205
Phosphate of potash, 68, 86; of lime, 285
Phosphatic acid, 94
Phosphaturia, 63, 143, 291

372

Phosphorus, 6, 7, 56, 108, 110, 269
Phrenitis, 185
Phthisis (*see also* Consumption and Tuberculosis), 9, 46, 180, 238, 252, 276, 316, 318; florida, 55; mucosa, 246
Physic, 184
Physical shock, 16; exhaustion, 242, 257
Physometra, 55
Phytochinin, 211
Phytolacca decandra, 58, 60, 218, 223
Pickoocker, 247
Pigeon berry, 223
Piles—*see* Haemorrhoids
Pile wort, 11, 73, 127
Pimpinella anisum, 217
Pimples, 172, 256, 293, 298
Pinheads, 80
PINK: pyrola, 228; root, 216, 246
Pinus strobus, 295, 296
Pinworms, 50, 65, 145
Pipperidge bush, 23
Pipsissewa, 216, 217, 228, 262
Pirey polzutchy, 98
Pishma, 280
Pityriasis, 23, 56
Placenta, adherent, 145
Plague, 5, 164, 165, 268
Plantago lanceolate, 220, 294, 313; major, 218, 220
Plantain, 218, 220, 294, 313
Plethora, 92
Pleurisy, 51, 88, 105, 176, 185, 186, 191, 197, 222, 223, 245, 246, 252
Pleurisy root, 155, 221, 222
Pleuritic adhesion, 106
Pleurodynia, 17, 74, 106, 223, 306
Pleuropneumonia, 68
Plumbagin, 267
Plumbago, 18
Pneumonia, 74, 111, 134, 147, 149, 150, 152, 163, 174, 185, 194, 210, 245, 246, 289, 297; acute, 55
Pocan, 223
Podophyllum, 192; emodi, 194; peltatum, 58, 105, 192
Podoroshnik, 220
Podsolnechnik, 270
POISON: ash, 129; ivy, 147; oak, 147, 201
Poisoned wounds, 113
Poisons, 66, 94, 151, 155, 166, 168, 184, 193, 195, 207, 223; to expel, 5, 153, 241, 311
Poisoning, 38, 40, 71, 122, 137, 147, 159, 187; gas, 224
POKE: 58, 60; root, 218, 223; weed, 184
Polecat weed, 251
Polin, 311; obiknovennaya, 202
Polygala senega, 100, 119, 244, 245; vulgaris, 261

Polygalic acid, 245
Polygonatum biflorum, 254; commutatum, 253
Polygonic acid, 18
Polygonone, 18
Polygonum hydropiper, 18; punctatum, 60, 294, 295
Polymnia uvedalia, 31
Polypodium vulgare, 124
Polypus, 25, 55, 281
Polysaccharide, 99
Polytrichum juniperium, 148
Polyuria, 220
Pool root, 239
Poplar, 225, 296
Poppy, 81
Populus balsamifera, 277; canadensis, 225, 277; tremuloides, 30, 225, 296
Post-influenzal debility, 174
Post-nasal catarrh, 75, 145, 281
Potash, 241, 285
Potassium, 6, 7 56, 134, 212, 270; chloride, 241
Potentilla rausch, 128, 129; tormentilla neck, 128, 129
Pot-bellied children, 240
Poultices, 19, 20, 34, 36, 51, 59, 64, 69, 71, 72, 81, 84, 88, 90, 92, 93, 97, 116, 119, 131, 133, 134, 159, 160, 164, 165, 176, 182, 183, 191, 195, 201, 204, 219, 229, 235, 243, 253, 254, 263, 266, 272, 276, 278, 288, 295, 297, 298, 300, 301, 304, 307, 312, 314, 315, 316, 318
Pregnancy, 10, 56, 130, 301; affections during, 55, 199, 263; albuminaria of, 66, 135, cough, 102; cramps, 101; disorders of, 56, 68, 82; imaginary, 281; morning sickness, 58, 186; pyrosis of 302; dropsy during, 240; vomiting of, 53, 96, 261
Precipitate lime, 279
Prenanthes serpens, 183
Priapism, 212
PRICKLY: ash, 218, 224, 231, 262, 284; ash bark, 226; ash berries, 226
Prickly heat, 172
Prim, 227
Primula officinalis, 99, 100; veris 122
PRINCE'S: feather, 11; pine, 217
Privet, 227
Privy, 227
Proctalgia, 150
Proctitis, 9, 194, 218, 263
Prolapsus, 20, 71, 120; ani, 63, 120, 207, 257, 288; uteri, 9, 63, 121, 260, 261, 288
Prolonging life, 141
Promote bile, 17, 95, 194, 198, 223, 311; digestion, 28, 55, 76, 145, 244, 275, 290; menstruation, 71, 81, 169, 215,

373

Promote—*cont.*
280, 299, 308; milk, 137; perspiration,
73, 105, 134, 136, 142, 149, 155, 156,
182, 215, 222, 227, 250, 283, 289, 313
Prophylactic, 95, 267, 309
Prostate affections, 108, 160, 224, 226;
disease of, 281; gland, 83, 97, 98,
143, 180, 244, 253; irritation, 218, 298
Prostatitis, 180, 194, 213, 218, 224, 295,
304
Prostration, 47, 135, 164, 246, 304
Protein, 63, 270
Protoveratrine, 149
Prulent cystitis, 97
Prunin, 86
Prunus serotina, 25, 177, 256, 296;
virginiana, 84, 85
Prurigo, 5, 316
Pruritus, 198; vaginae, 147; vulvae, 147,
263
Prussic acid, 235
Psilosis, 265
Psoas abscess, 94
Psora, 5
Psoriasis, 58, 88, 179, 186, 262
Psoriasism eczema, 90
Psychasthenia, 141
Ptelea trifoliata, 291
Pterygium, 218
Ptosis, 66, 135, 281
Puerperal convulsions, 132, 135, 150;
fever, 149; mania, 150, 180
Pulmonaria angustifolia, 188; officinalis,
186, 187
Pulmonary obscura, 188
Pulmonary, 34, 83, 185, 222; affections,
117, 119, 155, 172, 276, complaints,
165, 180, 185, 188, 203; consumption—
see Phthisis; difficulties, 269; disease,
125; system, 91, 117
Pulsatilla, 130
Pulse, reduced, 47, 149
Purgatives, 9, 20, 51, 70, 71, 74, 115, 124,
125, 135, 136, 163, 193, 288
PURPLE: angelica, 13; boneset, 146; clover,
233; coneflower, 113
Purpura, 17, 53, 307
Pushki, 110
Pussywillow, 302
Pustirnik serdechny, 200
Pustules, 194
Pyelitis, 95
Pyoemia, 113
Pyorrhoea, 107, 144
Pyrethrum, 125; parthenium, 125
Pyrola, 228; asarifolia, 228; elliptica, 228;
rotundifolia, 228, vivens, 228
Pyrosis, 55, 86, 302

Quaking aspen, 30, 225
Quay, 240
QUEEN: of the meadow, 146; Anne's, lace
298
QUEEN'S: delight, 261, 284; root, 261, 267
Quercus robur, 207, 208
Quick grass, 97
Quill, 240
Quinine, 39, 111, 189, 225, 291, 303, 313
Quinine cachexia, 22, 122
Quinsy, 55, 128, 161, 163, 311

Racoonberry, 192
Radiculitis, 168
Rage, 152
Ragged cup, 230
Ragweed, 253
Ragwort, 179
Ramel, Dr., 122
Ranula, 281
Ranunculus bulbosus, 105, 106
Raspberry, 230, 232, 302
RATTLE: bush, 163; root, 45
RATTLESNAKE: master, 119; root, 183, 244
Rectal conditions, 75; 266; haemorrhage,
266; irritation, 234; suppository, 253,
316
Rectum, 104; affections of, diseases of, 68,
145, 263; burning in, 58; cancer of,
224; cramp in, 240; pain in, 118;
prolapsed, 207, 288
RED: berry, 138; clover, 75, 233, 234;
cock's comb, 11; elm, 252; gum, 82,
276; lobelia, 184; maple, 194; milk-
weed, 43; pepper, 67, 68; puccon, 54;
river snake root, 289; root, 234, 235;
sarsaparilla, 240; top sorrel, 255
Reduce weight, 83
Reducing, 90
Refrigerants, 24, 35, 87, 89, 191, 255, 266
Regenerate the glands, 141
Relaxed bowels, 3, 129, 221; bladder, 15,
218; vagina, 104
Relaxants, 146, 184, 198, 225
Remittent chills, 291; fever, 39, 52, 61,
62, 135, 230, 291
Renal colic, 25, 95, 120, 146, 180, 205,
242, 302; conditions, 233, 244; con-
gestion, 212; torpor, 290; tract, 239;
weakness, 225
Repeinik, 63
Repeinoe maslo, 64
Reproductive glands, 244; organs, 239
Resolvent, 42, 57, 155
Respiration, abnormal, 224, 280
Respiratory conditions, 100, 122, 147,
187, 192, 246, 318; congestion, 277;
organs, 55, 86, 93, 159, 222, 267;
process, 84; tract, 161, 313

Restlessness, 39, 80, 153, 174, 249, 285
Restorative tonic, 77, 119, 209, 230
Retina, detachment of, 135,
Retinitis bulism, 66
Rhagades, 242
Rhamnus purshiana, 69
Rhatany, 164
Rheum, 265; palmatum, 52
Rheumatic conditions, 29, 38, 43, 89,
  151, 216, 256, 315; disease, 97; gout,
  40, 56, 68, 133; joints, 16, 82, 133;
  liniment, 225; neuralgia, 106; pains, 20,
  23, 38, 76, 152, 160, 164, 168, 204, 206,
  219, 227, 237, 242, 271, 300, 302, 318;
  swelling, 276; symptoms, 26
Rheumatism 5, 17, 23, 24, 25, 37, 38, 43,
  46, 55, 56, 58, 62, 63, 68, 69, 71, 74,
  75, 82, 83, 84, 87, 88, 97, 98, 99, 106,
  110, 115, 116, 121, 122, 126, 134, 135,
  136, 139, 143, 146, 147, 151, 156, 157,
  166, 172, 173, 182, 189, 190, 196, 197,
  199, 201, 205, 223, 240, 241, 243, 246,
  247, 251, 259, 262, 263, 266, 269, 277,
  278, 288, 291, 296, 302, 303, 304, 305,
  306, 307, 311, 312, 316, 317, 318;
  acute, 47, 61, 149, 222; chronic, 31, 61,
  112, 160; chronic muscular, 227; of
  deltoid, 205; gonorrhoeal, 218, 224,
  242, 281; inflammatory, 149, 196;
  syphilitic, 224; wandering, 41
Rheumatism root, 301
Rhubarb, 265; root, 52
Rhus cariaria, 266; glabra, 264, 265;
  glabrum, 237;
Rhus poisoning, 55, 60, 113, 147
Riabinka obiknovennaya, 280
Rich-weed, 263
Ricin, 71
Rickets, 54, 125, 173, 202, 210, 240, 250,
  273, 275, 281
Ringworm, 24, 53, 55, 62, 63, 65, 71, 74,
  153, 218, 224, 240, 241, 255, 276
Ripple grass, 218
Robin's rye, 148
ROCK: parsley, 212; polypod, 124; rose,
  131, 234
Rodent ulcer, 65, 224
ROMAN: camomile, 80; wormwood, 310
Romashka, 82
ROOT: of life, 141; of man, 141
Rosemary, 68
Rose pink, 76
Rossianka, 267
Rough-fruited cinquefoil, 128
ROUND: leaf, 266; leaved pyrola, 228;
  lobed hepatica, 170
Round worm, 312
Rubefacients, 67, 105

Rubus idaeus, 230, 232; strigosus, 302;
  villosus, 44
Ruddock, Dr. E. H., 49, 56, 89, 126, 132,
  156, 204, 224
Rue, 210
Rumex, 315; abtusifolius, 315; acetosa,
  254, 255; aquaticus, 315; britannica,
  315; cripus, 25, 58, 69, 218, 234, 262,
  314, 315; rumicis 316
Running sores, 74, 128, 147, 155, 191
Ruptures, 93, 169, 254
RUSSIAN: centaury, 77; lippa, 182
Ruta graveolens, 210
Rutin, 19, 295

Sabal, 243; serrulata, 98
Sabbatia angularis, 76
Sabur, 10
Sacred bark, 69
Sacrum, pain in, 9, 25
Saddle sores on horses, 143, 166
Saffron, 73
Sage, 152, 161, 237, 238, 311
Salad herbs, 100, 110, 143, 191, 249, 255,
  293
Salap, 243
Salicin, 303
Salicylate, 305
Salicylic acid, 303
Salisb, 277
Salivary glands, 317
Salivation, 58, 155, 224, 226, 227, 245,
  294; nocturnal, 82
Salix alba. 304; capra. 304; fragilis, 304;
  nigra. 302, 303, 305
Saloop, 242
Salpingitis, 113
Salseparin, 241
Salt rheum weed, 21
Salts of alumina, 245
Salves, 88, 234, 278, 281
Salvia officinalis, 237, 238,
Sambucus, 114; canadensis, 144, 313
Sandalwood, 98
Sang, 138
Sangree root, 289
Sangrel, 289
Sanguinaria, 54, 104; canadensis, 46, 54
Sanicle, 238, 239
Sanicula marilandica, 238, 239
Santalum album, 98
Santa root, 141
Saponaria, 81
Saponin, 130
Sapwood, 276
Sarsaparilla, 58, 71, 83, 240, 241. 261, 317
Sassafras, 241. 242, 296; albidum, 241;
  laurus, 296
Satin flower, 87

375

Skin—*cont.*
119, 122, 157, 164, 177, 179, 194, 209, 221, 226, 239, 240, 259, 265, 275, 283, 288, 307, 311, 315, 316; discolorations of, 100, 153, 210, 254, 265, 298, 300, 311; diseases of, affections of, 4, 33, 43, 44, 54, 65, 90, 110, 116, 133, 143, 153, 165, 172, 173, 203, 218, 222, 223, 229, 242, 247, 266, 284, 316, 317; eruptions, 38, 88, 133, 144, 172, 241, 243; freckles, 59, 89, 97, 100, 110, 116, 209, 254, 255, 280, 293, 298, irritations, 6, 66, 92, 154, 221, 272; itching, 119, 153, 154, 224; lesions, 9, 229; liver spots, 110; rash, 17, 119, 208, 265, 314; to soften, 80, 100, 116, 149; tonic, 225, 293; tuberculosis, 102, 143, 288; ulcers, 29, 95, 240, 259, 266; water blisters, 267
SKULL CAP: 101, 144, 155, 174, 185, 222, 248, 249, 285; helmet flower, 249
SKUNK: cabbage, 101, 251, 301; weed, 251
Sleep, disordered, 135, 152; dreamful 150; encourage, 50, 71, 286; producing, 50, 141, 151, 152, 153, 154, 215, 272, 285
Sleeplessness—*see* Insomnia
Slippery elm, 34, 67, 71, 201, 252, 266
Smallage, 75
Smallpox, 46, 73, 132, 144, 147, 163, 168, 246, 289, 307, 313
Small spikenard, 240
Smart weed, 294
Smell, illusions of, loss of, 55, 302
Smooth sumach, 265
Snake bites, 20, 47, 113, 114, 120, 160, 166, 183, 219, 220, 221, 245, 246, 250, 269, 289, 301
SNAKE: head, 21; lily, 57; milk, 195; root, 45, 238, 244
Snapping hazel nut, 306
Sneezing, fits of, 246; at end of cough, 246; with heat, 247
Snowball tree, 101
Snowdrop tree, 129
Snuffles, 50
Soapwort, 81
Sobachyi yazik, 159
Sodium, 26, 86, 110, 270
Soft pine, 296
Solanine, 133
Solanum dulcamara, 42; lacitum, 44; lacimiatum, 134; nigrum, 44, 132, 133; xanthocarpum, 44
Solar plexus, 123
Solidago canadensis, 141, 142; juncea, 141; missouriensis, 143
Solodka gladkaya, 179
Solomon's seal (American), 253, 254
Somnambulism, 202, 311

Sore breasts, 93; feet, 17, 92; gums, 144; mouth, 3, 5, 25, 38, 45, 104, 112, 144, 145, 229; nipples, 17, 144; throat, 3, 5, 28, 29, 36, 68, 104, 112, 121, 143, 145, 146, 161, 165, 171, 182, 192, 198, 203, 205, 207, 224, 228, 234, 235, 237, 240, 246, 256, 261, 266, 287, 296, 298, 316, 318
Soreness, 116
Sores, 11, 24, 29, 33, 36, 51, 54, 74, 97, 121, 128, 147, 153, 155, 186, 191, 208, 219, 231, 233, 236, 242, 259, 263, 266, 276, 278, 296, 298, 300, 318
Sorrel, 254, 255
SOUR: dock, 315; grass, 255
Sowthistle, 127
SPANISH: chestnut, 86; needles, 272
Spasms, 56, 74, 81, 82, 101, 132, 135, 149, 185, 187, 215, 233, 258, 268, 312; stomach, intestinal, 136, 180, 286
Spasmodic asthma, 123; cough, 123; croup, 185; diseases of bowels, 71, 136, 301; pains, 50
Spastic paralysis, 259
Spearmint, 68, 197, 278
Speech, affections of, 43, 82, 132
Spermatic cord, neuralgia of, 25; pain in, 180, 295; swelling of, 242
Spermatorrhoea, 108, 120, 135, 144, 174, 237, 242, 302, 304
Spice birch, 36
Spigelia marilandica, 216, 246
Spignet, 240, 256
Spikenard, 256, 296
Spinal centre, 249, 286; concussion, 259; congestion, 150; irritation, 106, 224, 258, 259, 302; meningitis, 135, 144; tabes, 314; tenderness, 203
Spindle tree, 292
Spitting of blood, 107, 133, 204, 219, 237
Spleen, 3, 5, 6, 9, 29, 44, 74, 75, 99, 117, 123, 125, 130, 194, 195, 212, 293; affection of, 19, 25, 57, 59, 122, 205, 208, 213, 236, 291, 295, 312, 315; congested, 150; enlarged, 31, 133, 164, 223, 230, 278; malfunction, 24, 130, 161, 235; obstructions of, 110; pain in, 53, 81, 147, 220, 224, 302; purifying, 89; suppressed, 14
Splenalgia, 17
Splinters, imbedded, 296
Spoonwood, 66
SPOTTED: alder, 306; comfrey, 187; cranesbill, 103; geranium, 103; lungwort, 187
Spotted fever, 62
Sprains, 16, 17, 68, 81, 94, 263, 311
Spreading sclerosis, 176; sores, 153; ulcers, 74

377

Sprue, 265
Sputum, bloody, 92
SQUAW: berry, 213; bush, 101; mint, 215; root, 45, 56; vine, 261, 302, weed, 179
Squill, 46
Squirrel corn, 283
ST. JOHN'S: grass, 257; wort, 257
St. Vitus dance, 39, 46, 126, 174, 250, 285
Stagbush, 47
Stagger weed, 283
Stamina, lack of, 137
Stammering, 43, 132; starting, 167
Starch, 46, 68, 228, 241, 251, 285
STAR: grass, 260; leaved gum, 276; weed, 87
Steam bath, 38
Stearine, 279
Steblelist moshny, 56
Stellaria media, 87
Stenocardia, 300
Stenocordid, 167
Steptic, 10
Sterility, 63, 96, 108, 146, 182, 193, 261
Sternutatory, 149
Sticklewort, 2
Stickwort, 218
Sticky heads, 146
Stiff neck, 43, 74, 224, 259
Stigmata maydis, 94, 95, 158
Stillingia, 131, 261, 262, 284; sylvatica, 261, 262, 267
Stimulants, 5, 14, 16, 19, 20, 22, 24, 28, 31, 37, 50, 55, 61, 67, 72, 75, 80, 82, 93, 101, 108, 111, 112, 115, 117, 122, 125, 136, 139, 142, 143, 145, 146, 155, 156, 161, 162, 163, 168, 180, 182, 183, 184, 189, 197, 209, 210, 211, 225, 227, 230, 231, 241, 243, 248, 251, 257, 267, 274, 275, 276, 277, 278, 279, 281, 289, 291, 293, 299, 305, 310, 317
Stings, 3, 17, 34, 164, 172, 205, 212, 240
Stinking balm, 215
Stinkweed, 166
Stitches in side, 117, 299
Stitchwort, 87
Stomach, 4, 22, 32, 33, 41, 48, 61, 76, 79, 99, 123, 139, 144, 182, 197, 218, 227, 242, 252, 255, 280, 291, 311; aches, 159, 318; acid conditions of, 14, 221, 225, 241; affections, complaints, conditions, disorders, sickness, trouble, 5, 35, 36, 68, 74, 77, 78, 82, 93, 102, 119, 130, 145, 161, 169, 173, 174, 176, 180, 188, 192, 196, 198, 199, 221, 249, 259, 274, 277, 280, 314, 316; bleeding, 34, 129, 158, 249, 278, 295; cancer, 83, 102, 252; chronic ills, 24; haemorrhages, 28, 107, 204, 255, 306; inflammation of, 88, 126, 129, 145, 221, 254; irrit-

ation, 27, 80, 185, 283; morbid matter, 9; neurosis of, 55; painful spasms of, 136, 258, 286; pain in, 38, 68, 78, 80, 134, 229; phlegm in, 88, 204; secretions, 156, 221; sour, 89, 274; toxic seepage, 28; tumours, 130; ulcers, 32, 38, 102, 144, 145, 152, 169, 228, 249, 252, 255, 311; unwanted mucus, 207; weakness of, 80, 111, 142, 169
Stomachic, 75, 80, 109, 137, 138, 155, 157, 179, 197, 274, 291, 310; bitter, 44
Stomatitis, 68, 194
Stoneroot, 262, 263
Stones, 37, 38, 44, 59, 81, 86, 89, 95, 142, 158, 160, 180, 202, 209, 212, 255, 263, 265, 299; to break, 20
Stools, clay coloured, 58
Strabismus, 120, 167, 194, 217, 280
Stramonium, 154
Strangury, 19, 23, 97, 146, 157, 242, 295
Strawberry leaves, 36, 128, 264
Stricture, 23, 71, 122, 144, 218
Struma, 114
Strychnine poisoning, 122
Styes, 63, 174, 288
Styptics, 103, 204, 259, 315
Succory, 88
Sudorifics, 59
Sugar diabetes, 29, 36, 141
Sugar maple, 194
Sumach, 237, 264, 265
Summer complaints, 45, 127, 228
SUN: dew, 266, 268; drop, 122; rose, 131
Sunburn, 9, 280
Sun headache, 66, 135, 167
Sunflower, 259, 268, 311
Sunstroke, 135, 150, 167, 187
Suppressed menstruation, 9, 73, 135, 180, 198, 199, 201; urine, 23, 125
Suppuration, 17
Suterberry, 226
Swallow wort, 221
SWAMP: beggar's tick, 272, 273; cabbage, 251; dogwood, 291; maple, 194; sassafras, 189;
SWEET: almond, 259; birch, 36; chestnut, 86; elder, 114; flag, 41, 273; grass, 273; gum, 276; rush root, 273; scented golden rod, 141; scented pond lily, 297; sedge, 273; wood, 177
Swellings, 11, 31, 33, 38, 71, 74, 88, 89, 92, 93, 97, 116, 128, 166, 182, 186, 188, 191, 201, 229, 242, 243, 280, 283, 288, 296, 298, 300, 306, 307, 311, 315. 318
Swollen breasts, 212, 224, 259, 287; feet, 16; glands, 43, 68, 112, 152, 212, 253; injuries, 19; legs and hands, 152; tonsils, 144, 224, 236; tongue, 208, 265, 317

378

Tonsilitis, 43, 127, 296, 309; follicular, 163
Tonsils, inflamed, acute, 203; swollen, 144, 224, 236, 211; ulcerated, 93
Toothache, 75, 81, 82, 118, 132, 135, 147, 152, 157, 176, 182, 198, 218, 220, 224, 227, 240, 243, 275, 281, 283, 288, 302, 313
Toothache tree, 226
Tormentilla erecta, 128, 129
Toxic waste, 28
Trachea, affections of, 182, 316; tickling in, 68
Trailing arbutus, 14
Trauma, 210
Traumatic fever, 17
Tree of life, 281
Tree primrose, 122
Trefoil, 233
Trembling, 99, 284
Tremors, 47, 135, 167
Trifolium pratense, 233, 234
Trillium erectum, 33; pendulum, 33
Trismus, 167
Triticum, 96, 97; repens, 97, 158
True unicorn root, 260
Trumpet weed, 146
Tsuga canadensis, 134
Tubercular cough, 50; lungs, 99, 102, 137, 173, 200, 202, 206 208, 221, 249, 280, 311, 314, 316; skin, 102, 143
Tuberculosis (see also Consumption and Phthisis), 54, 56, 75, 79, 142, 154, 159, 163, 172, 182, 209, 251, 288, 296; anaemia, 259; of bones, 78; early stages, 24; incipient, 117, 307
Tuber root, 221
Tumeric root, 143
Tumours, 1, 17, 20, 25, 34, 43, 51, 55, 74, 88, 92, 96, 107, 116, 122, 131, 133, 134, 159, 194, 201, 210, 224, 239, 252, 255, 280, 281; of breast, 55, 218, 259, 315, 316; of eyes, 281; fungoid, 55; indolent, 90; inflamed, 203, 287, 307; malignant, stomach, bowel, 130; painful, 43, 307; uterine, 130; of womb, 253
TURKEY: aloes, 8; corn, 94, 283
Turnera aphrodisiaca, 108
Turn hoof, 5
Turpentine, oil of, 23, 278, 294
TURTLE: bloom, 217; head, 21
Tussilago farfara, 91, 182, 185, 256, 302
Twitch grass, 97
Tympanites, 23, 132
Typhoid fever (see also Enteric fever), 23, 28, 44, 61, 80, 105, 110, 112, 113, 114, 122, 132, 150, 193, 291
Typhus fever, 24, 112, 137, 145, 164, 167, 168, 249, 275

Tzicory, 89
Tzitzin, Prof. N. B., 98

Ulcerated sores. 278
Ulceration of bladder, 39, 104, 144, 207, 228; of bowels, 228; of cervix uteri, 30; of cornea, 194; of ears, 228; of kidney, 93; of lungs, 5; of mouth, 10, 13, 32, 56, 68, 88, 128, 131, 224, 228, 266, 298, 316; of skin, 29, 95, 240, 259, 266; of stomach, 32, 38, 102, 144, 145, 152, 169, 221, 228, 249, 252, 255, 280, 311; of throat, 10, 13, 56, 88, 128, 145, 228, 237, 316; of tongue, 131, 164, 281; of tonsils, 93; of womb, 298
Ulcers, 1, 6, 9, 14, 19, 24, 33, 36, 43, 49, 51, 54, 59, 63, 71, 74, 75, 78, 79, 82, 90, 93, 94. 95, 97, 104, 114, 121, 122, 131, 132, 133, 143, 144, 145, 147, 152, 157, 159, 160, 162, 163, 164, 179, 180, 202, 203, 206, 211, 219, 221, 224, 225, 226, 227, 229, 230, 231, 237, 240, 242, 243, 249, 259, 263, 275, 276, 284, 295, 298, 300, 307, 312, 314, 315, 316; aphthous, 131; chronic, 266; duodenal, 255, 280; gangrenous, 158; gastric, 177, 307; indolent, 4, 34, 104, 147, 165, 186, 227, 234, 276, 304; inward, 110; malignant, 102, 218, 233; offensive, 34; putrid, 19
Ulmus alata, 292; fulva, 34, 201, 252, 266
Unicorn root, 104
Upland cranberry, 29
Uremia, 23, 197, 205
Urethra, carbuncle, 122; inflammation, 94; irritation, 218, 231; stricture of, 71, 122, 186
Urethritis, 29
Uric acid accumulation, 94, 119, 169, 263, 281; deposits, 146, 306; disorders, 256
Urinary affections, difficulties, disorders, 15, 23, 25, 30, 50, 68, 95, 110, 146, 157, 199, 213, 218, 226, 228, 250; cramps, 199; obstruction, 148, 225; organs, disease and irritation of, 14, 15, 29, 89, 121, 151, 160, 204, 218, 264; release, 5, 94, 100; retention, suppression, 23, 75, 95, 118, 125, 143, 146, 148, 156, 158, 201, 212, 220, 258; system, 176; tract, 231, 242, 248, 252—inflammation, 29, 121, 160
Urine, 94, 258; with blood, pus, 15, 92, 207, 208, 218, 228, 249, 258; difficulty in passing, 44, 157; flow of, 75, 153, 155, 164, 169, 196, 228, 299; incontinence of, 44, 75, 98, 108, 120, 146, 160, 193, 203, 313; mucus in, 248; scalding, 89, 218, 266
Urogenital organs, 71

380